THE
SOURCEBOOK
OF
MEDICAL
ILLUSTRATION

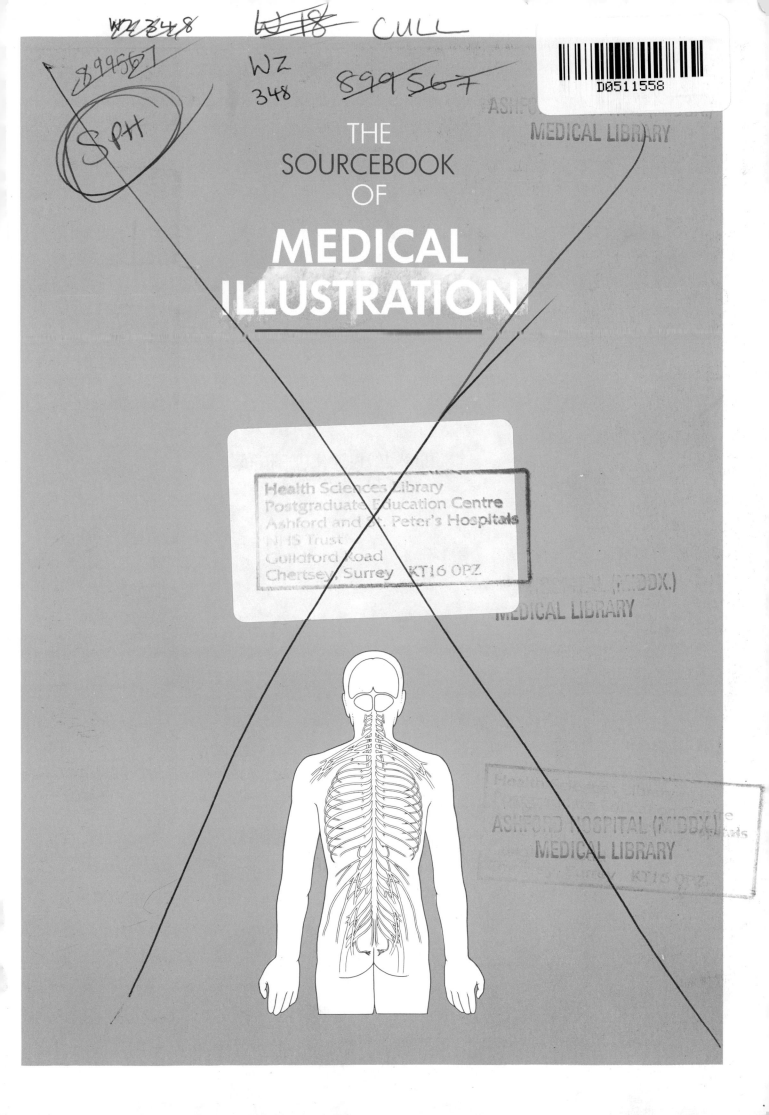

THE
SOURCEBOOK
OF
MEDICAL
ILLUSTRATION

Over 900 anatomical, medical and scientific illustrations available for general re-use and adaptation free of normal copyright restrictions

Edited by Peter Cull, FMAA, Hon FIMBI
Director, Education & Medical Illustration Services
The Medical College of St Bartholomew's Hospital
London, England

Drawings by
Lois Hague, BA Hons, MMAA, AIMBI
Andrew Bezear, MMAA
Joanna Cameron, BA Hons, MMAA
Wendy Proctor, BA Hons
Sandra Hill, BA Hons
Anne Clayton, MMAA
and other staff artists

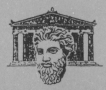

The Parthenon Publishing Group
International Publishers in Science & Technology

Casterton Hall, Carnforth,
Lancs, LA6 2LA, U.K.

120 Mill Road, Park Ridge,
New Jersey, U.S.A.

Published in the UK by
The Parthenon Publishing Group Limited
Casterton Hall, Carnforth,
Lancs, LA6 2LA, England

British Library Cataloguing in Publication Data
The sourcebook of medical illustration.
  1. Medicine
  I. Cull, Peter   II. Hague, Lois
  610
  ISBN 1-85070-255-1

Published in the USA by
The Parthenon Publishing Group Inc.
120 Mill Road,
Park Ridge,
New Jersey 07656, USA

Library of Congress Cataloging-in-Publication Data
The Sourcebook of medical illustration.
    1. Anatomy, Human--Atlases.   I. Cull, Peter.
II. Title: Medical illustration.   [DNLM: 1. Anatomy,
Artistic--atlases.   2. Medical Illustration--atlases.
WZ 17 S724]
QM25.S677   1989   611'.0022'2   89-3358
ISBN 0-940813-72-6

First published in 1989
This paperback edition published 1991

Printed and bound by
Dotesios Printers Ltd, Trowbridge, UK

Section 16. Bacteria, Yeasts, Protozoans, Helminths, Viruses and Arthropods

Section 17. Graph, Chart and Layout Guides

Section 18. Scientific Symbols, Pictograms, Animals

Section 19. Maps

Section 20. Freehand Lettering Guides

Introduction

The communication of medical and scientific information is a 'growth industry' which in recent times has created an unprecedented demand for visual support materials. Artwork and graphics of every description and degree of complexity are used in printed form, as projected images, in posters and exhibitions, video tapes and films, with the aim of improving the communication process. Some medical institutions employ artists and designers to produce these materials and this is the ideal situation since, without doubt, close collaboration between client and specialist medical artist will usually result in a superior and more effective product. By no means however is this universal practice and many scientists are forced to create their own diagrams etc. Even where illustrators are employed the demand for their services is such that anything which contributes to increased speed and volume of production is welcome.

This collection of simple, commonly used medical illustrations and graphics has been designed therefore to assist amateur and professional alike by providing a source of reference and copyable images which are free from restrictions on use.*

*The contents of the collection remain copyright to the Medical College of St. Bartholomew's Hospital, London, but this is not intended to deter the legitimate scientific user from copying, modifying or publishing them. Permission need not be sought and no fee is required from such users other than the purchase of the collection. The contents however must not be reproduced, published or resold in similar collections, or as syndicated works of any kind without the permission of the copyright owner. When illustrations are used in publications, films etc, we would appreciate, though not require, the usual acknowledgements.

SOME GENERAL ADVICE ON USING THE DIAGRAMS AND CREATING GRAPHICS

The diagrams have been prepared to help you create graphics for slides, overhead projection transparencies, television, posters and publication etc. In many instances they will be useful as they appear but often some modification will be necessary, such as changing the size, adding or subtracting detail and text, or combining with other diagrams to create a 'scheme' or layout. Some advice on how to do this is given below and in some cases examples are shown of how the diagrams and guides can be used and adapted.

Proportion and size

It is important to create artwork of the correct proportion for the intended presentation medium and that the best use is made of the working area it provides. 35mm slides are of the proportion 2:3; television screens on the other hand are rather more square, having a proportion of 3:4. Overhead projectors have two basic sizes of aperture: 10x10 inches square, or A4 which is roughly of the proportion 2:3. It may be helpful to bear in mind that this collection of diagrams is printed on sheets of A4 size, a suitable proportion for slides or OHP transparencies.

If the artwork is to pass through a camera process, e.g. made into slides, prints or recorded on video tape, *in theory* it doesn't matter what size the artwork is providing it is of the correct proportion. *In practice* however there are a number of factors which influence choice of size and these will be considered under the relevant headings.

Reduction and enlargement

Often it will be found that the diagrams as printed do not meet your precise requirement for size and will therefore need to be enlarged or reduced. There are three main ways of doing this; firstly, by photographing the illustration and having a print made of the correct dimensions. This is the most expensive method. Secondly, most institutions nowadays possess an electrostatic (plain-paper) photocopier capable of enlargement and/or reduction, and most 'photocopy shops' also offer this service. Providing the copier produces a high quality, clean and undistorted print, this is the cheapest and quickest method. Thirdly, you can use (if available to you) an artists optical enlarger/reducer — an advanced form of 'camera lucida' on which one can trace the enlarged or reduced image. Some of the more elaborate versions called PMT machines or repro cameras are equipped to produce immediate photographic prints of the image.

If your diagram required modification it is much easier to do this *before reduction.*

Modifying the diagrams

You will probably wish to keep the original drawings in your collection unsullied and in good condition for future use. It is therefore wise to make modifications on a good quality photocopy. Use a smooth white paper for this, better than the normal photocopying paper since this is often highly absorbent and ink tends to spread. Try using a paper called 'Proofing Chromo'; it has a thin china clay surface coating which permits the correction of errors by scratching away with a fine blade, and it is excellent for ink work.

Removing detail or 'blocking-out' can be done by brushing over with artists 'process white'. Alternatively, one of the various grades of "TIPP-EX" type correction fluids can be used. There are two general purpose grades, one of which is water-based and easier to thin out. 'Fotocopying' is a special grade which will not dissolve the toner in photocopies and thus prevents smears. 'Manuscript' is the grade recommended for covering ink, pencil, ballpoint and felt-tip pen.

Adding detail is best done with 'india ink' using a 'Rotring' type pen. These have a tubular nib and produce a line of constant thickness and they are available in a range of sizes. Some high quality fibre or felt tip pens can be used for this purpose but one needs to choose carefully. Ask for advice — and try them out — at your art material supplier. It is important that all lines should be dense black.

An entirely different approach is to trace the diagram, making the required modification in the process. Tracings can be made on a good quality tracing material such as Frisk K-Trace — this is a dimensionally stable film with an excellent surface for inkwork from which errors can be erased with a blade. Despite the translucency of the material it photocopies well.

Perhaps the best tracing method however is to use a light-box or x-ray viewing box to transilluminate your work. This permits you to work on good white paper or 'proofing chromo' providing an opaque surface which takes ink, stencilling, typewriting and dry-transfer lettering well. Some excellent small drawing boards incorporating a light-box with built-in set and 'T' squares are available and well worth a modest investment.

Creating lettering and text

For maximum legibility and clean appearance choose a simple type style without 'serifs' (the curly bits at top and bottom of letters). 'Univers' and 'Helvetica' are both excellent typefaces in this respect and anything which comes close to these will be adequate.

Contrary to what many people think, words composed of all capital letters are not as readable or legible at a distance as a combination of upper-case (capitals) and lower-case (small) letters.

Providing letters are correctly aligned and spaced the most professional effect is obtained by using dry-transfer rub-down lettering such as 'Letraset'. These materials are however expensive and setting them can be a time-consuming task if a lot of text is involved.

If well done, pen-stencilled lettering using 'UNO', 'MARS' and similar equipment, can be quite effective and quick to produce.

The electric typewriter has become a very popular method of creating text but a number of points need to be borne in mind: on standard typewriters each letter occupies the same space so that M's, W's etc become squashed and I's occupy more space than they deserve. This creates an uneven look to the text and reduces legibility. Many modern machines however, have proportional spacing in which each character occupies its proper space and this is preferable, both from the point of view of appearance and legibility.

High density (blackness) and clarity of impression in typewriting is also important and this is best provided by machines using a disposable, single-use, carbon ribbon.

As we pointed out earlier, the final presentation method (slide, print, video etc) has an influence on the shape and size of the artwork we create as will be seen later when the special needs of each are discussed. When using dry-transfer lettering or stencilling we are able to vary the size to match the needs of the medium in relation to the size of the drawing. When using a typewriter to create text the position is reversed; the size of the artwork and drawings have to be modified to match the size of the lettering. Further guidance on this point will appear later and sheet No. 17.11 will be found particularly useful.

Unless you are a real expert, hand lettering is rarely acceptable for slides, publication, posters or video, whereas with the overhead projector it is not only acceptable but in many cases preferable. Perhaps this is because we look upon the OHP as an 'instant' visual aid, a sort of extension of the blackboard. Although we may create sets of stock transparencies which we use over and over again in our teaching, the great bulk of work produced for the OHP is expendable; used once and thrown away. Nevertheless, to be effective, lettering needs to be neat and legible and for this reason, sheets 20.1 to 20.22 will be found useful. The group comprises a set of lettering grids for the OHP with distance/legibility guides and a range of sample alphabets of different 'weights' and styles to suit each grid. The samples are there simply as guides and it is not intended that you should trace over the letters — though of course you may if you wish!

Creating a 'scheme' or a 'layout'

This entails putting together a number of elements; drawings, lettering, arrows etc, by means of the 'paste-up' technique. The elements are usually photoprints or photocopies of diagrams combined with dry-transfer or typewritten text and lines or arrows which can be created with ink work, dry-transfer, or 'graph-tapes'. The latter, of which there are several varieties on the market, comprise reels of self-adhesive tape, solid black or colour, or patterned (dots, dashes etc.) ranging from around 1mm to 10mm in width.

First, sketch out your rough layout on tracing paper laid over one of the various graph grids in the collection (Section 17) and a light-box. Use good firm lines preferably made with a felt tip pen. The finished work should be carried out on a good white paper or 'proofing chromo' laid over both grid and rough sketch on the light-box. The grid will help you keep the various elements straight, level and positioned accurately.

When cutting out any photocopied elements don't cut too close to the outer edge line because it's usually wise to paint over the cut edge with some process white or Tipp-Ex when the element has been glued in position. This helps keep the edges invisible in subsequent photography or photocopying.

Whatever adhesive is used to glue down the elements it should allow for easy positioning (and repositioning if necessary) and it should not wrinkle or stain the paper. Scotch Spray Mount is ideal and only the lightest application is necessary.

Other Graphic Aids

A wide variety of aids are available to help you create high quality graphics without recourse to ink and pen. The 'graph-tapes' mentioned earlier can be used to generate graphs and charts etc, and the flexible variety can be employed where curves are involved. Manufacturers of dry-transfer lettering also make sheets of various symbols: open and closed circles, squares, triangles, arrows and so forth, in various sizes and ideal for plotting graphs etc. Filling in the columns of bar charts, diagrams etc, with various patterns of cross-hatching is easily done with sheets of self-adhesive 'mechanical tints' available from the manufacturers of dry-transfer lettering and colour can be added in the same way.

These are just a few items from the extensive range of materials and aids currently available. The list is too great to cover here and new ideas and methods are always emerging, so arm yourself with manufacturers catalogues and discuss your needs with a reputable supplier.

Computer Graphics

Finally a brief word about this 'new' technology that is fast revolutionizing the production of graphics. User-friendly machines like the Apple Macintosh and others now permit those with no drawing skills to produce immaculate graphs and charts, lettering and typography etc. With certain programmes and using regular shapes like rectangles, circles, ellipses and lines it is possible to create simple diagrams with shading and, depending on the machine, add colour etc. Other programmes/ machines permit free-hand drawing and painting of a very high standard but the operator does need the basic art skills. It is possible however to overcome this problem with the aid of a computer/scanner which will digitise and insert existing photographs, drawings etc into the computer for further processing. The illustrations in this series can be utilized and adapted this way; they can be enlarged, reduced, modified, shaded and colourised; they can be incorporated into schemes and layouts with the addition of typography etc for output in the form of laser prints on paper, slides, OHP transparencies and video tape. Regular users may find it convenient to scan and store the whole or parts of the collection on disc, thereby creating their own computer graphics library. It should be pointed out however that the copying of these illustrations and further distribution by gift or sale would contravene the copyright conditions under which the collection is published.

THE PRESENTATION MEDIUM
Artwork for Publication

The first rule is to READ AND FOLLOW THE PUBLISHER'S INSTRUCTIONS to contributors since these usually dictate how artwork is to be presented. Next, look at previous editions of the publication to which you are submitting, and assess the style of presentation of graphics, how the illustrations are placed on the page and the size of lettering used in the figures. Many journals have a 'house-style' and it is as well to match it.

Many publishers will demand that lettering should never be smaller than 2mm in capital height when reduced and printed (roughly the same as typewriting), and this requirement may well dictate the size of artwork. Most professional designers work to either twice or three times the printed size using lettering of 4 or 6mm respectively; though good quality same-size artwork is perfectly acceptable.

Use a good quality white paper or 'proofing chromo', not larger than A4 size since anything bigger causes difficulties in postal transmission. Finished work must be clean and free from blemishes and remember that if you wish to retain the original, a high quality, electrostatic photocopy is as good as a photographic print to send to the publisher — but it *must* be really good.

Artwork for Slides

The commonest complaint about many of the slides we see is that either the lettering is too small for it to be seen clearly on the screen, or that too much information has been included. There are some simple rules which can help avoid these problems:

1. If possible, always design your slides to the horizontal or 'landscape' format to the proportion 3 units across and 2 units vertical. The following rules are based on this format.

2. Text Slides: Never use more than 6 words in a single line title; never more than 8 words to the line for subsidiary text; never more than 8 lines in height.

3. Tables: Never use more than 5 columns in all and never more than 8 lines in height (including the title).

4. Bar Charts: (Sometimes termed histograms, with bars either vertical or horizontal). Never use more than 8 bars (or columns).

5. Line Graphs: Never include more than 4 different lines or curves.

6. Pie Charts: Limit the number of wedges to no more than 7.

If you are using a typewriter to create the text use the guide on sheet 17.11.

Always produce the finished artwork on good white paper or 'proofing chromo', never on graph paper since it creates difficulties in photography. Once again the use of a light-box in combination with one of the graph-grids in Section 17 will help.

Artwork for Television

Because television pictures are constructed of lines and dots the images we see on the screen are poorly defined and any artwork we produce needs to take account of this problem. In general terms this means that drawings need to be bolder and simpler, lines thicker and lettering larger with rather more space than usual between individual letters, words and lines of text. It is almost certain that you will need to create your artwork in colour and the methods of doing this are too numerous to review here. Remember however, that very effective graphics in colour can be created with the aid of a photocopier: For example, copying a diagram on coloured paper, cutting it out and mounting it on to a different coloured background.

When choosing colours remember that tonal contrast is as important as colour contrast, Red on Blue of similar tone (or density) will be ill-defined, whereas Pink on Blue will be well defined. A good rule is to use lighter colours for the items of interest (diagrams, lettering etc) and darker colours for backgrounds. Having said all that it is important to add that very high contrast (white or very light colours on black or very dark colours) should also be avoided.

The proportions of the television screen are, as pointed out earlier, 4 units across and 3 units vertical and a good working size for the artwork image is 12″ × 9″ (30cm × 23cm). In addition to this one needs to allow space around the image of about 10%. A further 10% of safety space needs to be added to allow for difference between the camera image and that shown on the television screen and another 10% for handling by the camera operator. So our final artwork will be on a background measuring 16″ × 12″ (40cm × 30cm) with the image confined to 12″ × 9″.

Lettering needs to be simple in style (e.g. Univers) and bolder in size than for slides. Working to the above dimensions the *absolute minimum* capital height is 10mm with no more than 30 characters to the line (counting spaces between words as one character).

Artwork for Overhead Projection

The overhead projector is an extremely versatile teaching aid, offering a host of novel ways in which to present information in an interesting and highly effective manner. Exploiting the potentials of the OHP goes beyond the scope of these notes but it is well worthwhile looking into the possibilities with the aid of one of the booklets listed below.

The subject of size and proportion for OHP was dealt with earlier but it is worth mentioning that most people find A4 the most convenient and practical size to work with. Allowing for some 'air' around the illustration or diagram it is suggested that artwork should be confined within a space of 6.5″ × 8.5″ (17cm × 22cm).

There are two basic ways of making a transparency for the overhead projector. The first is by simply drawing directly onto the transparency, the second involves the creation of an illustration or scheme on paper then transferring this to a transparency by means of photocopying. A special type of transparency material is required for photocopying.

Two types of pen are available for creating the 'hand-made' transparencies: Permanent (spirit-based ink) and non-permanent which will wash off with water. They are available in various sizes and colours and the Staedtler Lumocolor series is one of the several types manufactured specifically for OHP work. Areas of transparent flat colour can be added by means of self-adhesive colour film manufactured by Staedtler, Letraset and others.

Diagrams can be traced directly or after reduction/enlargement by photocopy etc as described earlier. There is a range of grids, plotting guides, symbols etc in the collection which will help you plan the more complex schemes or simply plot graphs and charts. Several examples in which these grids etc have been used are included in the collection.

The lettering grids and samples will be found particularly useful and the legibility factor will help you choose appropriate sizes. Transfer, rub-down lettering (e.g. Letraset) can be used but remember to use the special transparent variety when introducing colour. Finally keep the quantity of text to the minimum.

Artwork for Posters

We refer here to posters used for presenting data at scientific meetings; not those used in advertising.

There is no accepted standard for the size or format of scientific posters so one must create the material according to the specific instructions issued by the organisers.

Always consider the problems of transporting your poster to the display location and think about breaking down the allocated space into manageable flat pieces, which can be neatly and easily reassembled on site. At all costs, avoid transporting the poster in a roll. Remember that unlike a lecture slide, your poster will be competing with many others for the attention of the audience, therefore in addition to being informative it also needs to be bold, and attractive.

Posters are intended to be read by an audience 'on the hoof' so that main headings need to be legible at least 5 metres (15 feet) away and nothing should be so small as to be illegible at 1 metre (3 feet). To achieve this, lettering for headings should never be less than 25mm in capital height, subheadings not less than 10mm, and general text not smaller than 5mm.

In order to create a smart, clean presentation, assembling the various graphic and text elements by the paste-up method, and producing the final work from this in the form of photographic prints or photocopies is probably the best regime. This also permits working the original layout to a smaller scale (say ½ or ⅓ size) which in turn allows text to be generated directly on a typewriter.

Most of the techniques mentioned earlier will be found useful in preparing your artwork. Colour will be important and there are various ways of introducing it. Self-adhesive transparent sheets can be applied over certain areas of the finished print and material such as 'Pantone' will be found suitable. Alternatively some elements could be photocopied onto coloured paper. Pantone can be used to fill columns on bar charts; the plot points in line graphs can be joined by coloured graph tapes or felt-tip pen.

Useful Reference Material

Listed below are several extremely useful small publications which will help you improve both the design and production of artwork, and get the most out of the presentation medium. Some are available free.

"Charts and Graphs" Edited by Doig Simmonds for the Institute of Medical and Biological Illustration. Published by MTP Press Ltd, Falcon House, Lancaster.

"A Guide to Better Slides" Published by Boehringer Ingelheim, Southern Industrial Estate, Bracknell, Berks.

"A Guide to Better Posters" Published by Boehringer Ingelheim, Southern Industrial Estate, Bracknell, Berks.

"Overhead Projection Handbook" Published by Staedtler (U.K.) Ltd, Portyclun, Mid-Glamorgan.

"Bright Ideas" (OHP Guide) Published by Bell & Howell Ltd, Wembley, Middlesex.

ACKNOWLEDGEMENTS

In preparing the drawings for this series we have been helped enormously by many members of the academic and medical staff at St. Bartholomew's Hospital and Medical College. They have advised us on the selection of illustrations, given guidance on the content and checked the accuracy of work at various stages of production. In so doing they have given generously of their time and we would wish to acknowledge our indebtedness and record our gratitude to those whose names appear below.

Prof. J.A.H. Wass, MD, FRCP

R.A.J. Spurrell, MD, FRCP

K. Jones, MD, MRCP

P.D. Fairclough, MD, FRCP

C.N. Hudson, FRCS, FRCOG

L.N. Dowie, FRCS

Stella Barnass, MD, MRCPath

A.P. Hopkins, MD, FRCP

D. Harper, PhD

P.C.A. Grint, MB, BS, MRCPath

D.G. Lowe, MRCPath

W.R. Cattell, MD, FRCPE, FRCP

A.W.F. Lettin, MD, FRCS

R.J. Davies, MD, FRCP

Parveen Kumar, MD, FRCP

W.F. Hendry, ChM, FRCS

R.A.F. Whitelocke, FRCS

J.D.T. Kirby, FRCP

A. Nistri, MD

C.J. Ronalds, FIMLS

H. Kangro, PhD

Prof. R.B. Heath, MD, FRCPath

T.B. Boulton, MD, FRCP

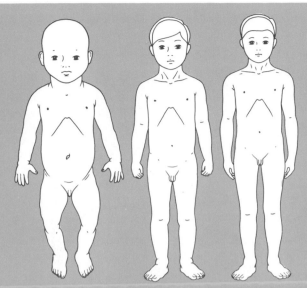

Section 1

Body Outlines

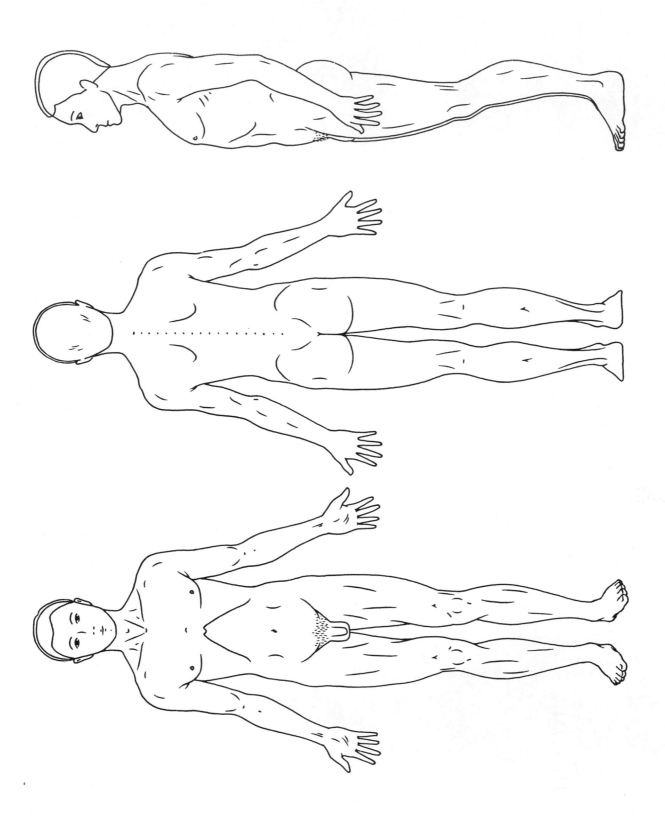

Fig. 1.1 Male figures, AP, PA, lateral, adult

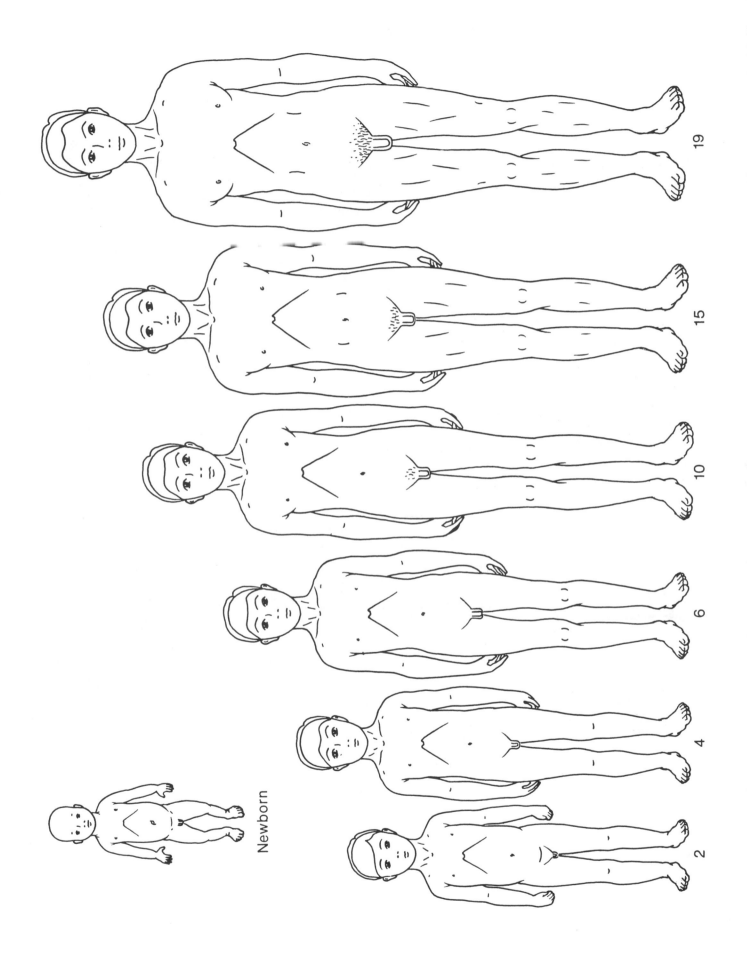

Fig. 1.2 Male figures, AP (size related) at birth, 2, 4, 6, 10, 15, 19 years

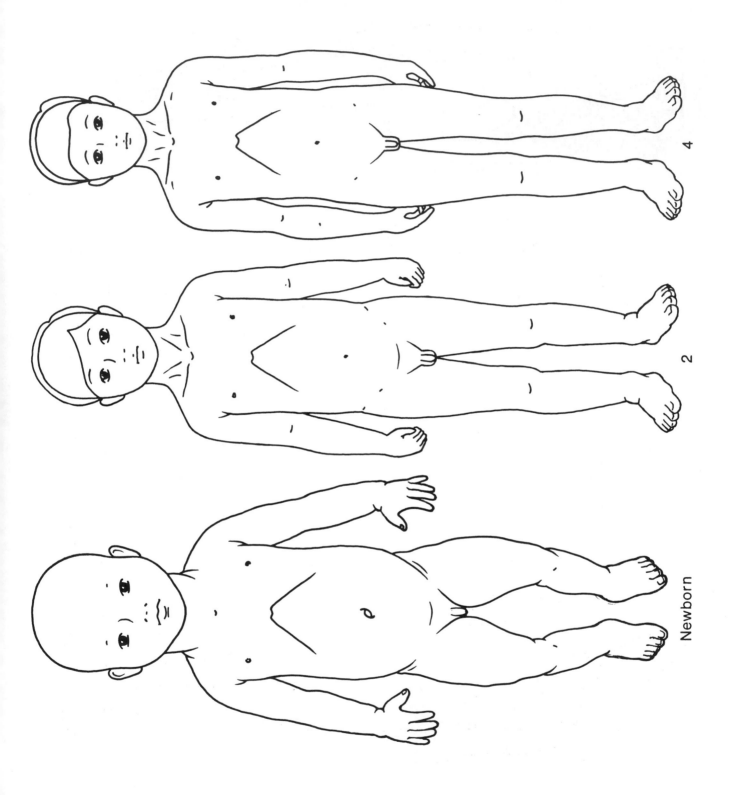

Fig. 1.3 Male figures, AP (proportion related) at birth, 2, 4 years

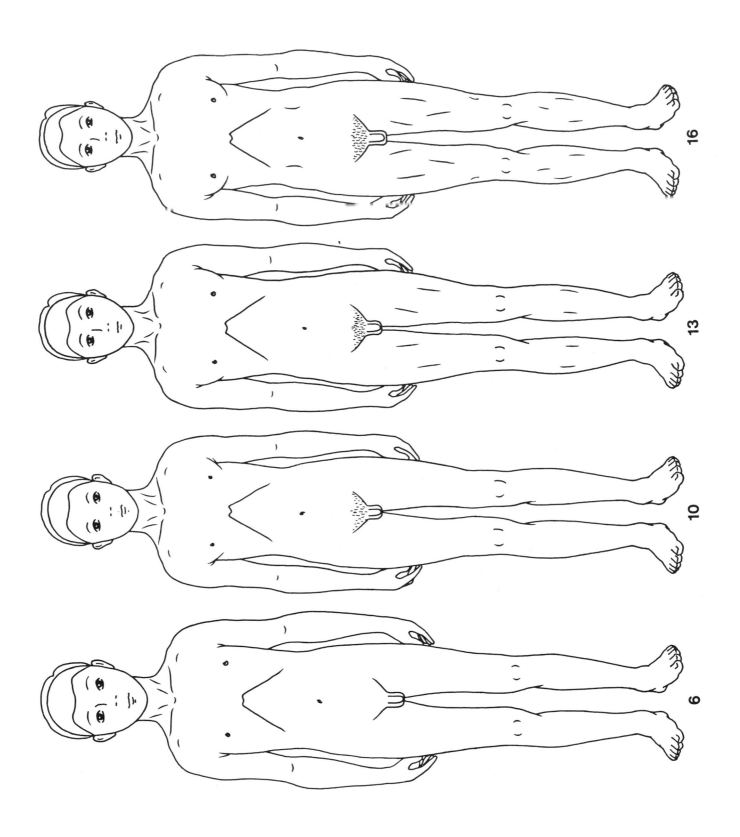

Fig. 1.4 Male figures, AP (proportion related) at 6, 10, 13, 16 years

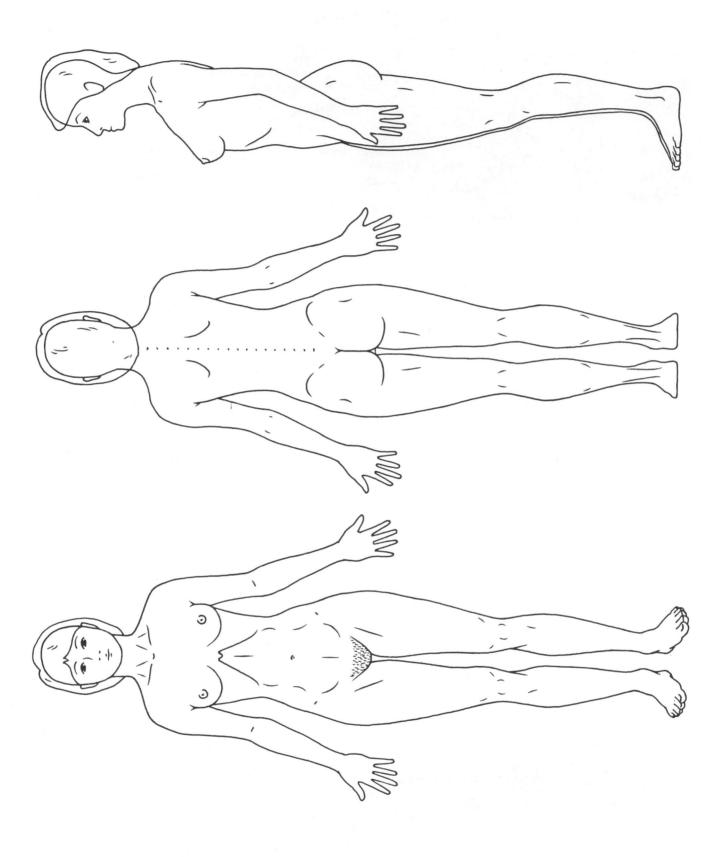

Fig. 1.5 Female figures, AP, PA, lateral, adult

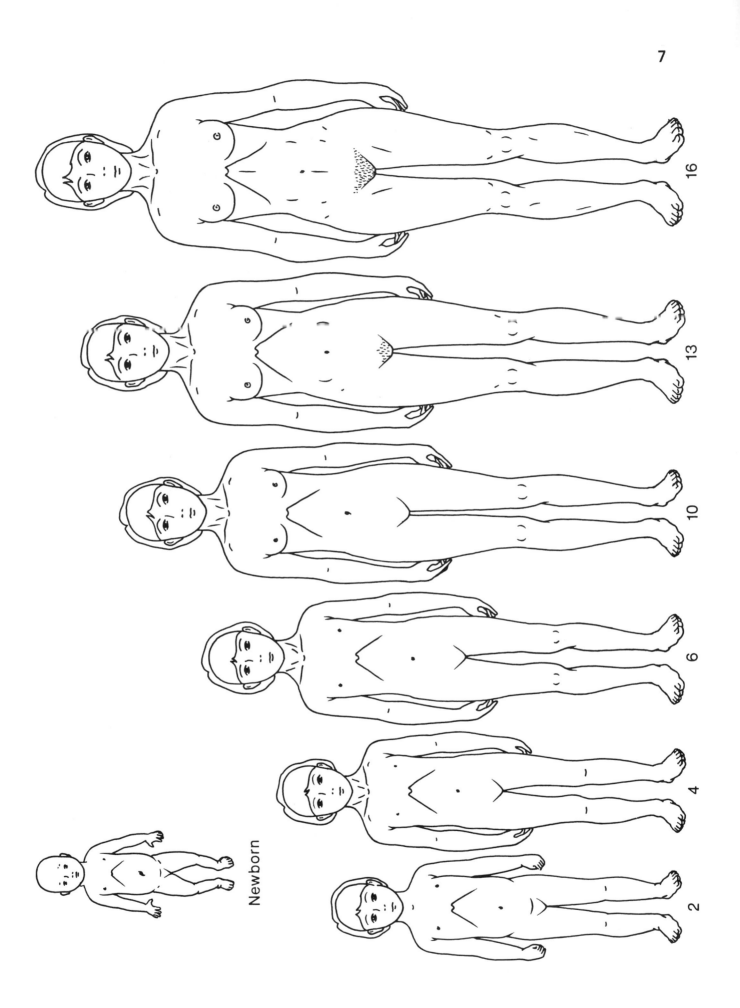

Fig. 1.6 Female figures, AP, (size related) at birth, 2, 4, 6, 10, 13, 16 years

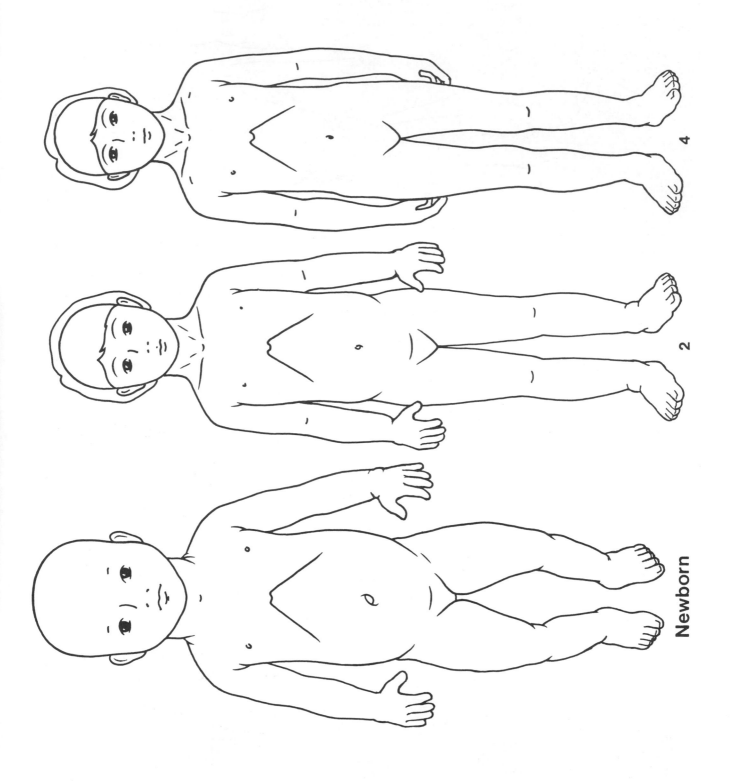

Fig. 1.7 Female figures, AP, (proportion related) at birth, 2, 4 years

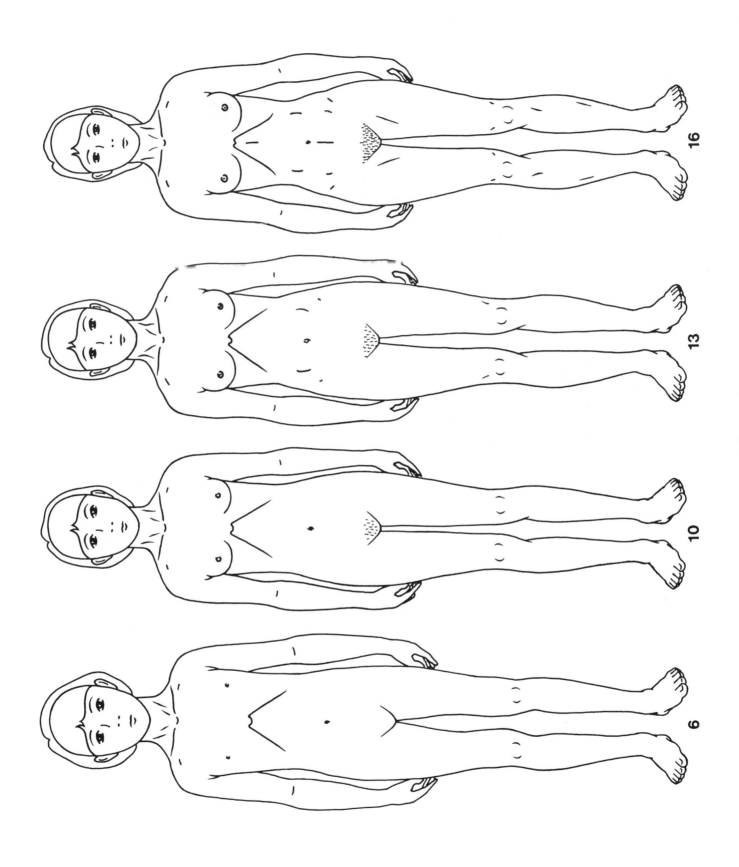

Fig. 1.8 Female figures, AP, (proportion related) at 6, 10, 13, 16 years

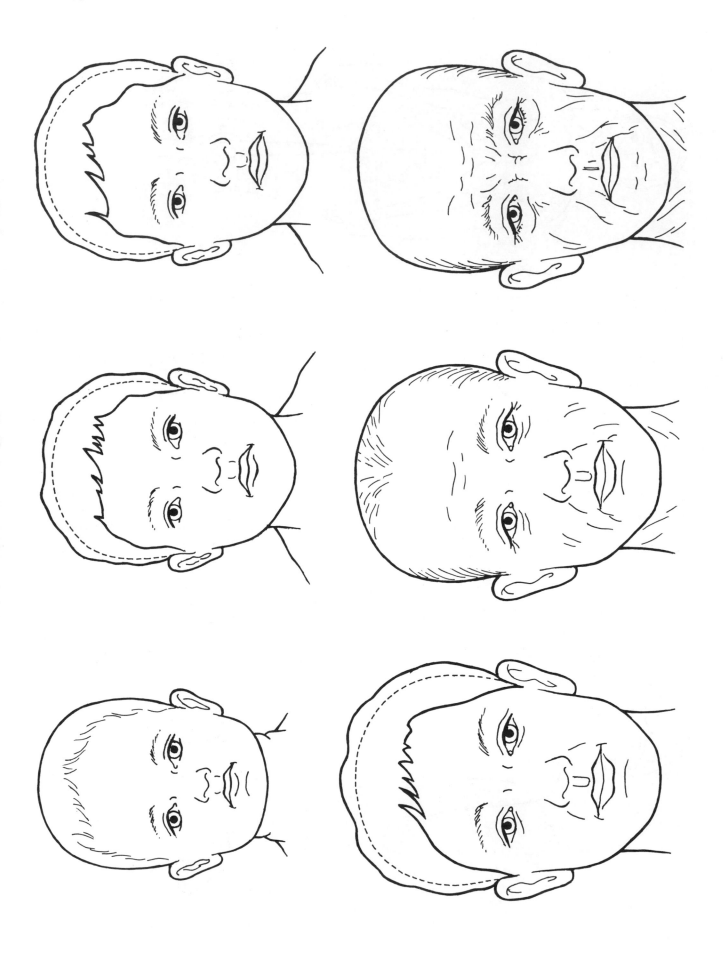

Fig. 1.9 Male faces (6) AP, infant to elderly

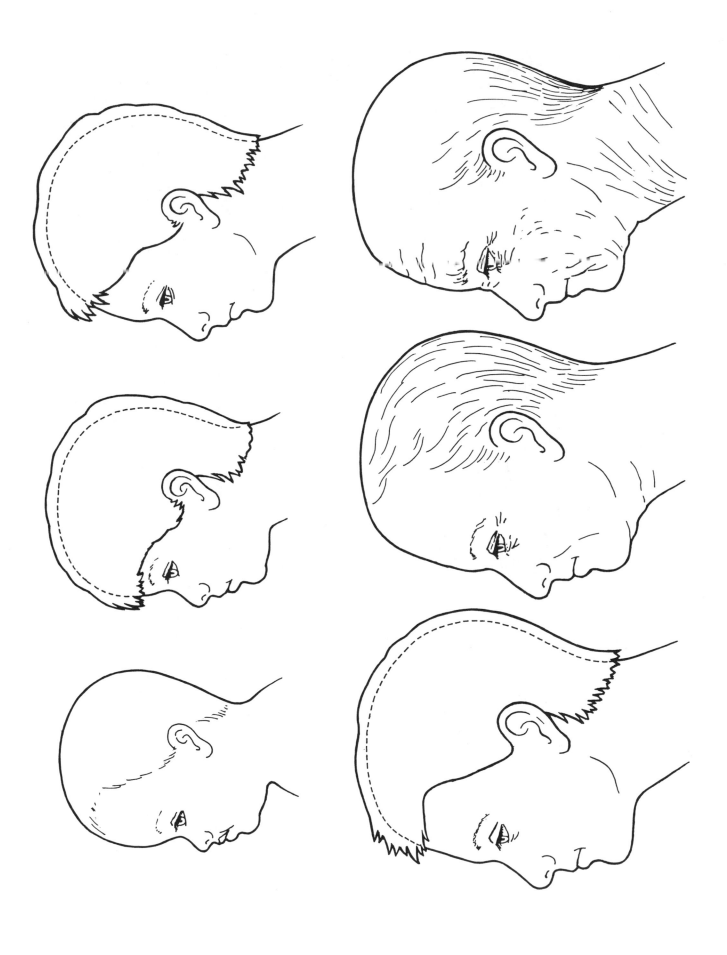

Fig. 1.10 Male faces (6) lateral, infant to elderly

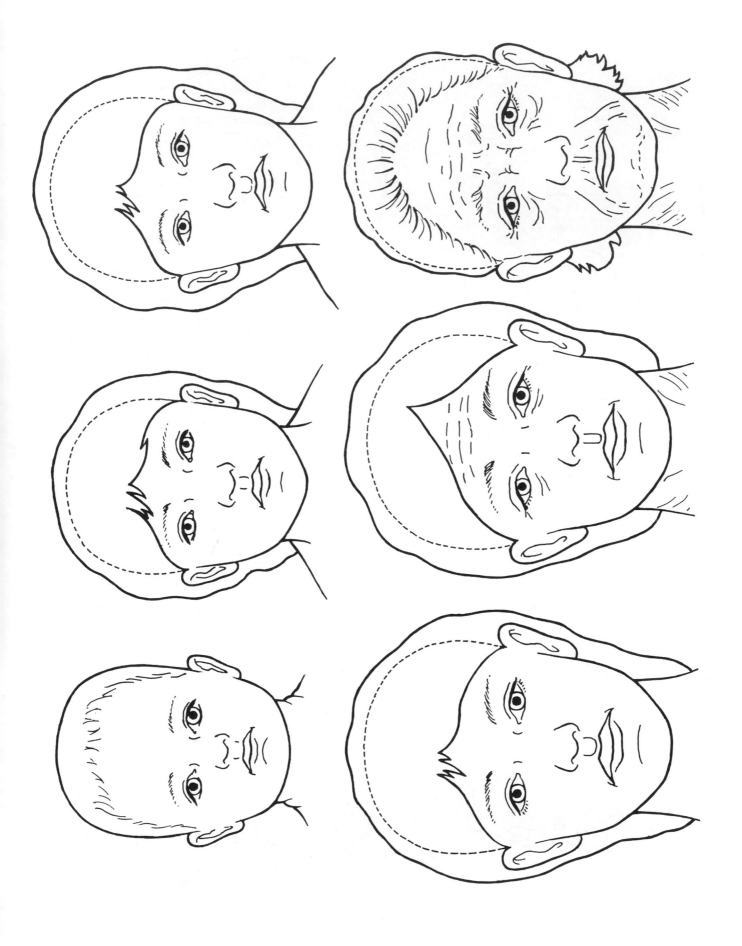

Fig. 1.11 Female faces (6) AP, infant to elderly

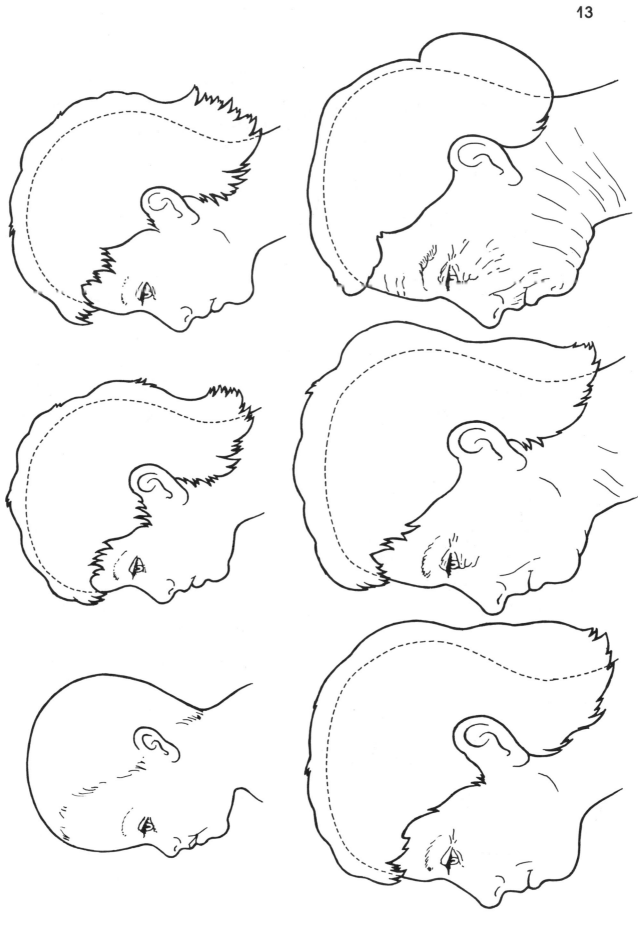

Fig. 1.12 Female faces (6)lateral, infant to elderly

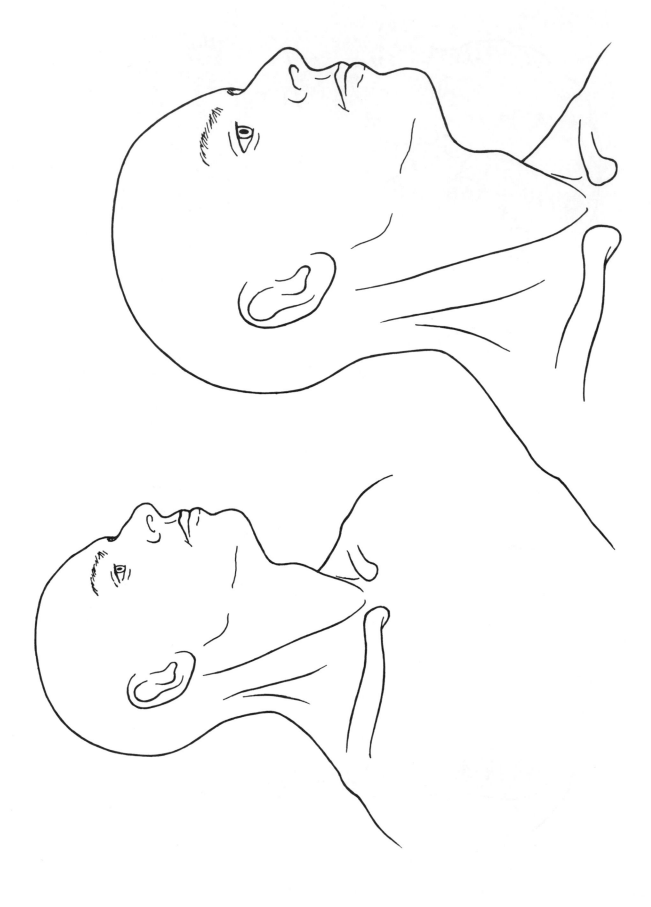

Fig. 1.13 Head and neck, lateral

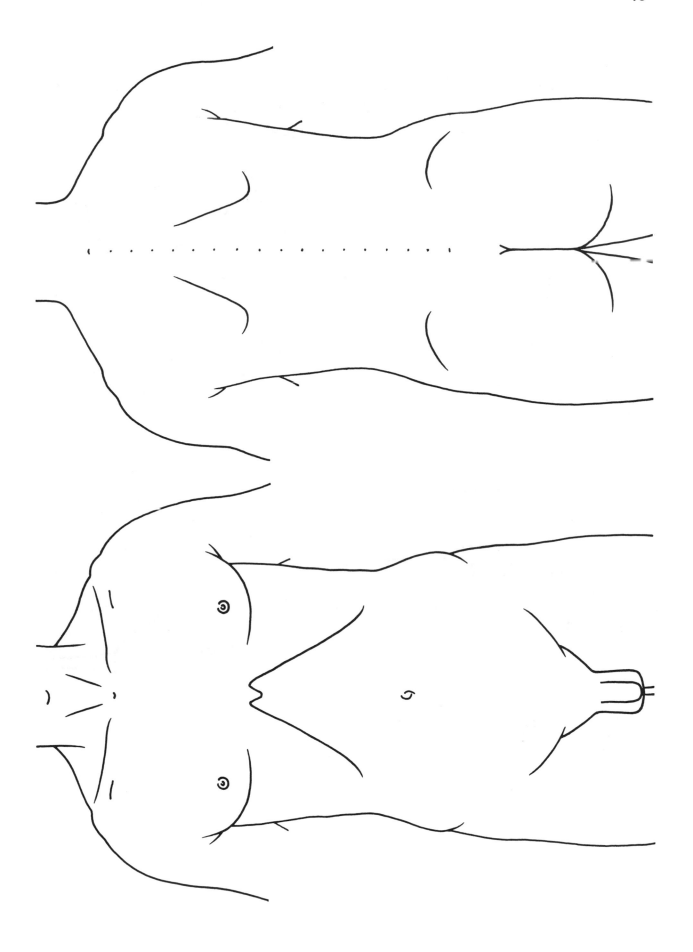

Fig. 1.14 Male torso, AP, PA

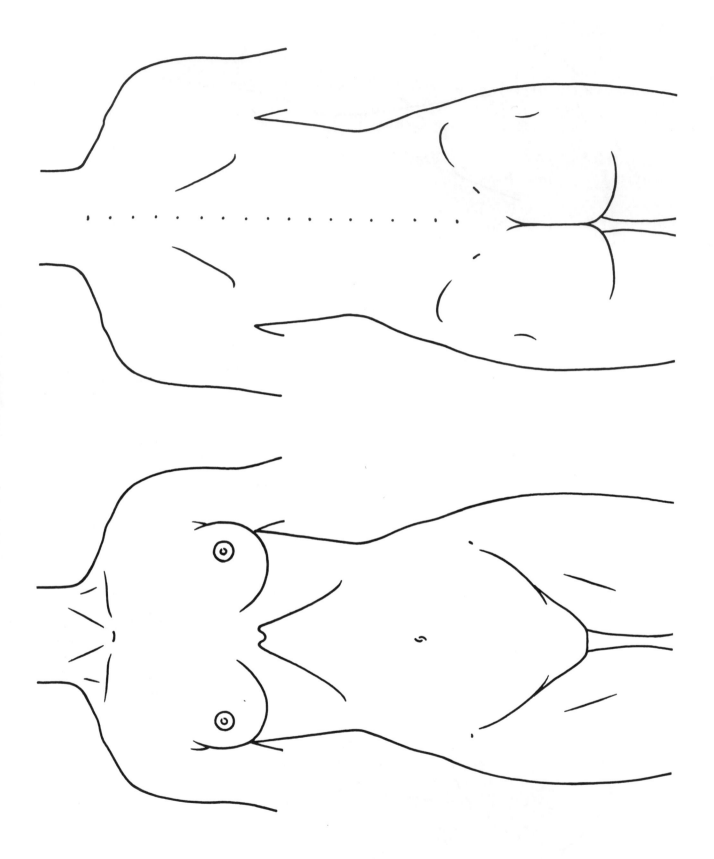

Fig. 1.15 Female torso, AP, PA

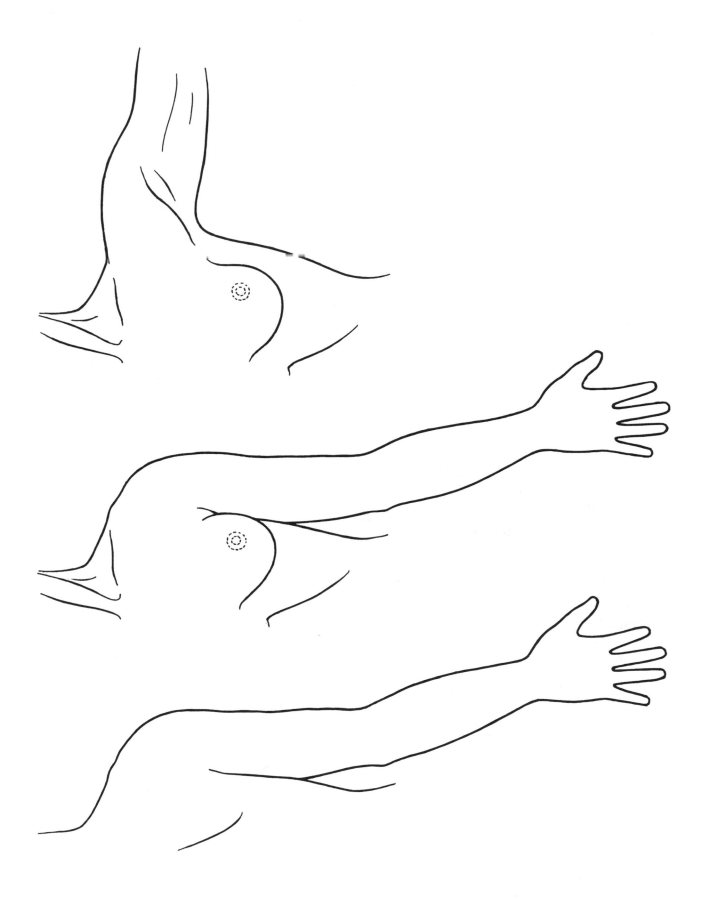

Fig. 1.16 Female thorax, shoulder, arm, PA, AP, axilla

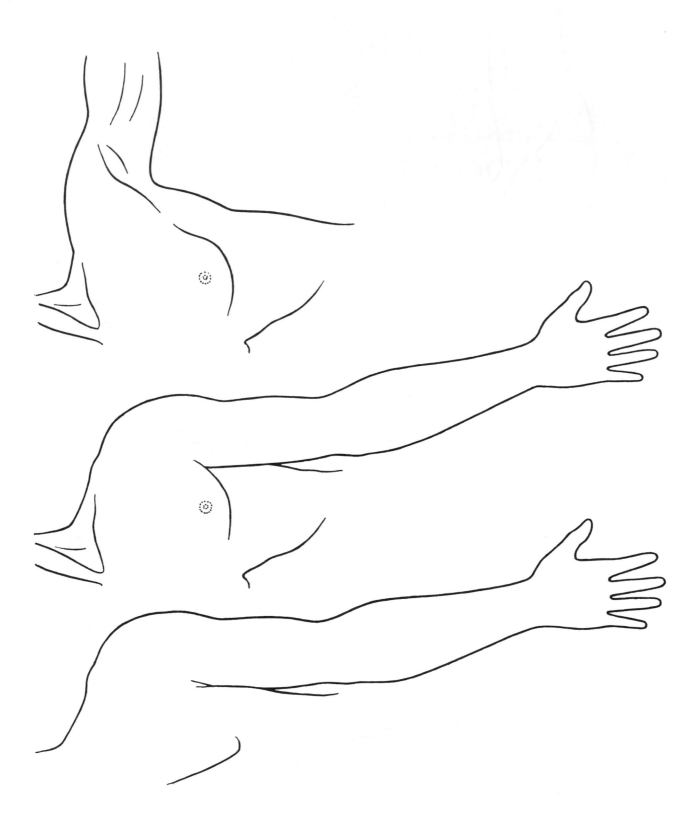

Fig. 1.17 Male thorax, shoulder, arm, PA, AP, axilla

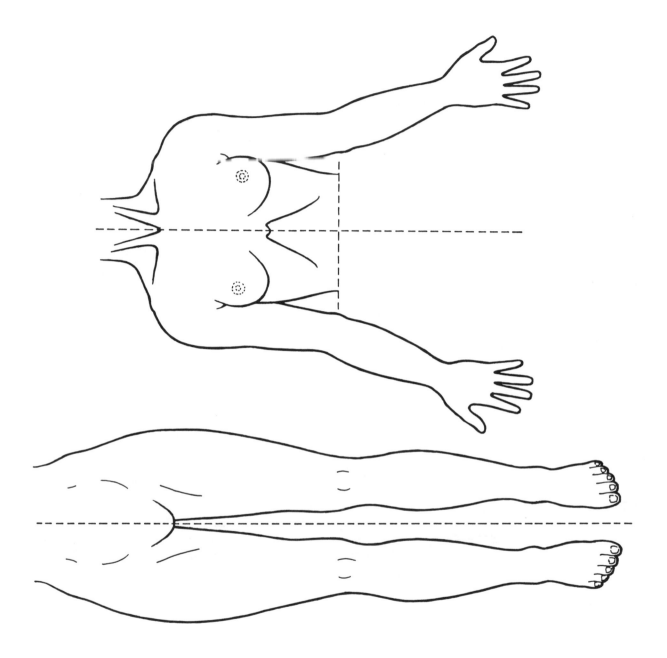

Fig. 1.18 Female thorax/arms, abdomen/legs AP

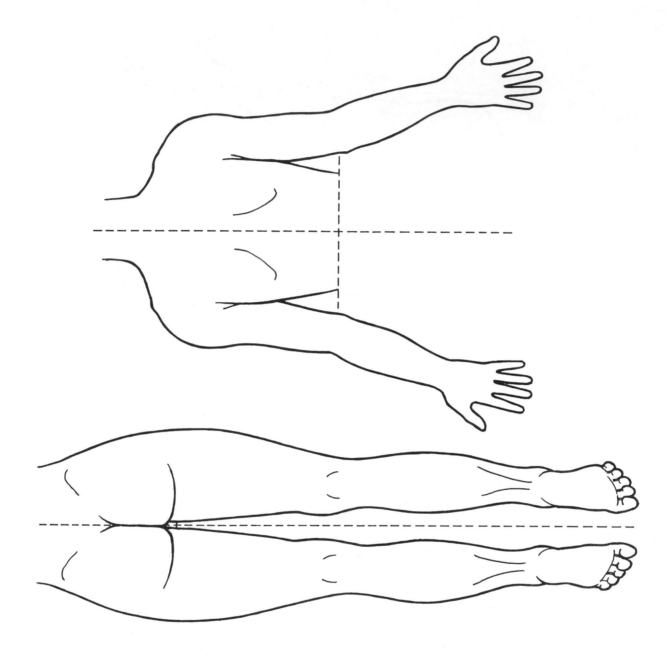

Fig. 1.19 Female thorax/arms, abdomen/legs PA

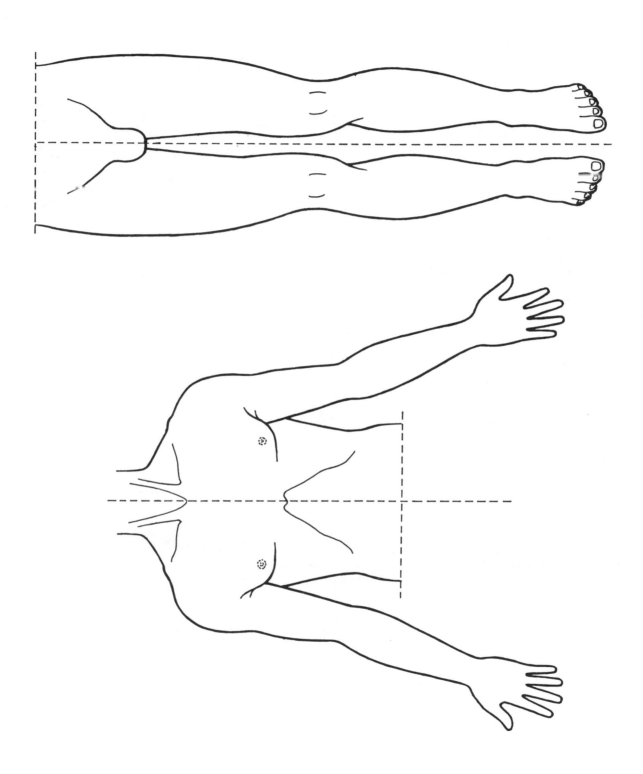

Fig. 1.20 Male thorax/arms, abdomen/legs AP

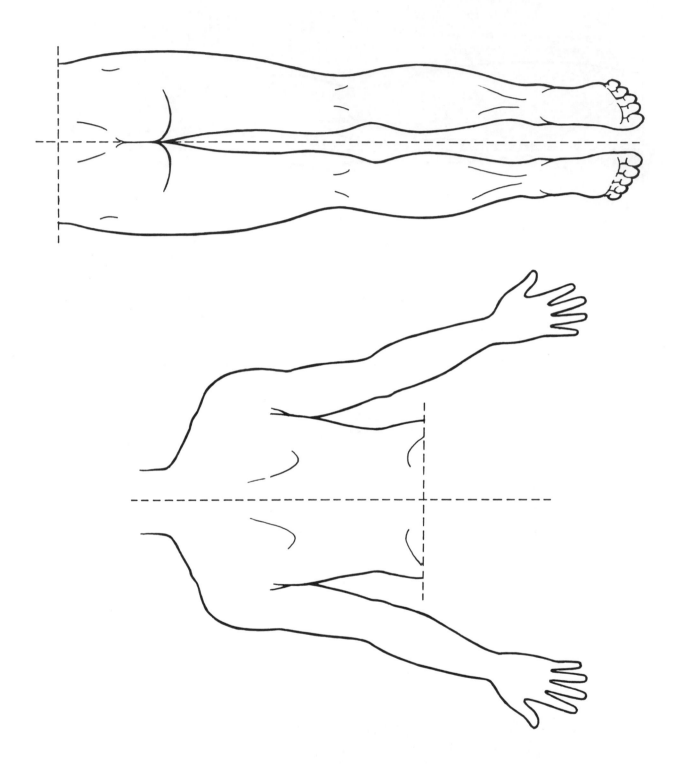

Fig. 1.21 Male thorax/arms, abdomen/legs PA

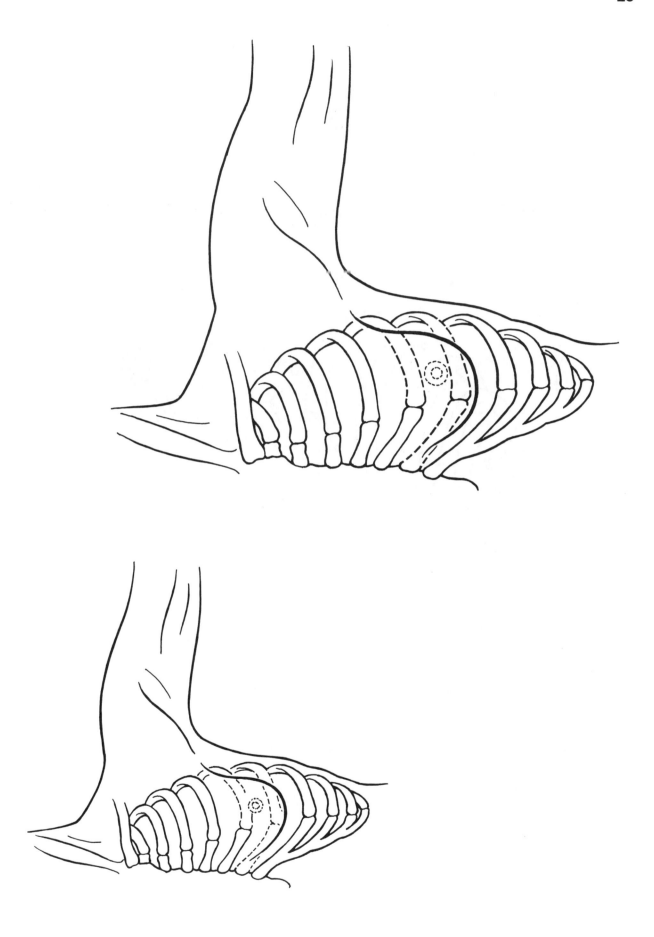

Fig. 1.22 Female ribs, axilla AP

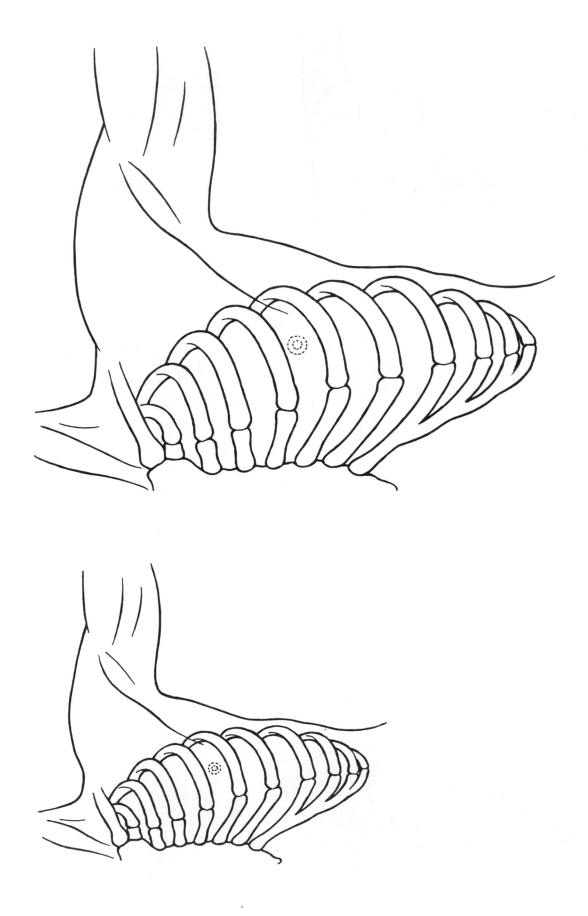

Fig. 1.23 Male ribs, axilla AP

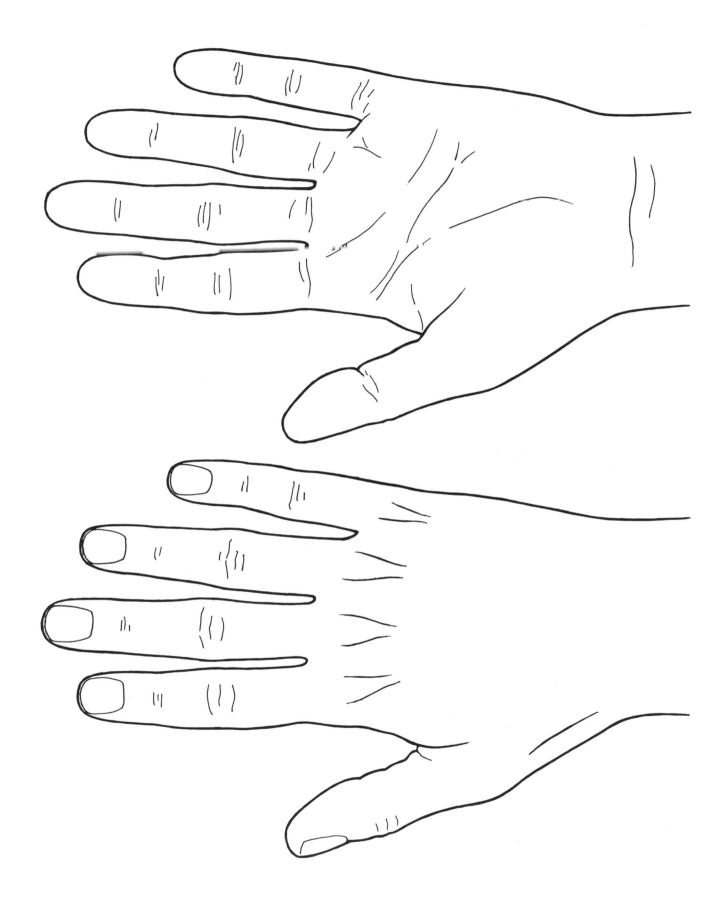

Fig. 1.24 Hands, palmar, dorsal

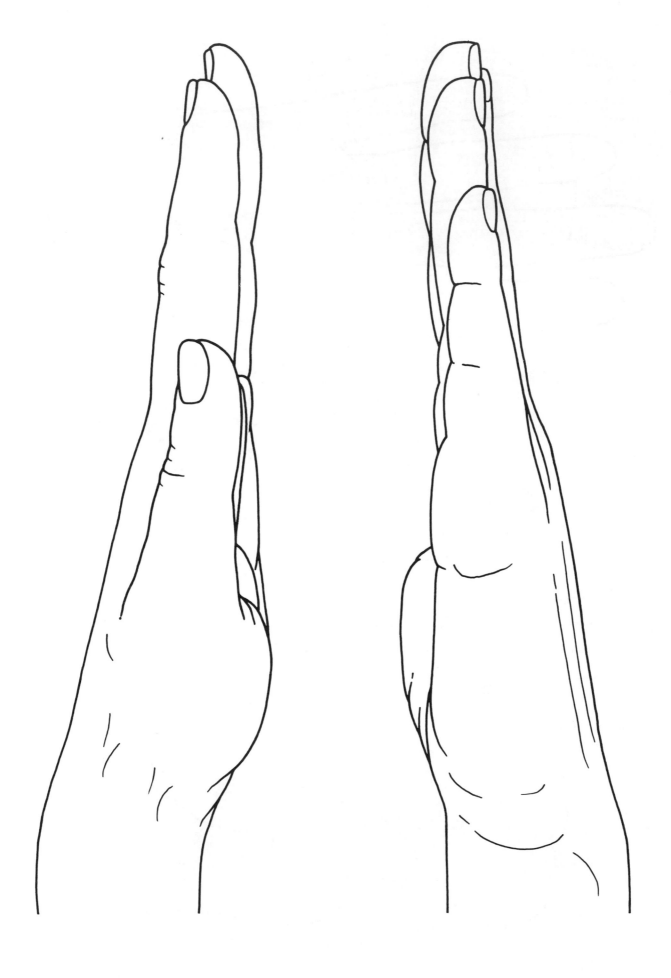

Fig. 1.25 Hands, lateral, medial

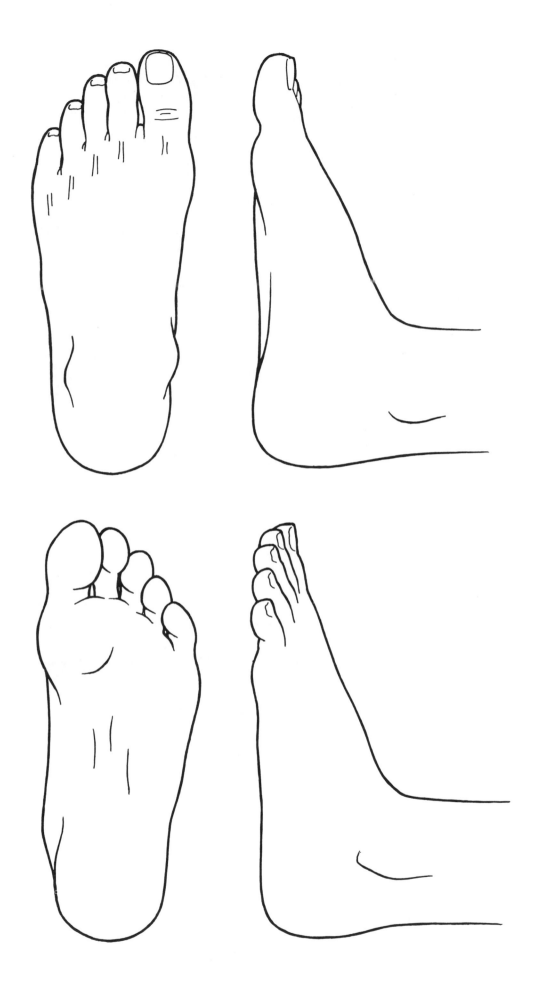

Fig. 1.26 Feet, medial, lateral, dorsal, plantar

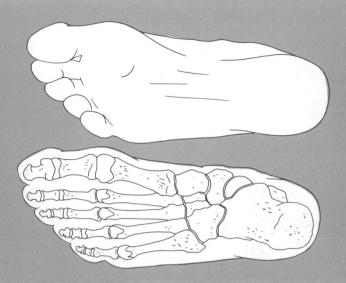

Section 2

Bones and Joints

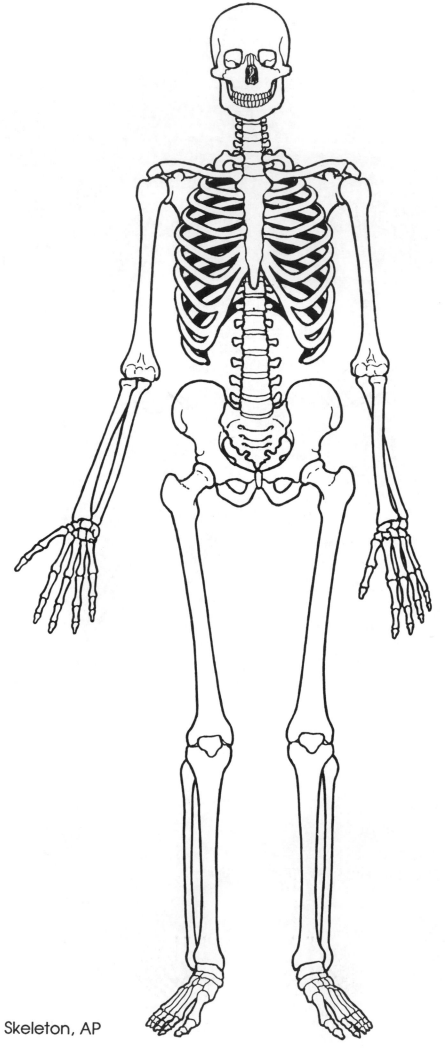

Fig. 2.1 Skeleton, AP

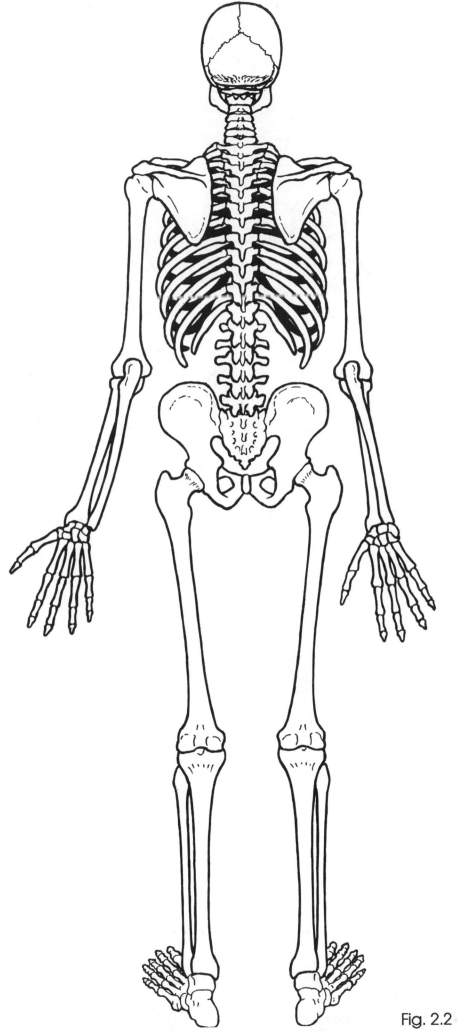

Fig. 2.2 Skeleton, PA

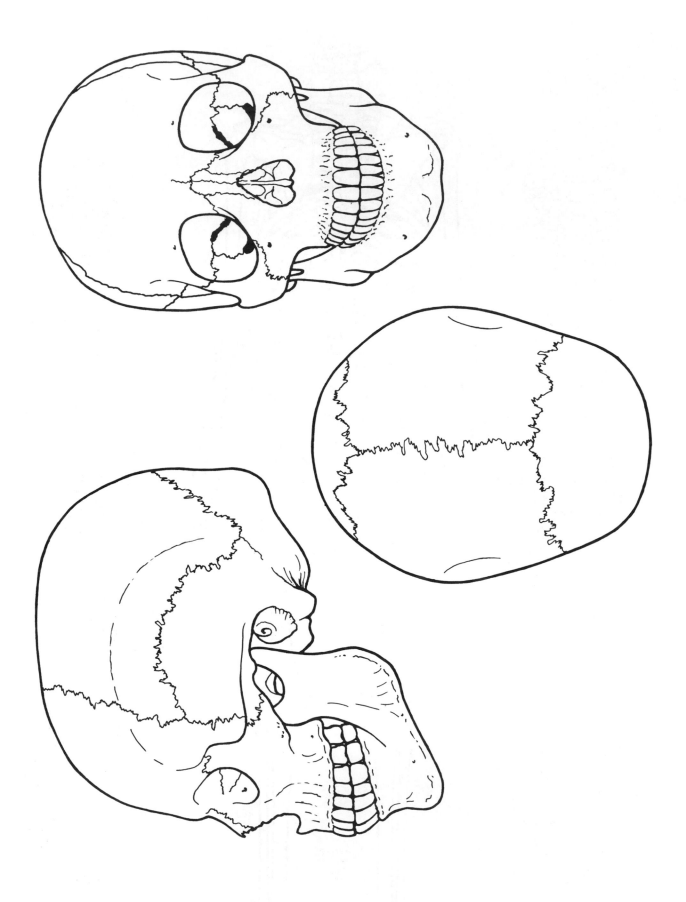

Fig. 2.3 Skull, AP, lateral, superior

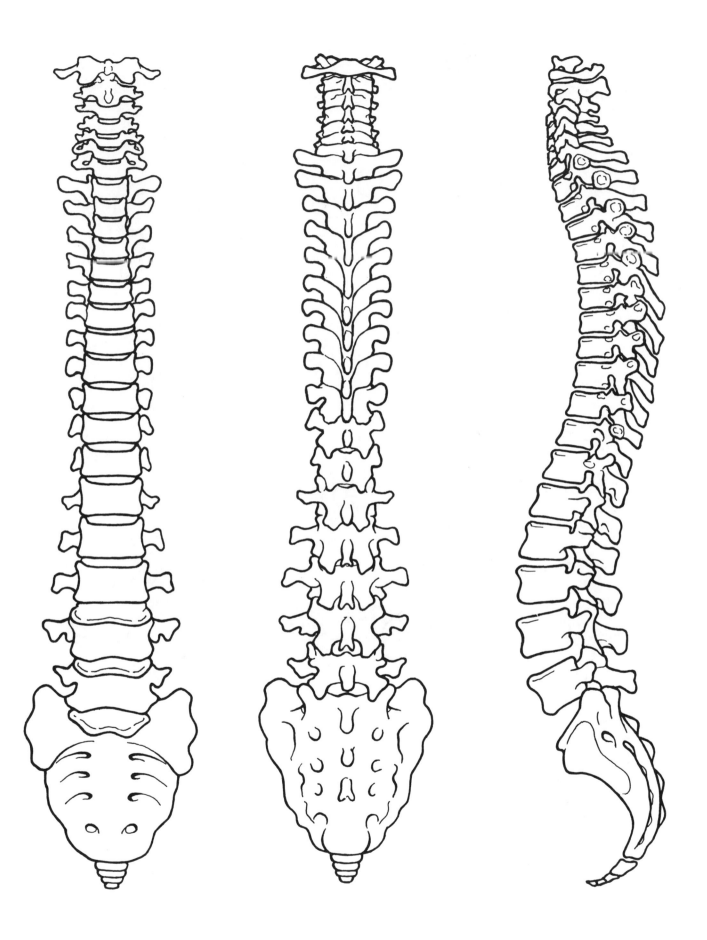

Fig. 2.4 Spine, AP, PA, lateral

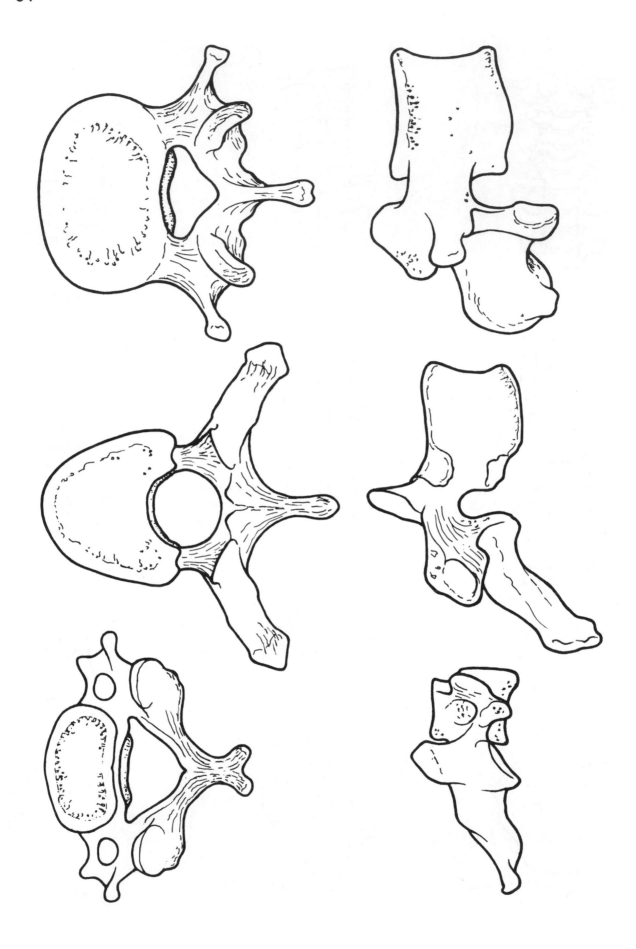

Fig. 2.5 Vertebrae, Cervical/ Thoracic/Lumbar, superior, lateral

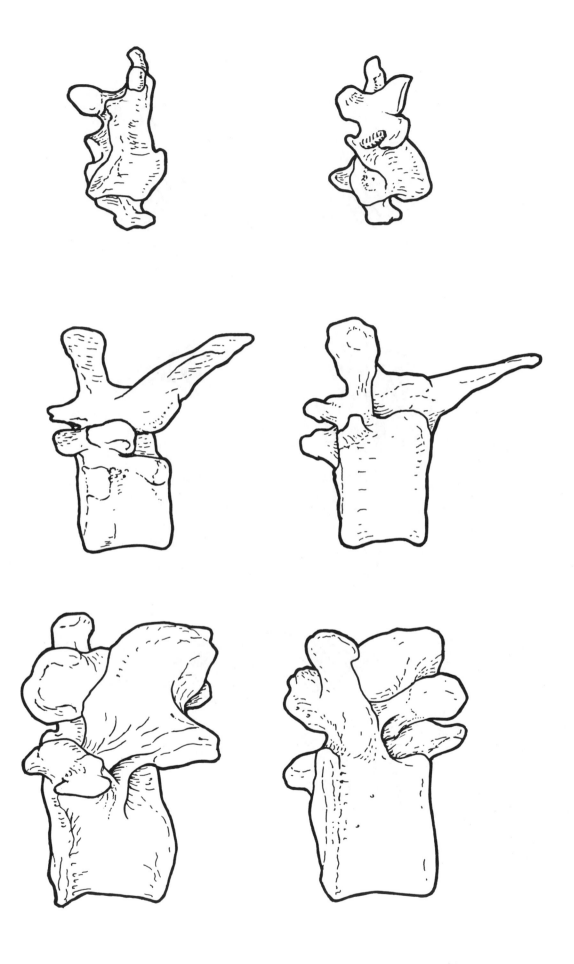

Fig. 2.6 Vertebrae, Lumbar/Thoracic/Cervical,PA oblique,AP oblique

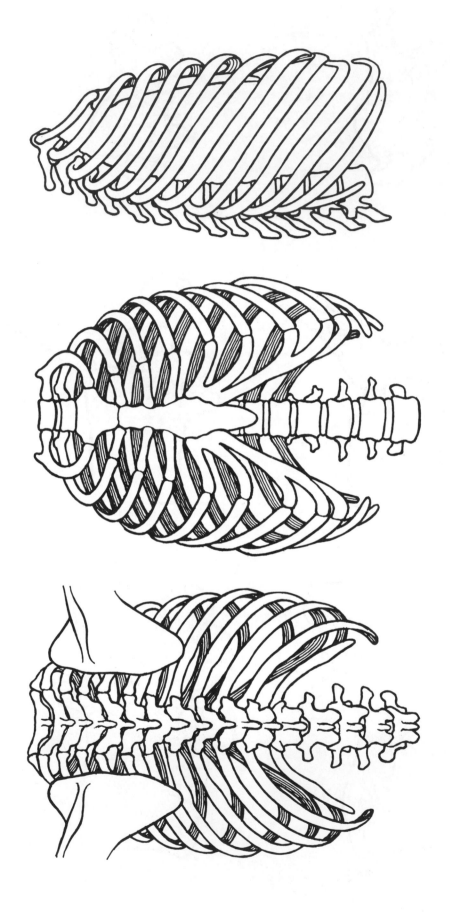

Fig. 2.7 Thorax, PA, AP, lateral

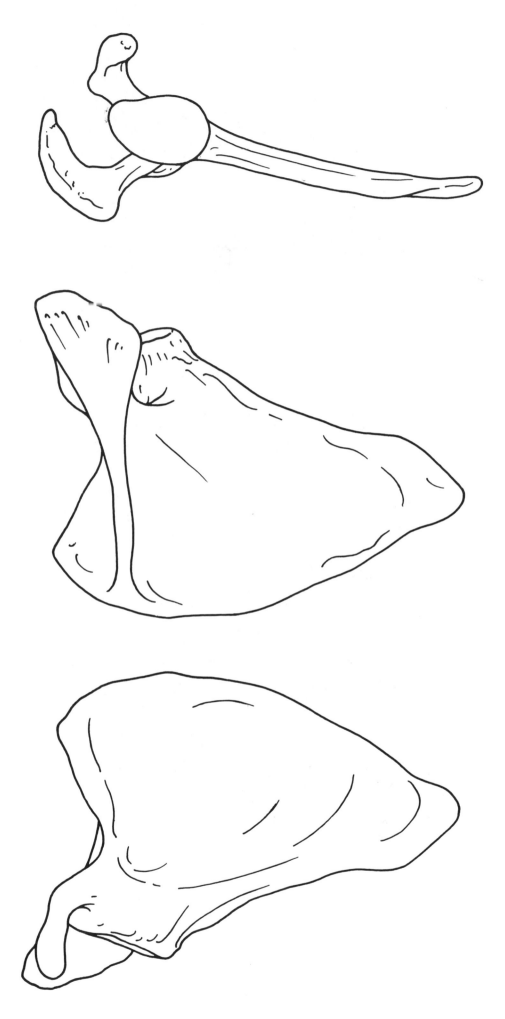

Fig. 2.8 Scapula, Costal,Dorsal, lateral

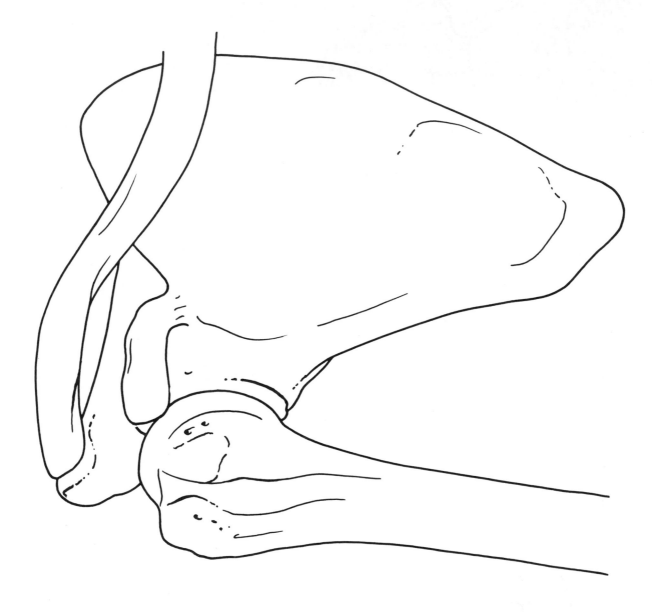

Fig. 2.9 Shoulder, AP

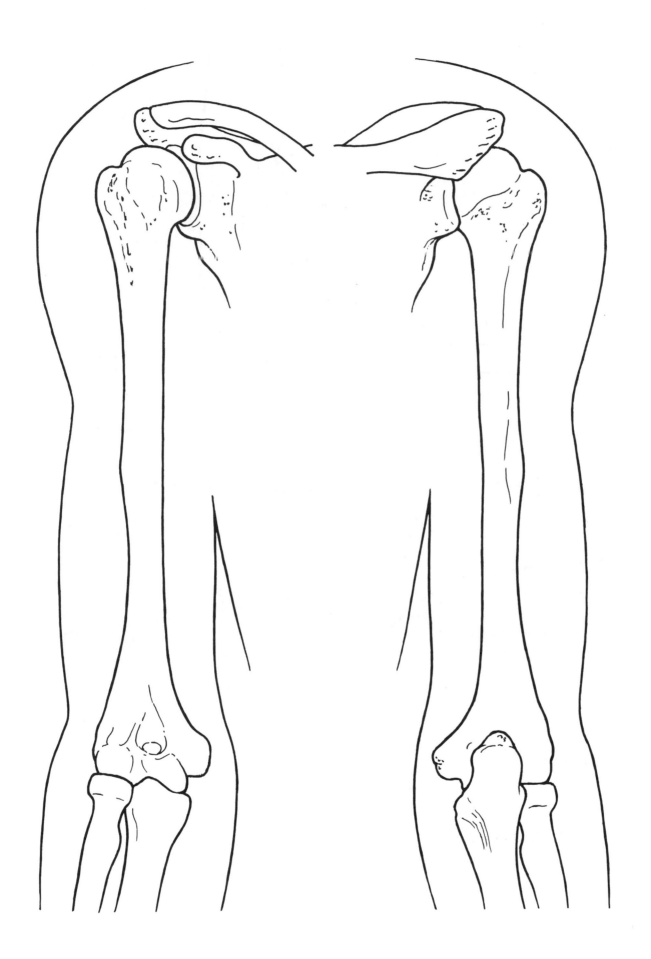

Fig. 2.10 Upper arm, AP, PA

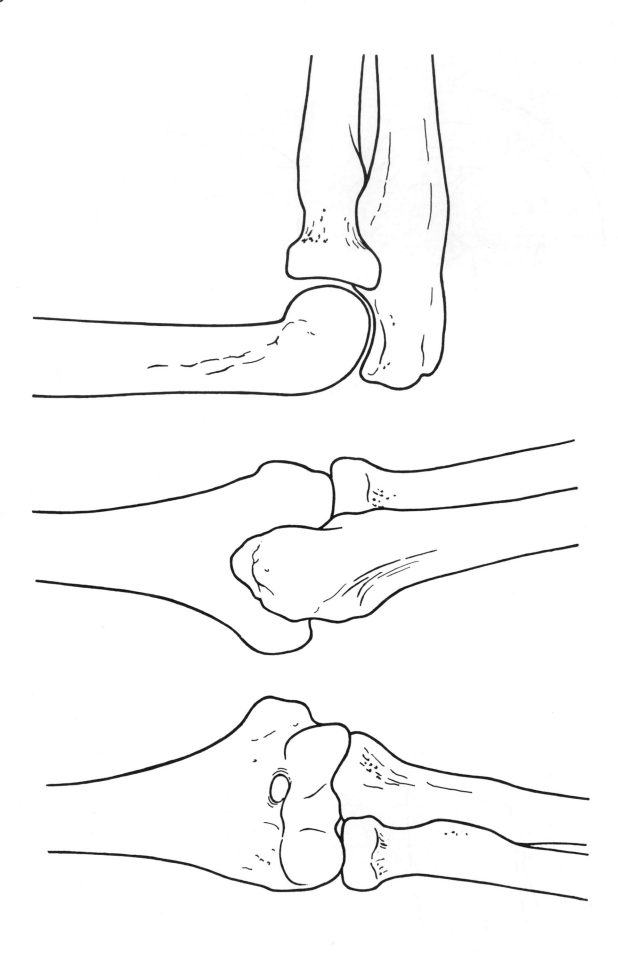

Fig. 2.11 Elbow, AP, PA, lateral

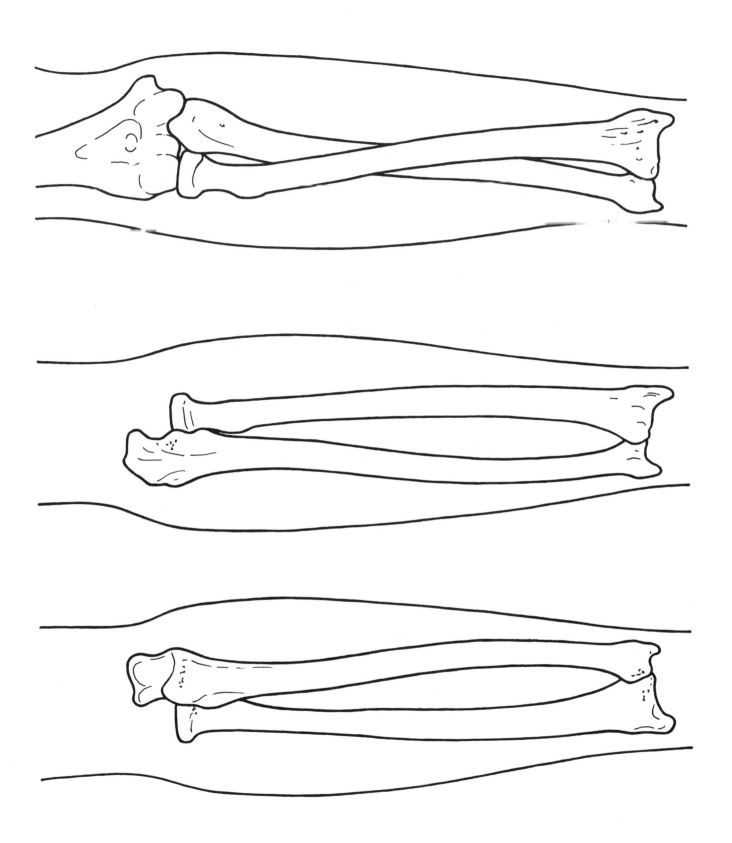

Fig. 2.12 Lower arm, AP, PA, pronated

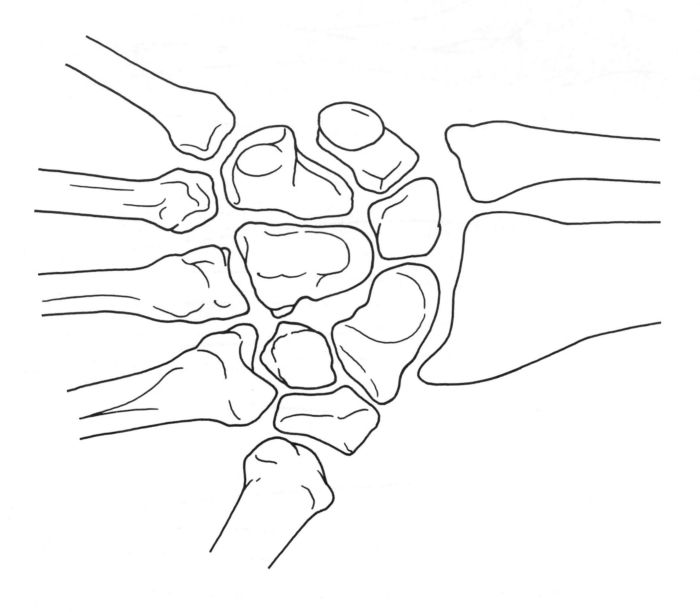

Fig. 2.13 Wrist, palmar

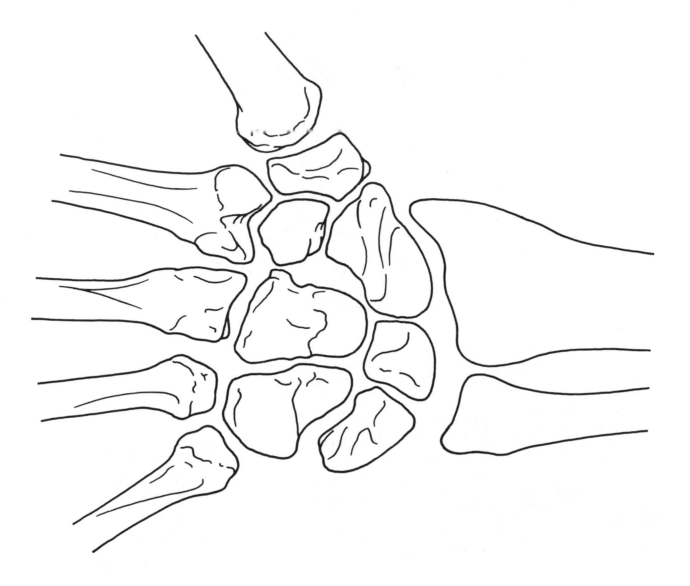

Fig. 2.14 Wrist, dorsal

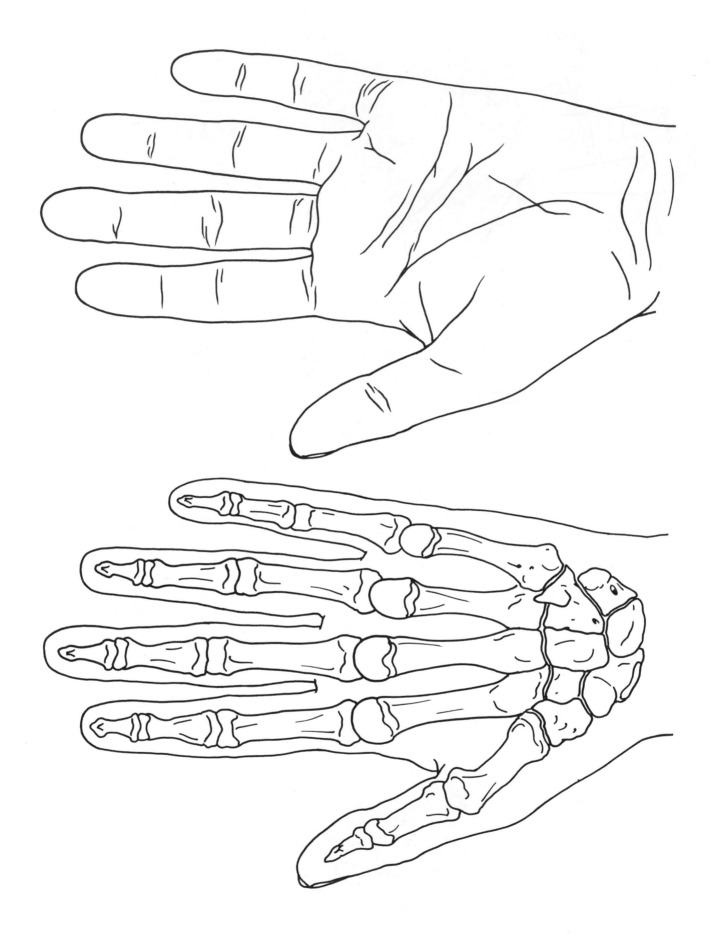

Fig. 2.15   Hand, palmar

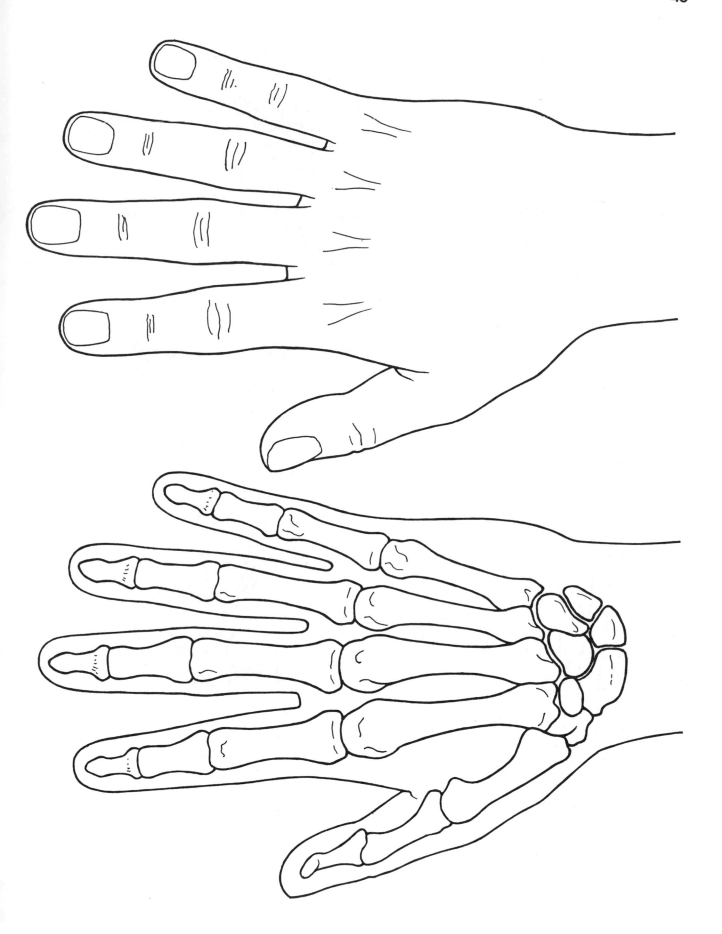

Fig. 2.16 Hand, dorsal

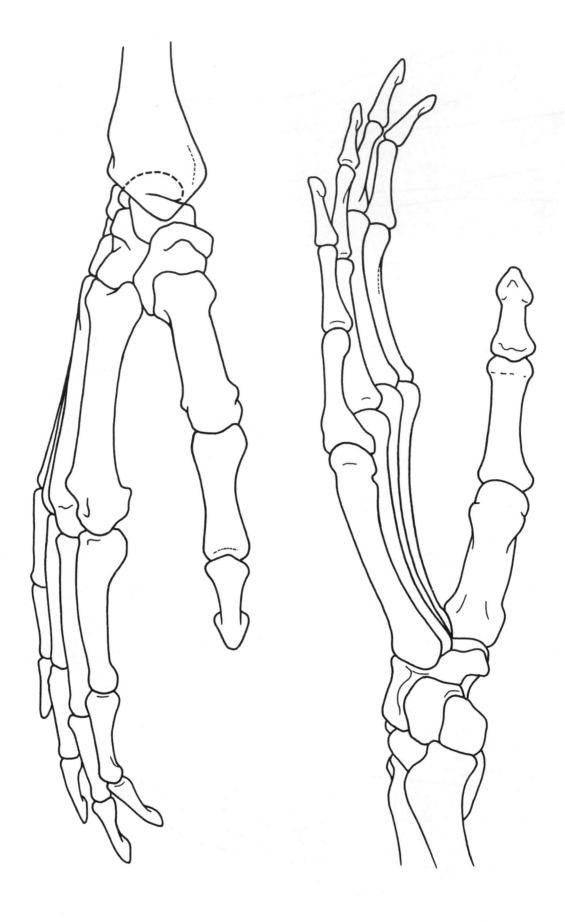

Fig. 2.17 Hand/Wrist, lateral, medial

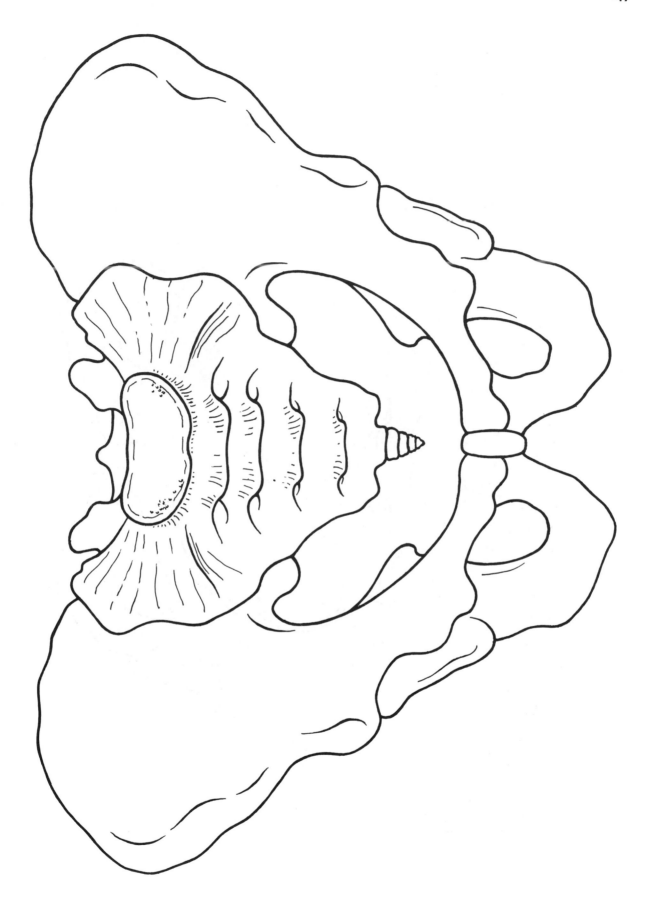

Fig. 2.18 Pelvis - Male, AP

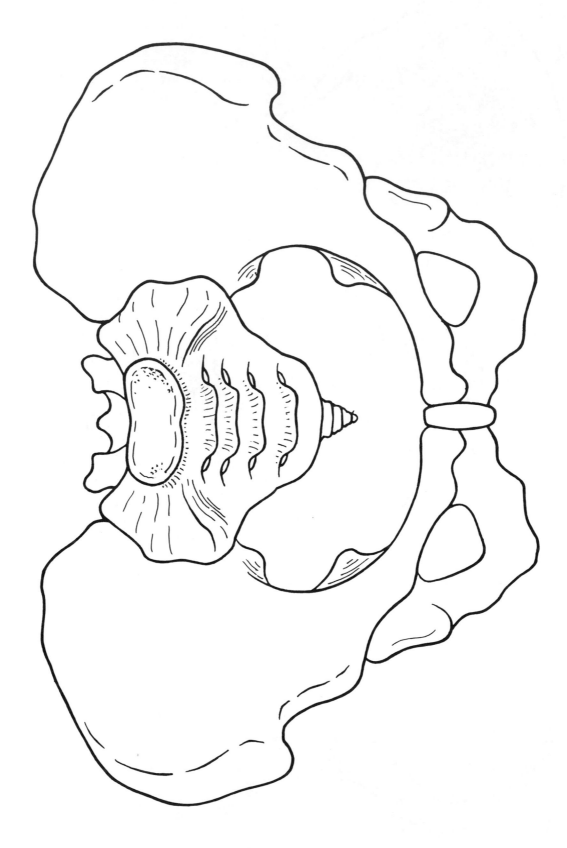

Fig. 2.19 Pelvis - Female, AP

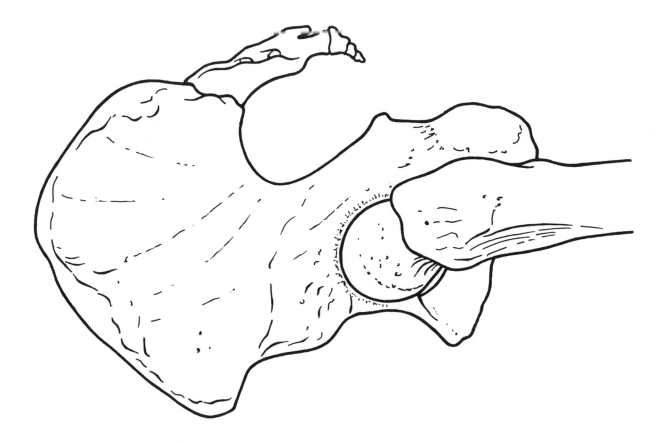

Fig. 2.20 Hip, lateral

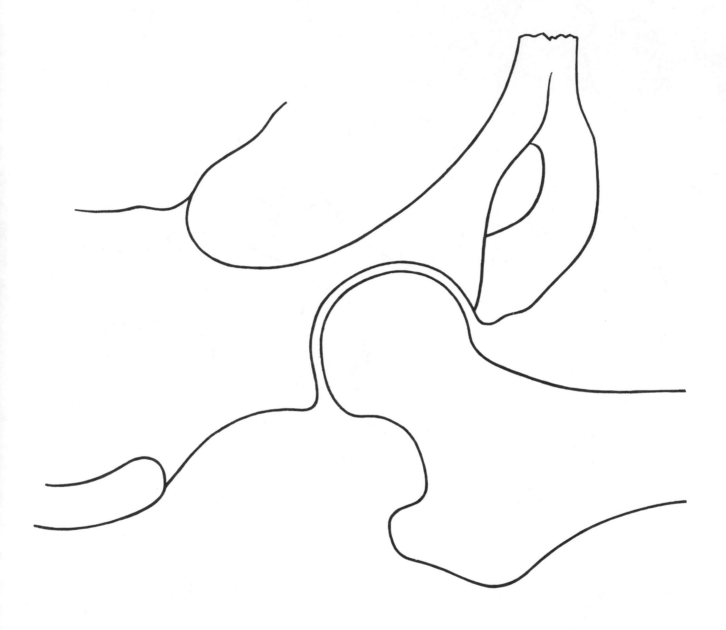

Fig. 2.21 Hip, AP

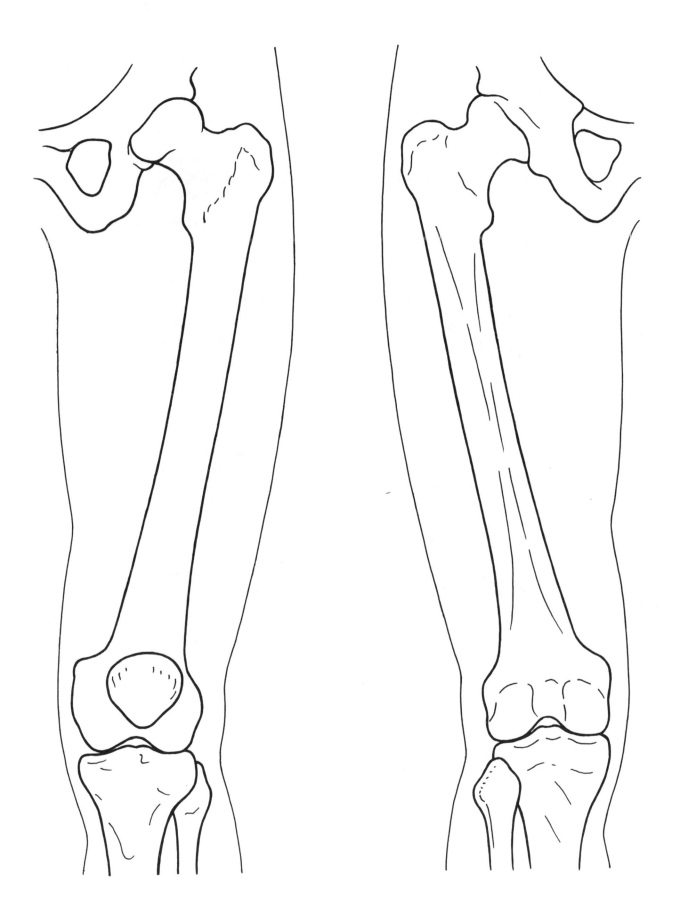

Fig. 2.22 Upper leg, AP, PA

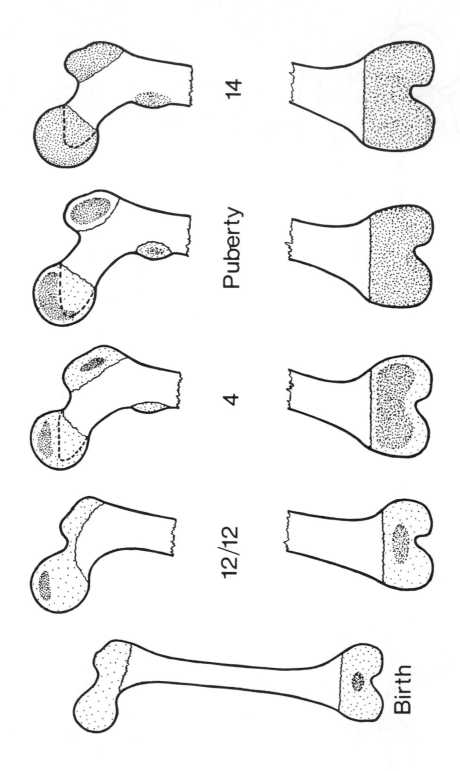

Fig. 2.23 Femur, ossification

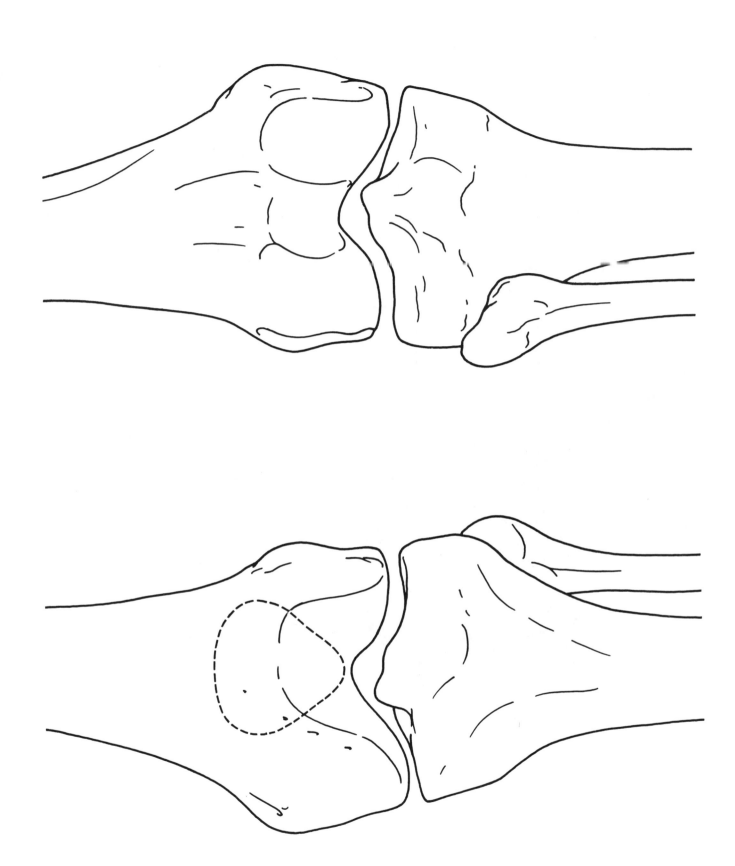

Fig. 2.24 Knee, AP, PA

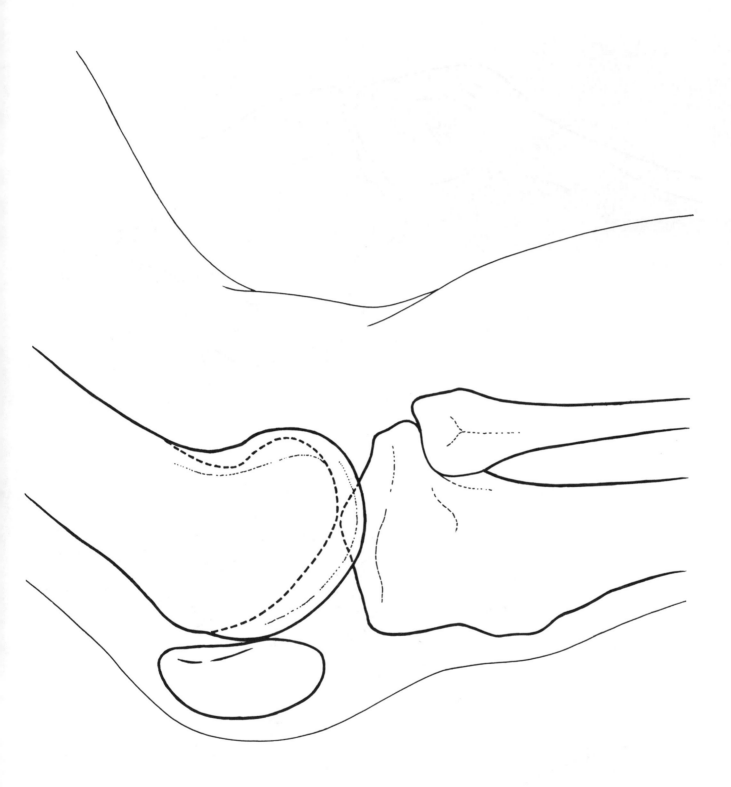

Fig. 2.25 Knee, lateral

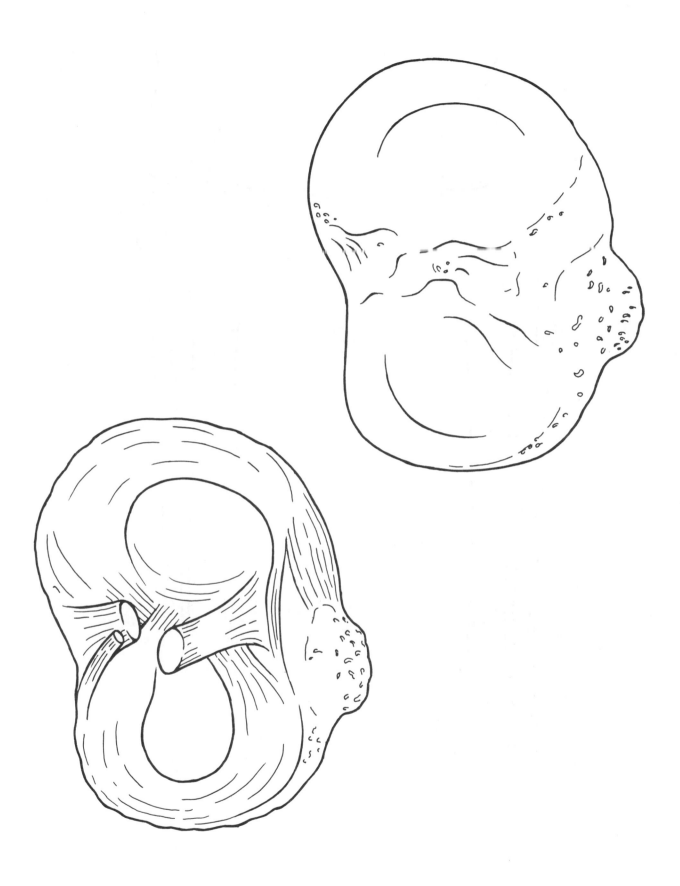

Fig. 2.26 Tibia head, superior views, menisci

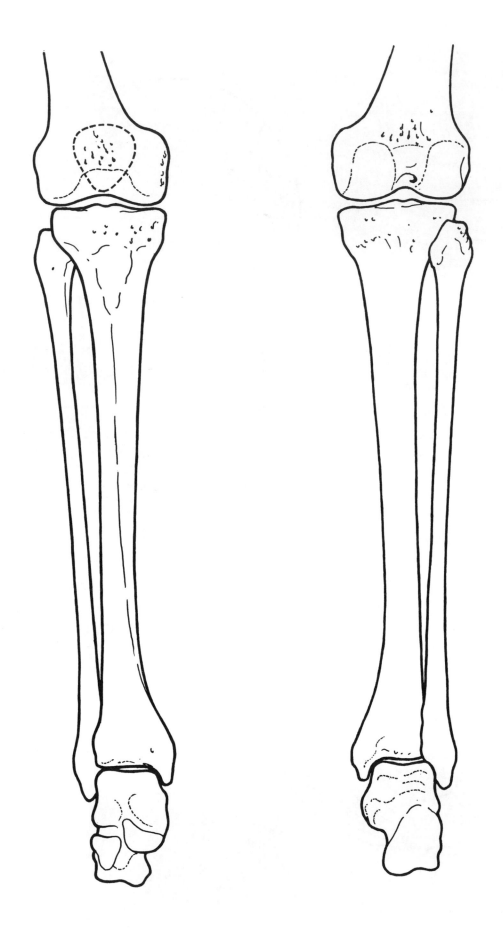

Fig. 2.27 Lower leg, AP, PA

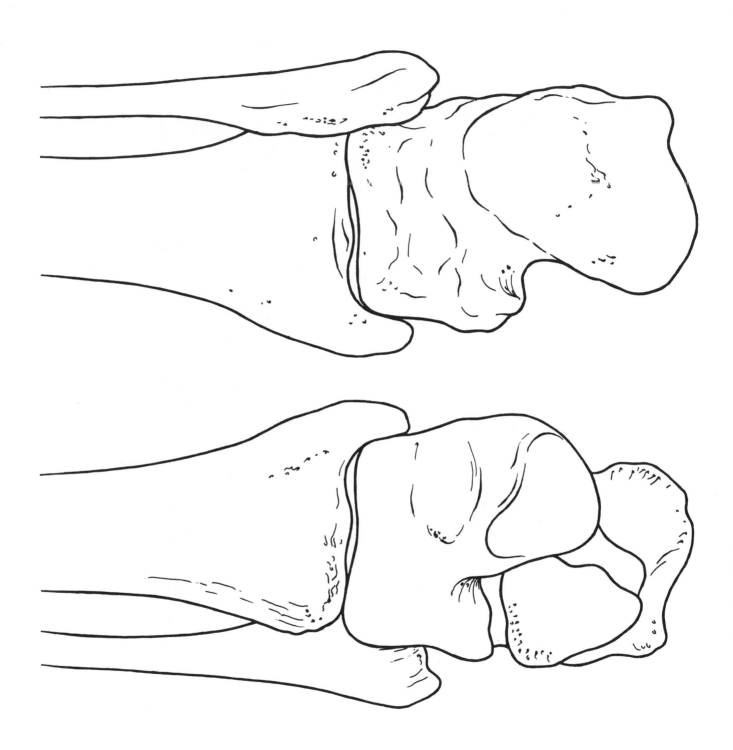

Fig. 2.28 Ankle, AP, PA

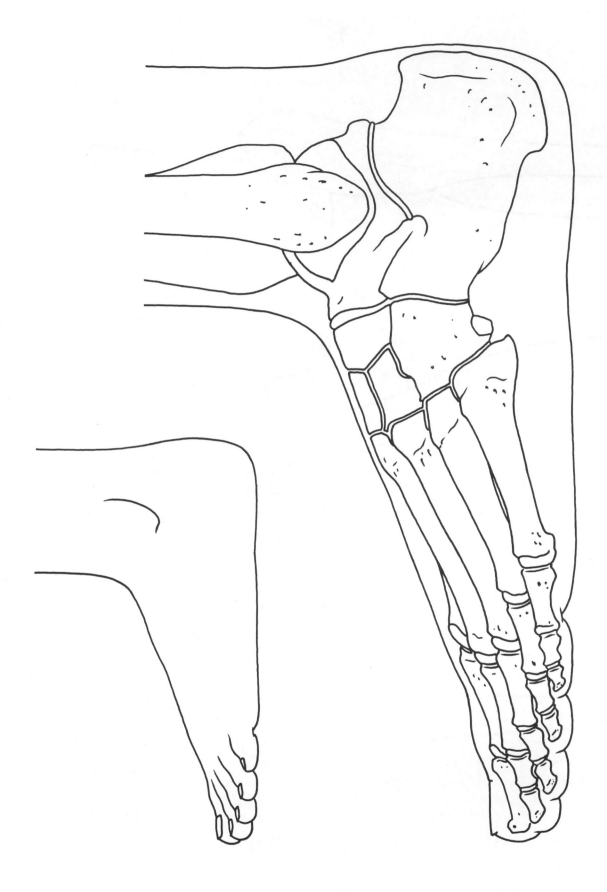

Fig. 2.29 Foot, lateral

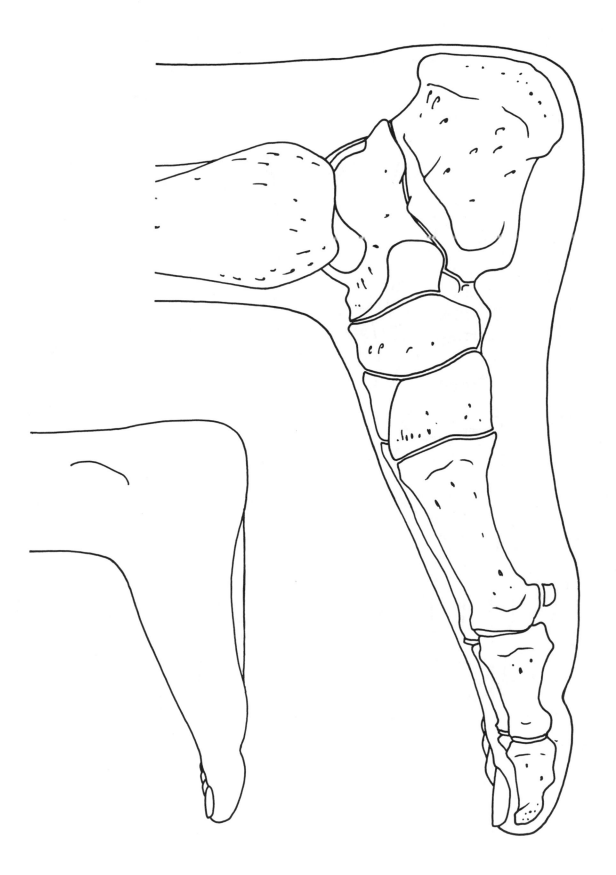

Fig. 2.30 Foot, medial

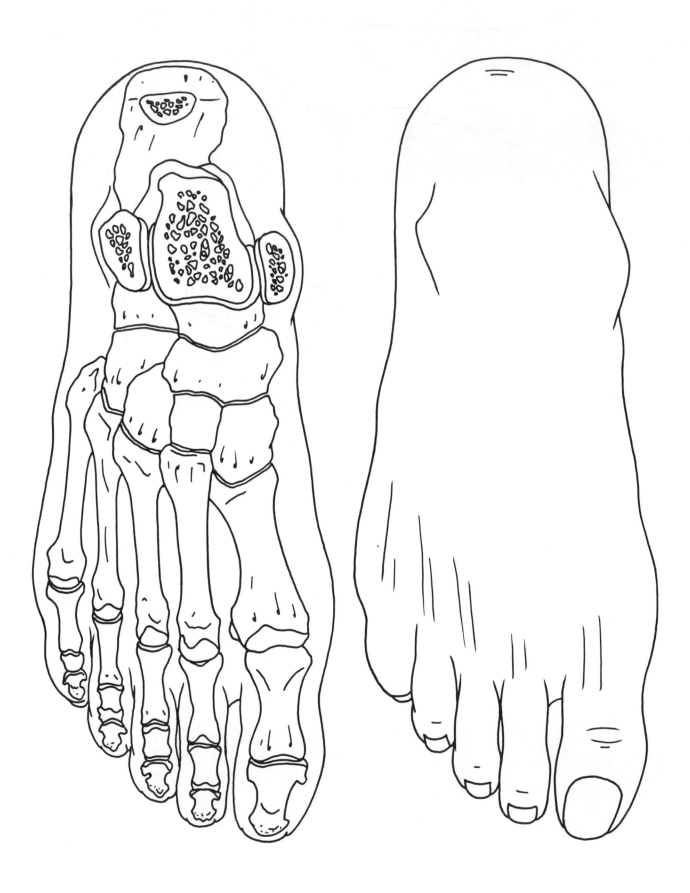

Fig. 2.31 Foot, dorsal

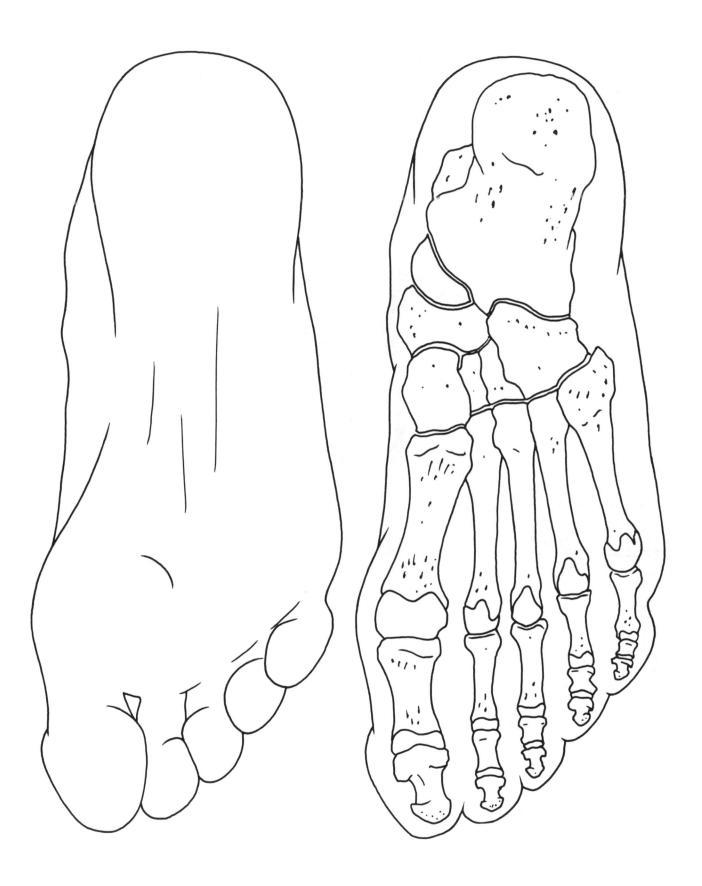

Fig. 2.32 Foot, plantar

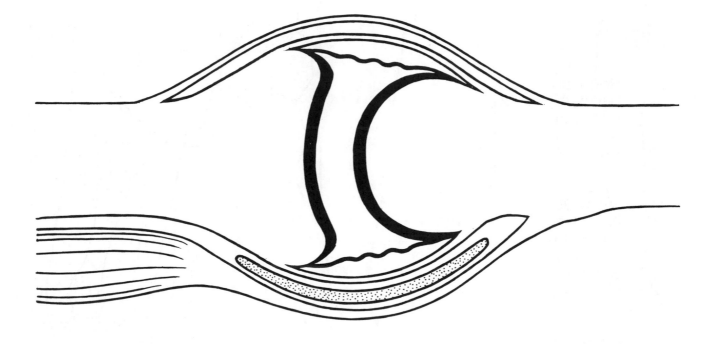

Fig. 2.33 Synovial joint, scheme

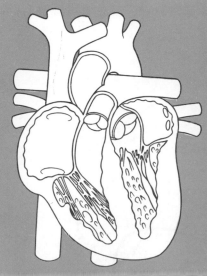

Section 3

Heart, Lungs and Circulation

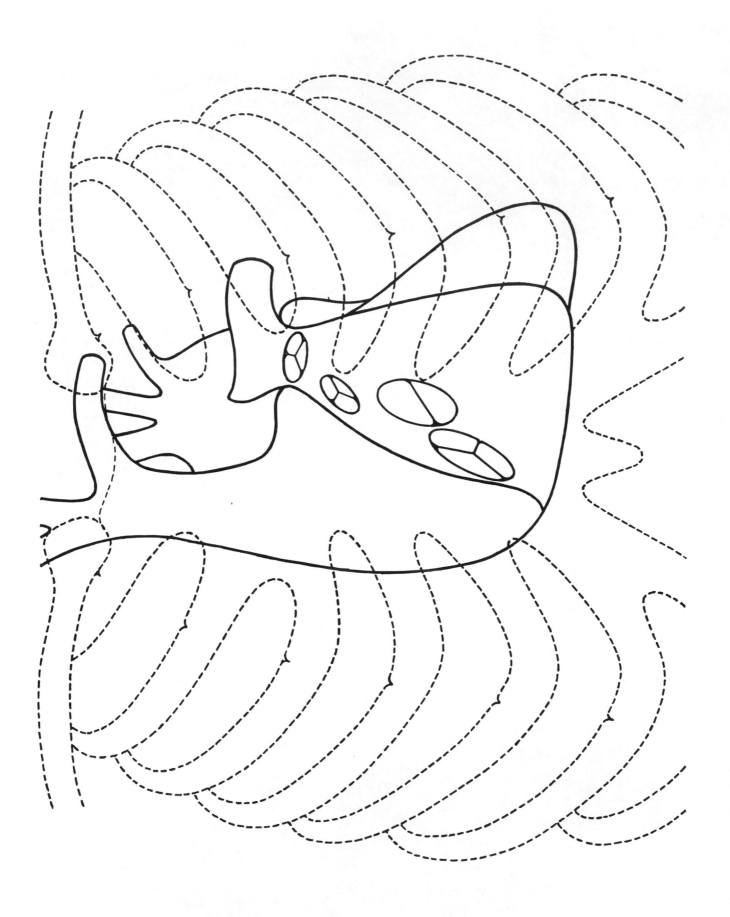

Fig. 3.1 Heart and valves, position in rib cage

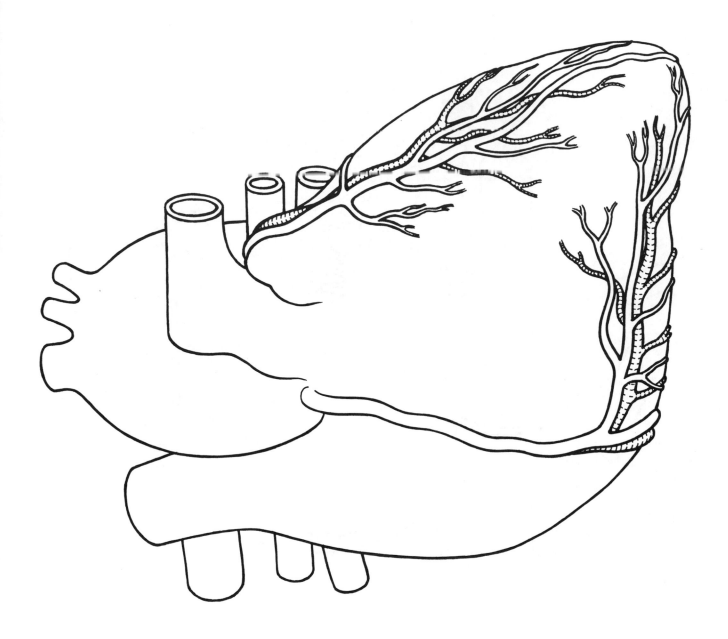

Fig. 3.2   Heart, AP

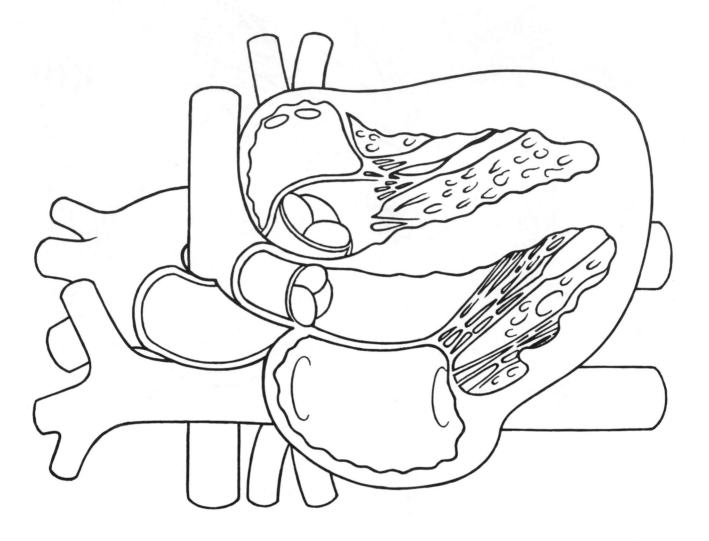

Fig. 3.3 Heart, coronal section, AP

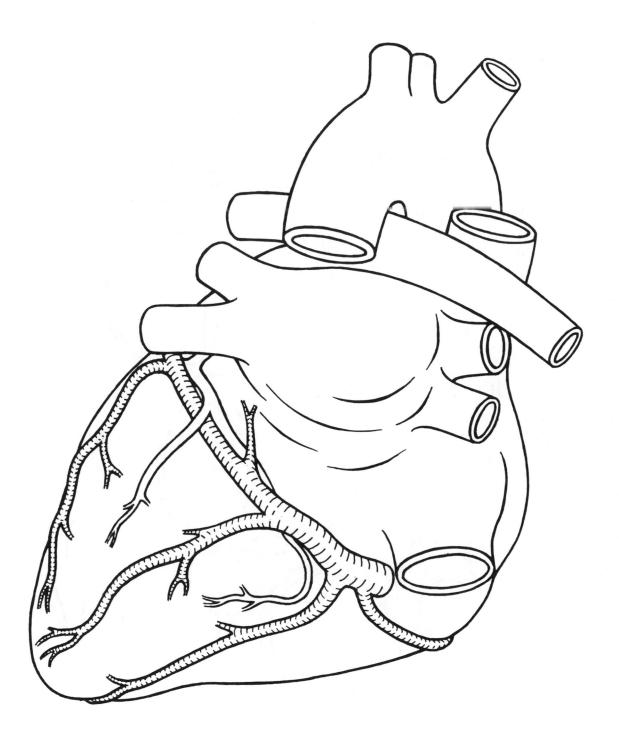

Fig. 3.4 Heart, PA

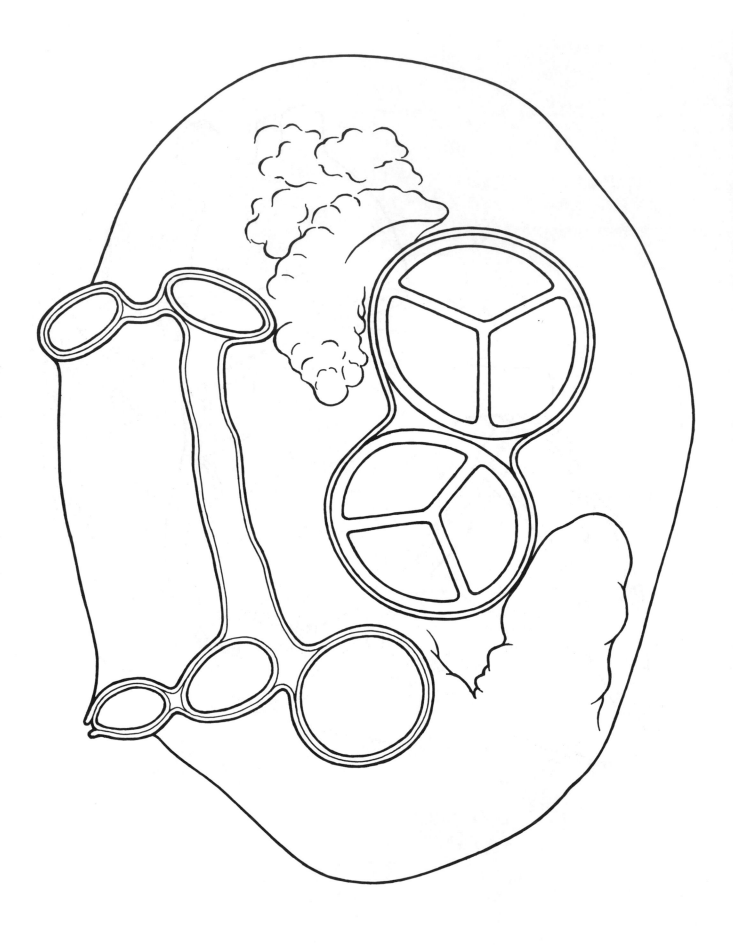

Fig. 3.5 Heart, superior view

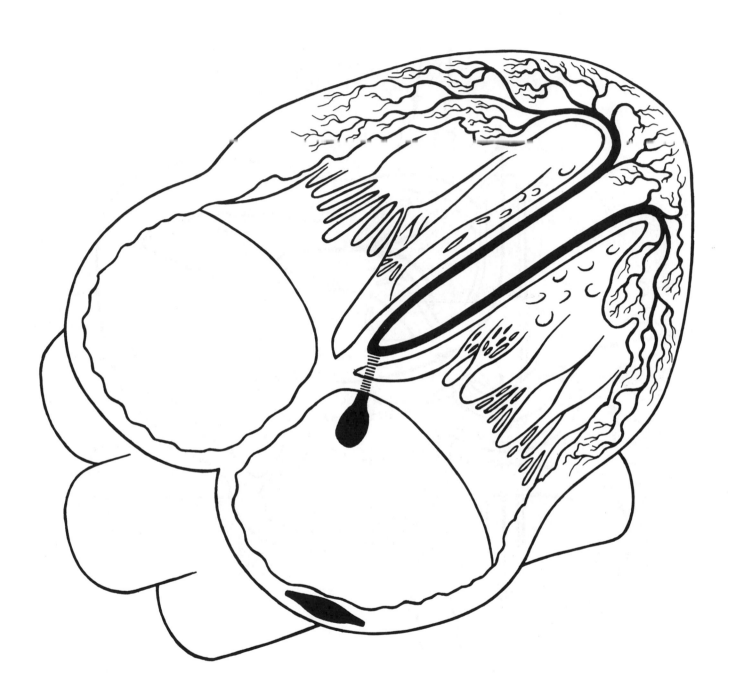

Fig. 3.6 Heart, conducting fibres

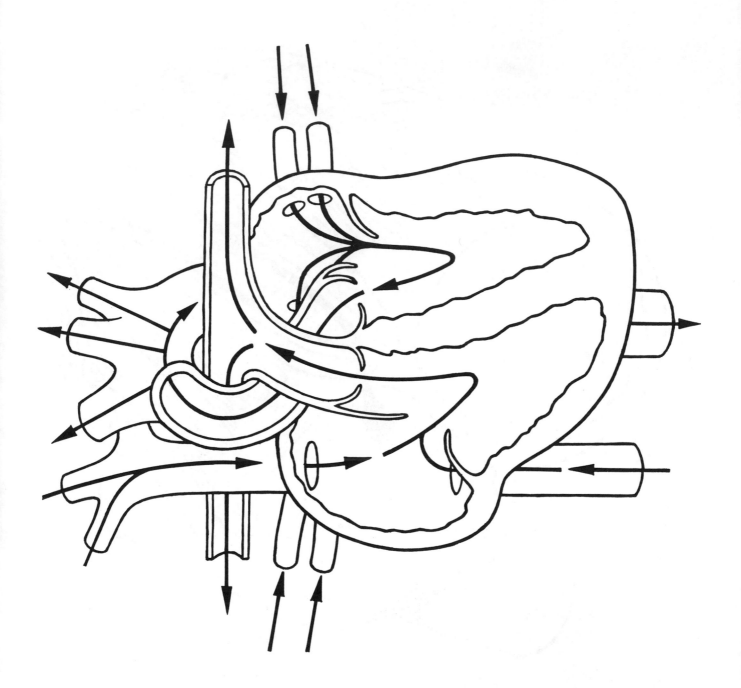

Fig. 3.7 Heart, direction of blood flow

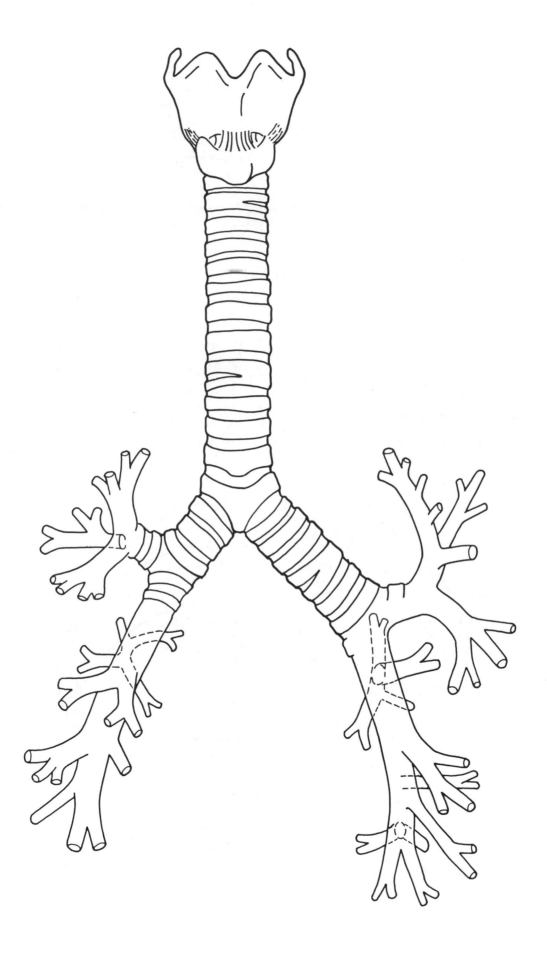

Fig. 3.8 Bronchial tree

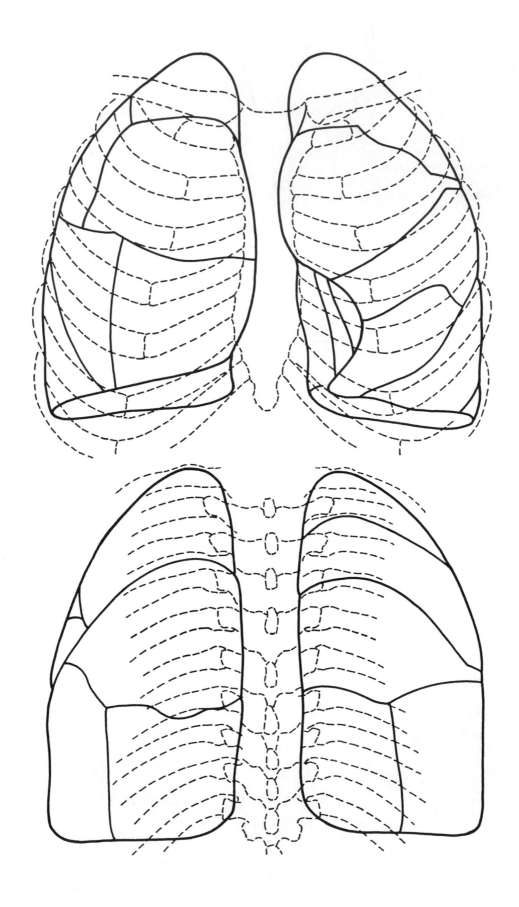

Fig. 3.9 Broncho-pulmonary segment in relation to ribs, AP and PA

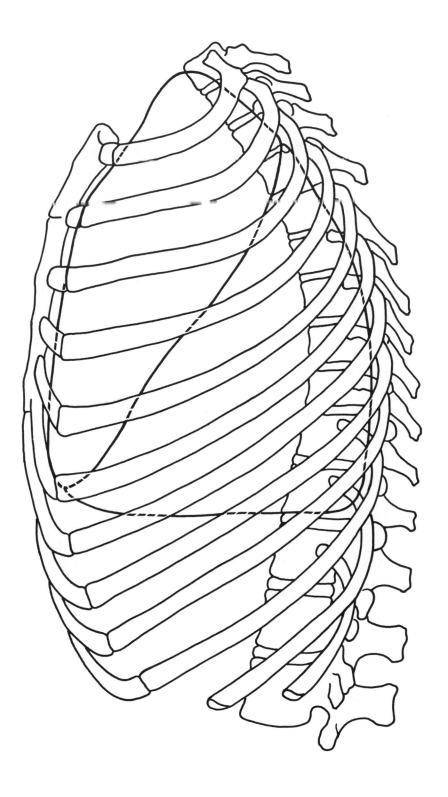

Fig. 3.10 Surface relation of lobes of left lung, lateral

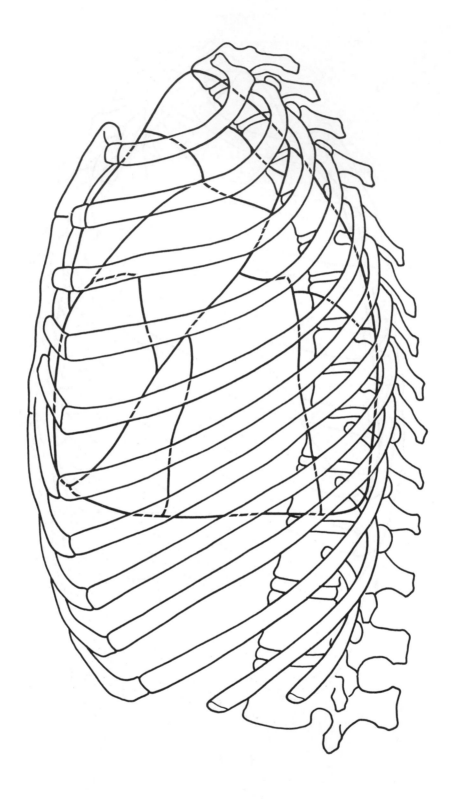

Fig. 3.11 Left broncho-pulmonary segments, lateral

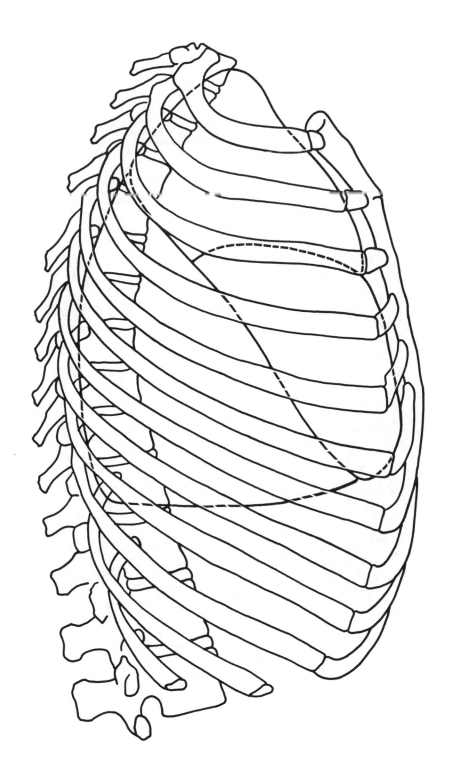

Fig. 3.12 Surface relation of lobes of right lung, lateral

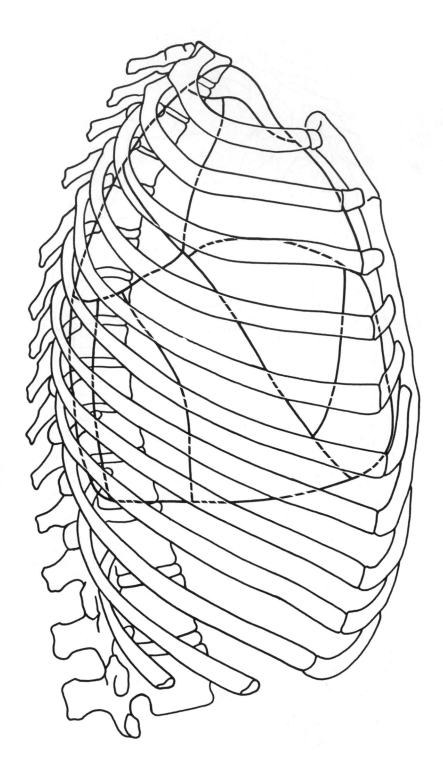

Fig. 3.13 Right broncho-pulmonary segments, lateral

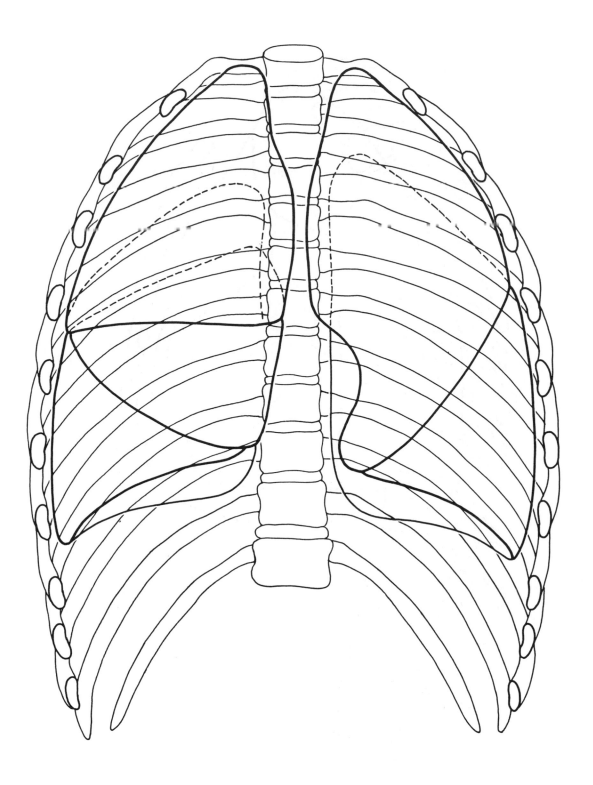

Fig. 3.14 Lungs in rib cage, lobes, AP, (lobes PA dotted)

78

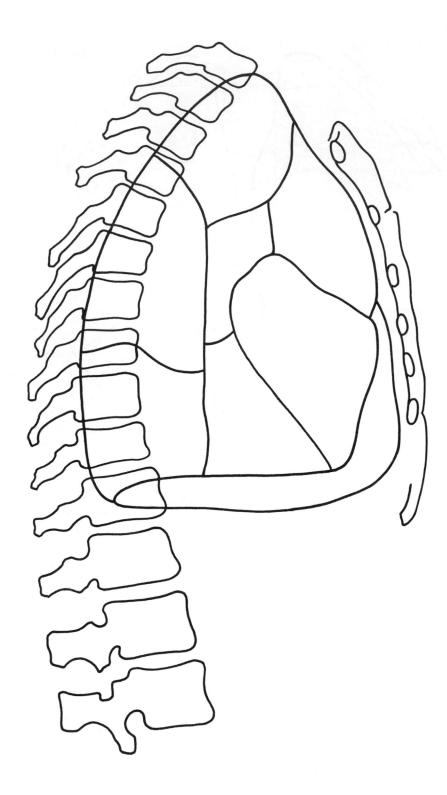

Fig. 3.15 Left broncho-pulmonary segments, medial

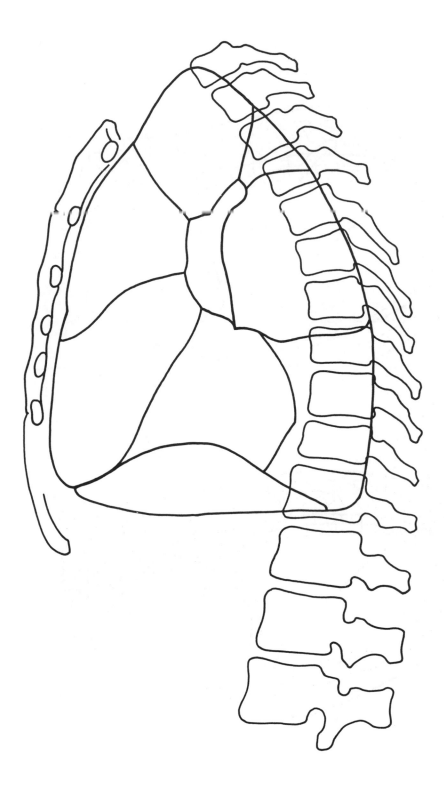

Fig. 3.16 Right broncho-pulmonary segments, medial

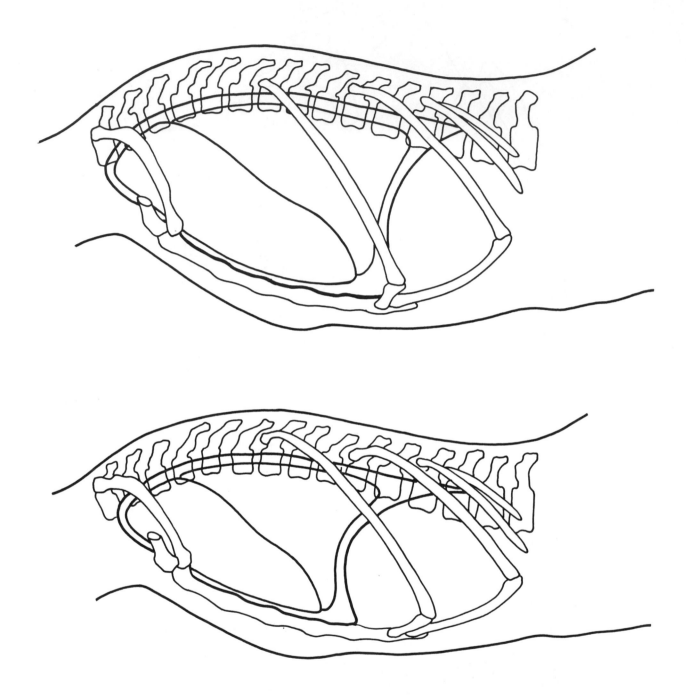

Fig. 3.17 Expiration and inspiration, left lateral

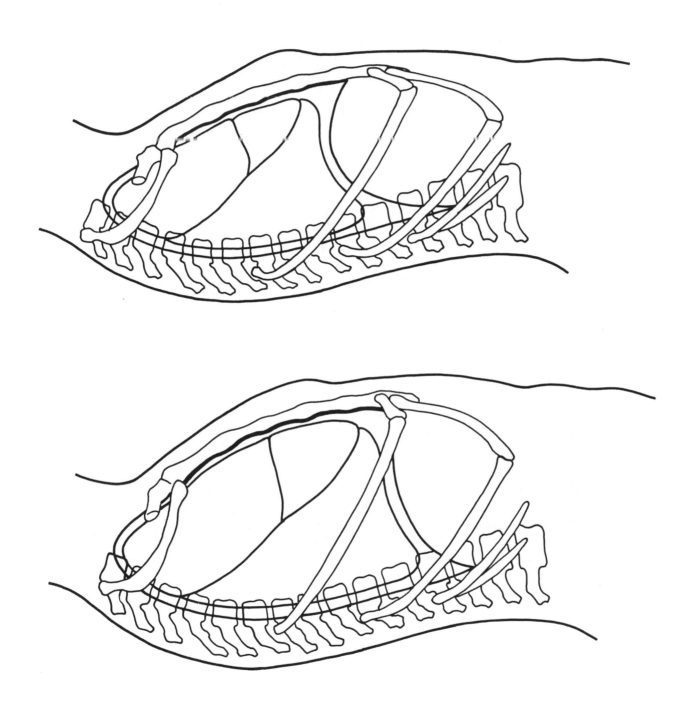

Fig. 3.18 Inspiration and expiration, right lateral

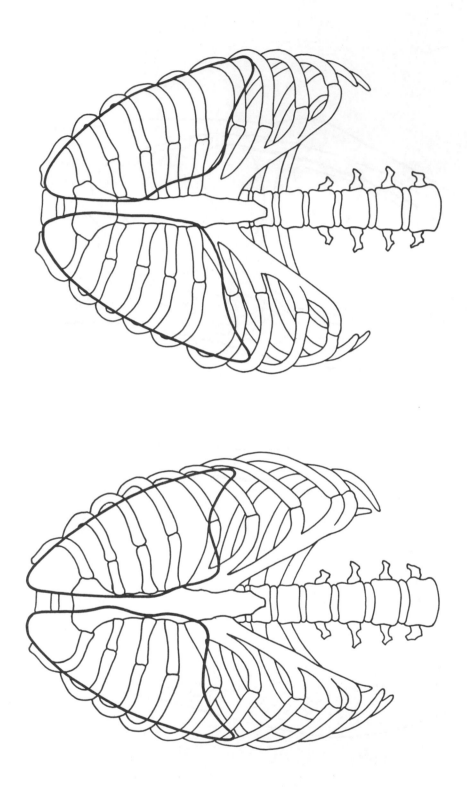

Fig. 3.19 Quiet respiration and full inspiration, AP

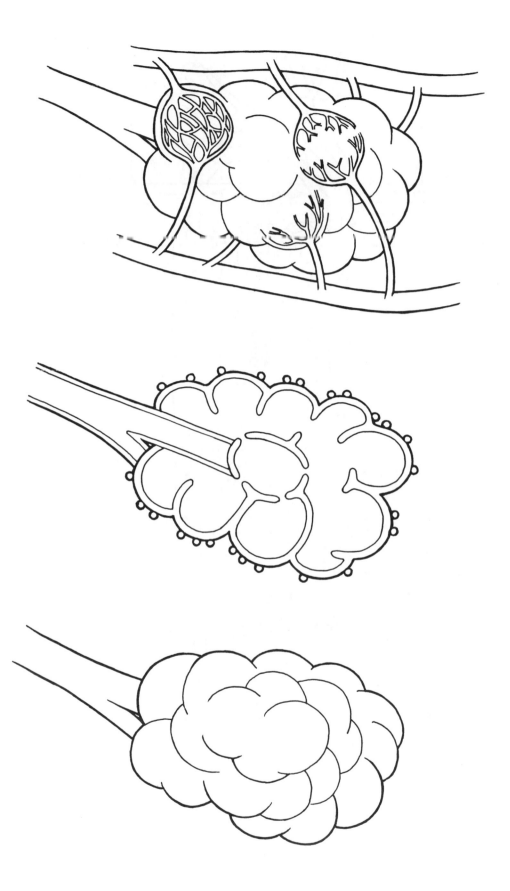

Fig. 3.20 Bronchiole, alveoli

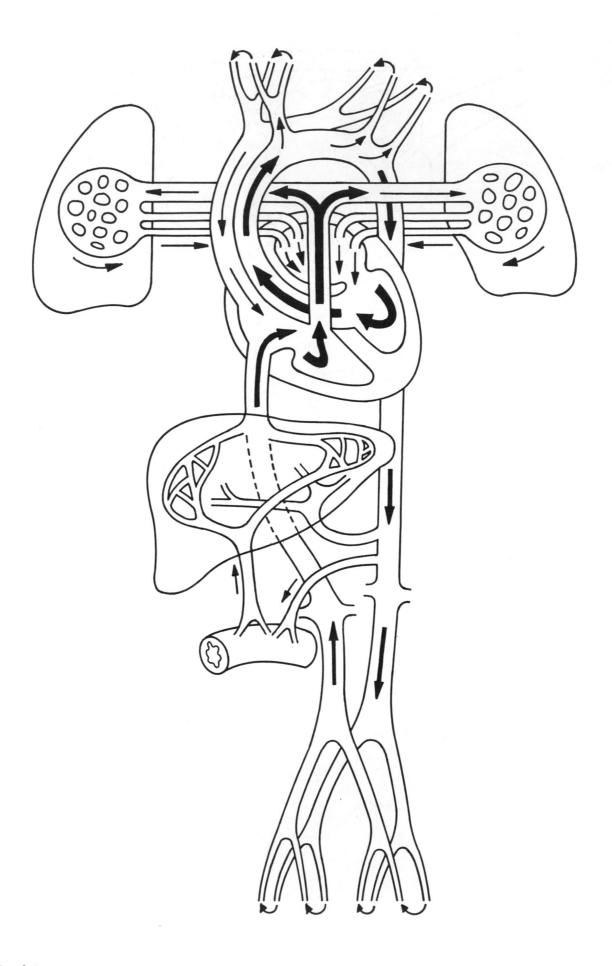

Fig. 3.21 Scheme of circulation, adult

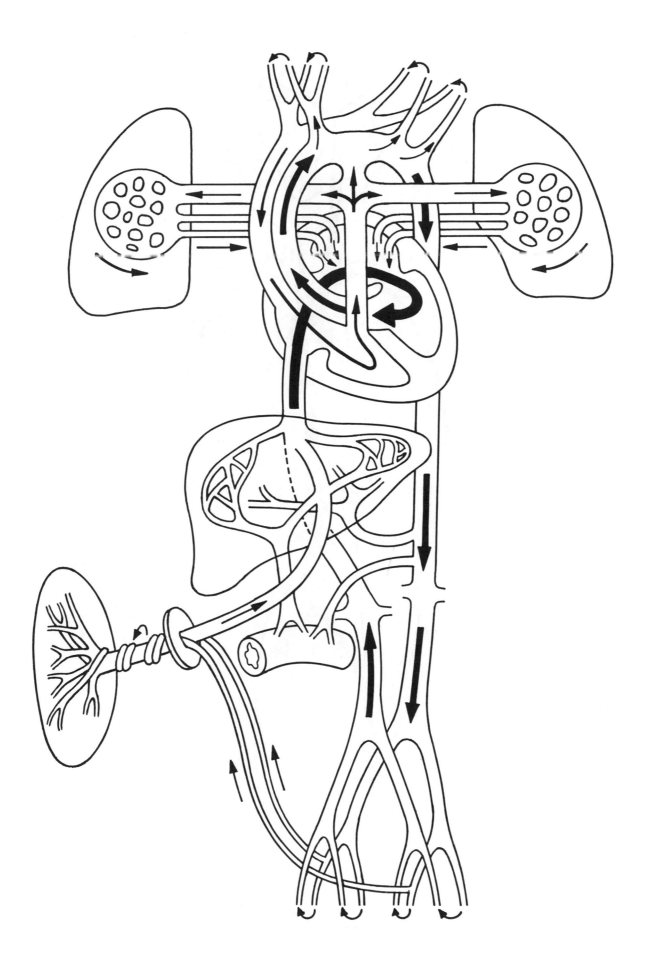

Fig. 3.22 Scheme of circulation, fetus

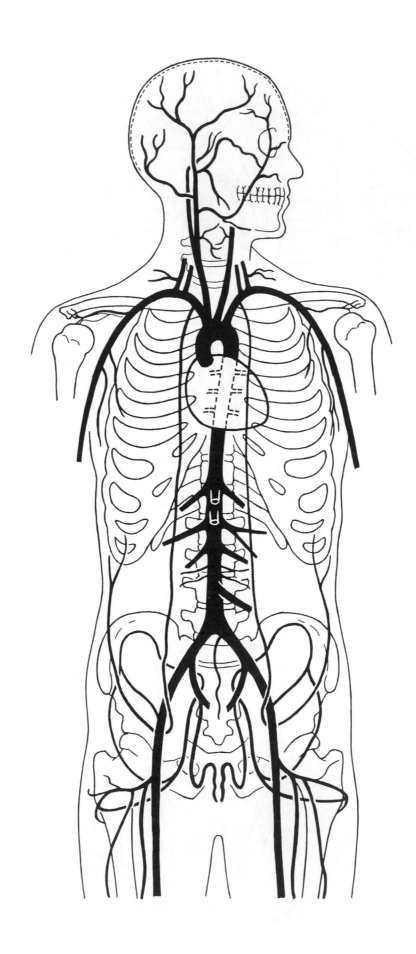

Fig. 3.23 Principal arteries - torso

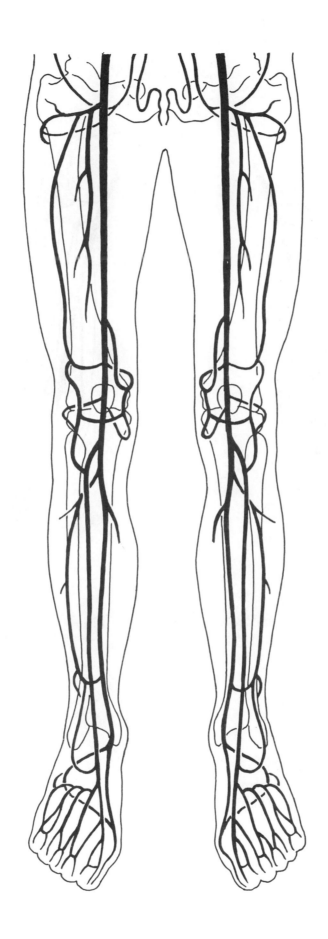

Fig. 3.24 Principal arteries - legs

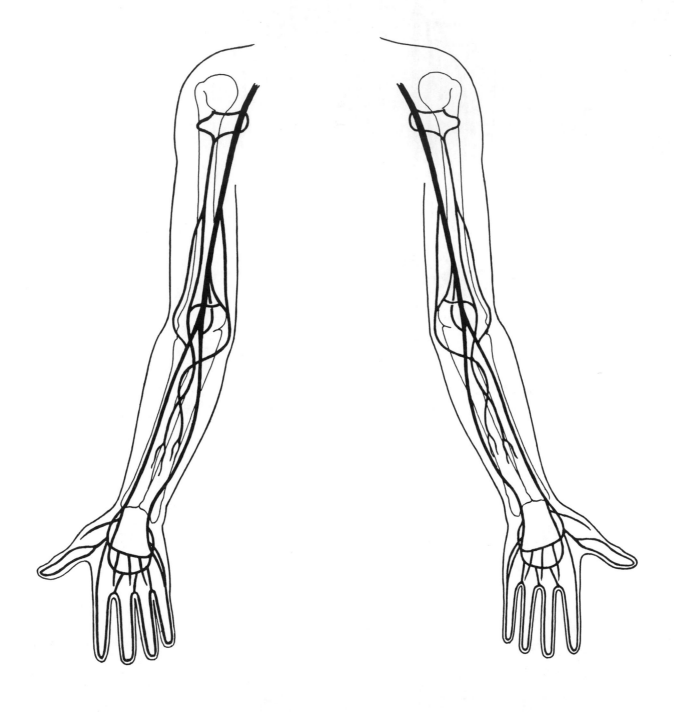

Fig. 3.25 Principal arteries - arms

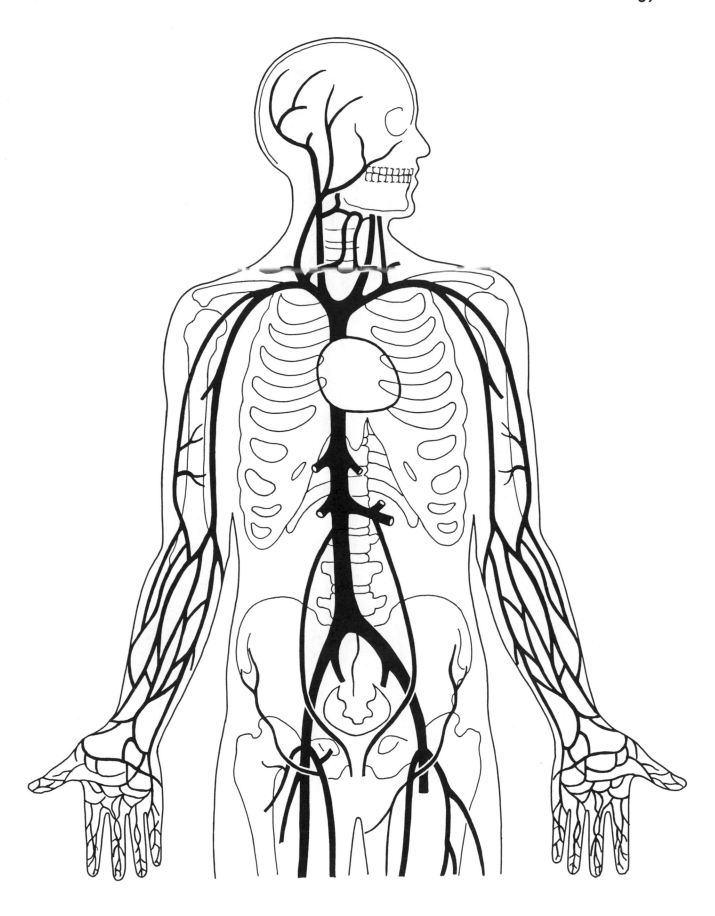

Fig. 3.26 Principal veins - torso

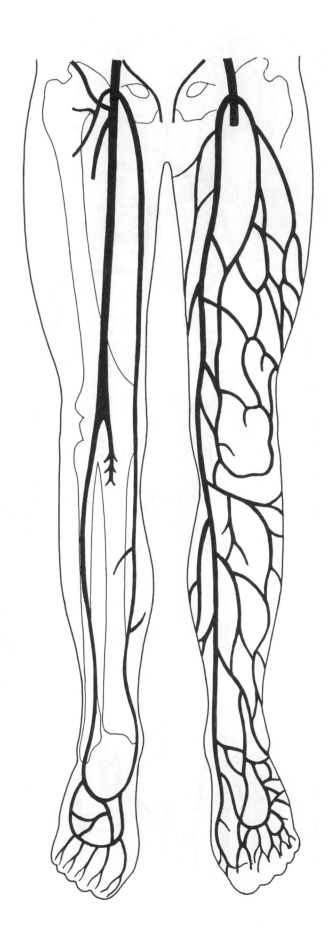

Fig. 3.27 Principal veins - legs

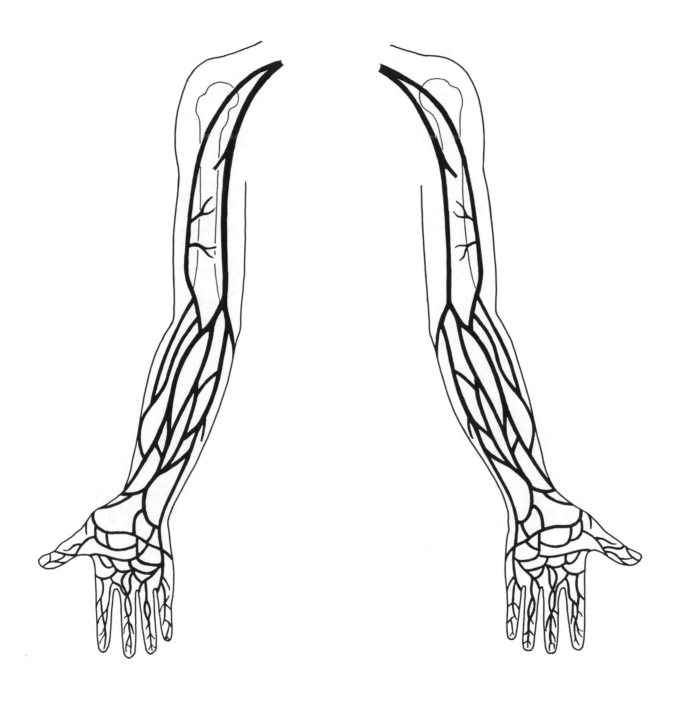

Fig. 3.28 Principal veins - arms

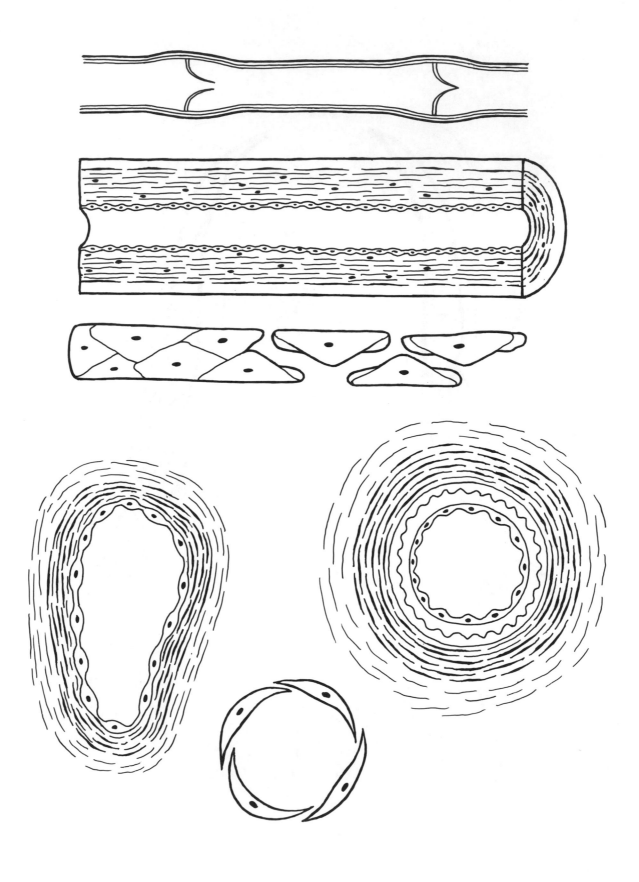

Fig. 3.29 Blood vessels, sections

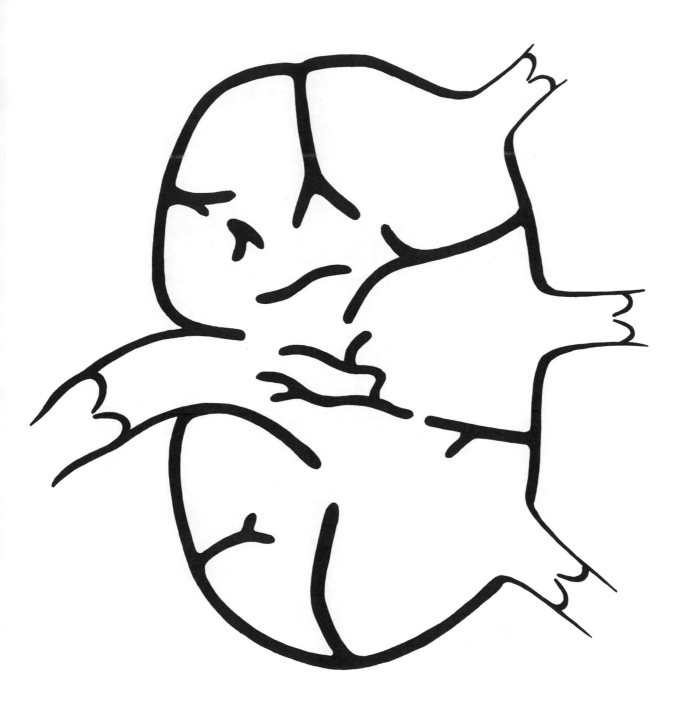

Fig. 3.30 Lymph gland, section

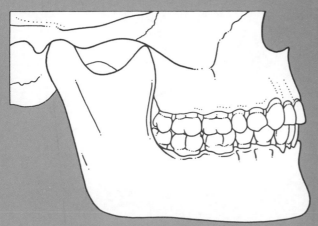

Section 4

Digestive Tract

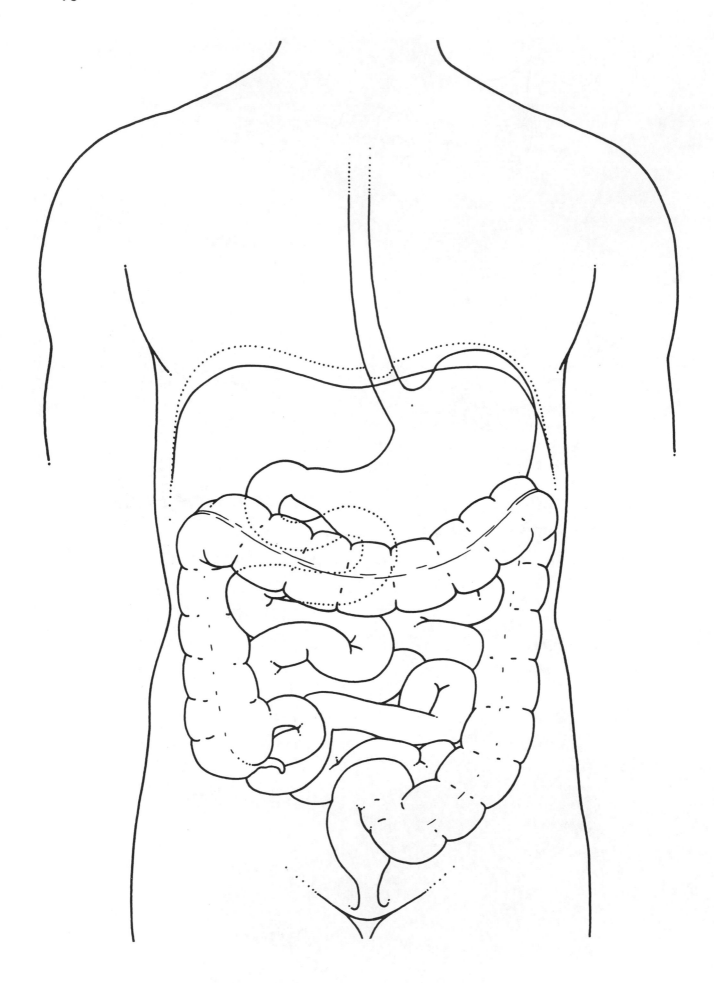

Fig. 4.1 Digestive tract in body outline

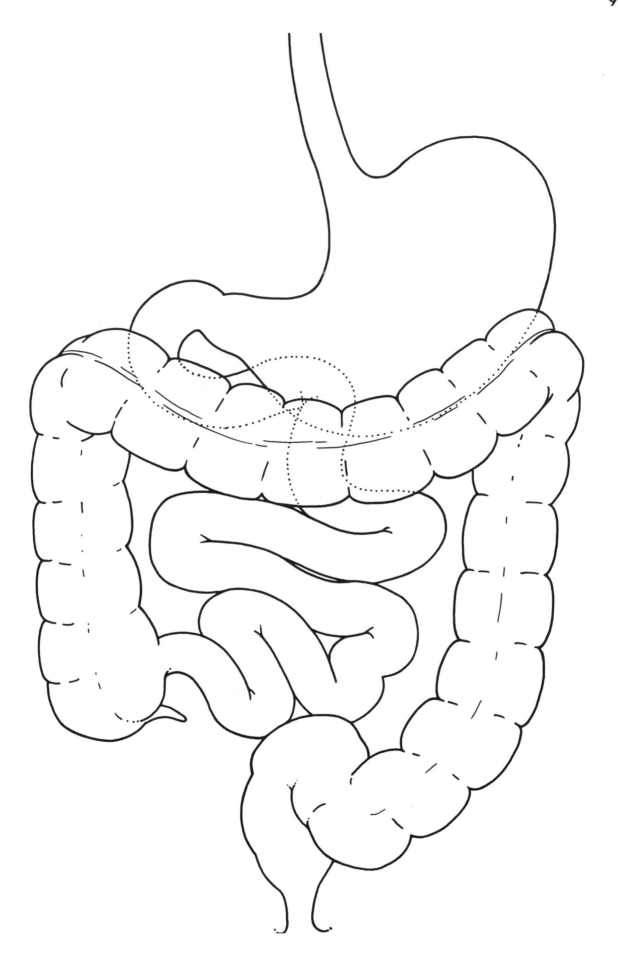

Fig. 4.2 Digestive tract - scheme

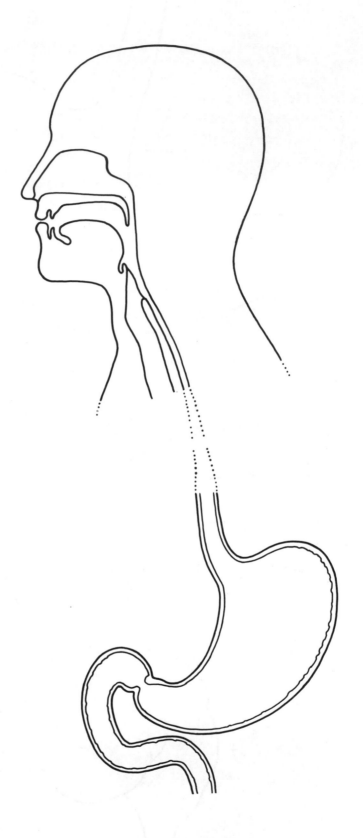

Fig. 4.3 Mouth, oesophagus, stomach - sections

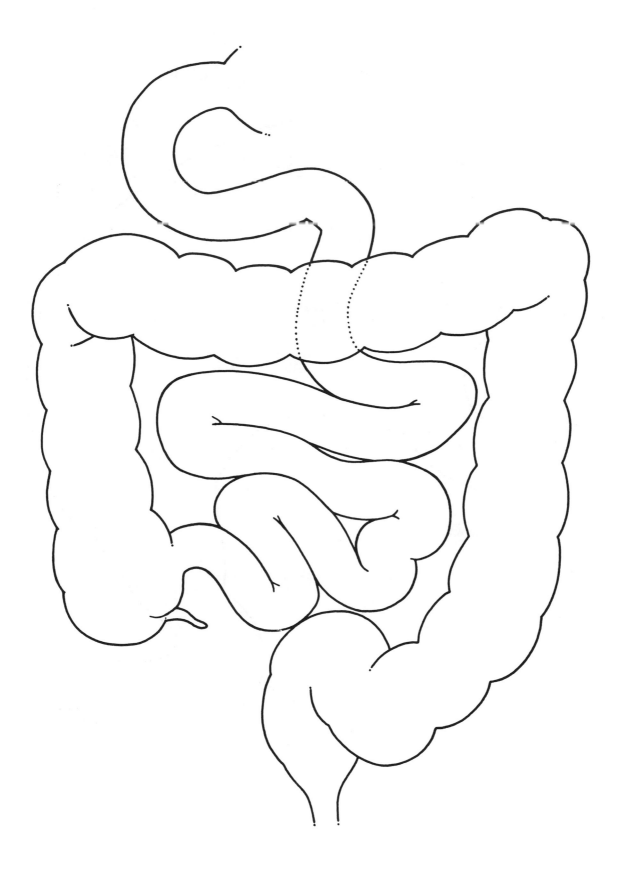

Fig. 4.4 Small and large bowel - scheme

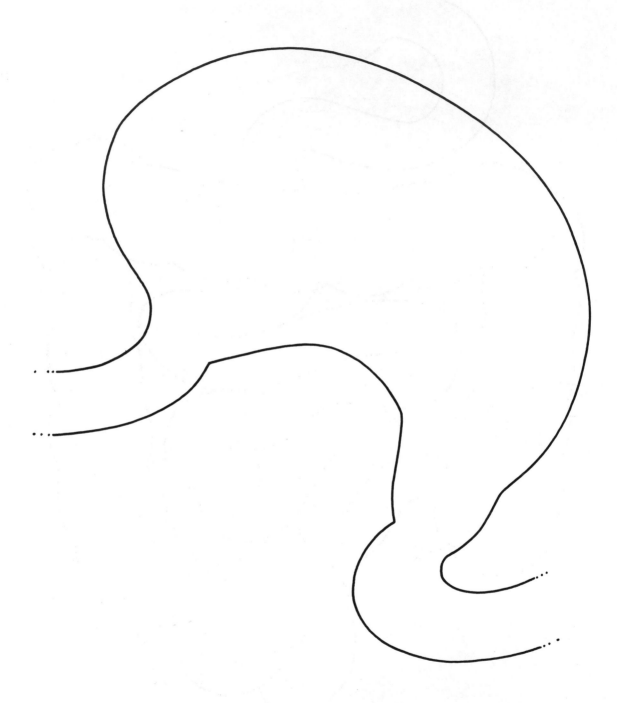

Fig. 4.5 Stomach - outline

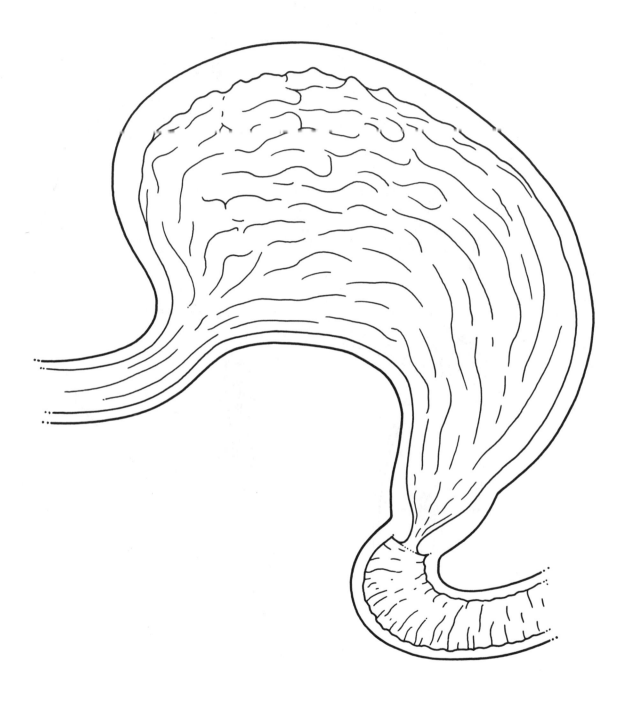

Fig. 4.6 Stomach - section

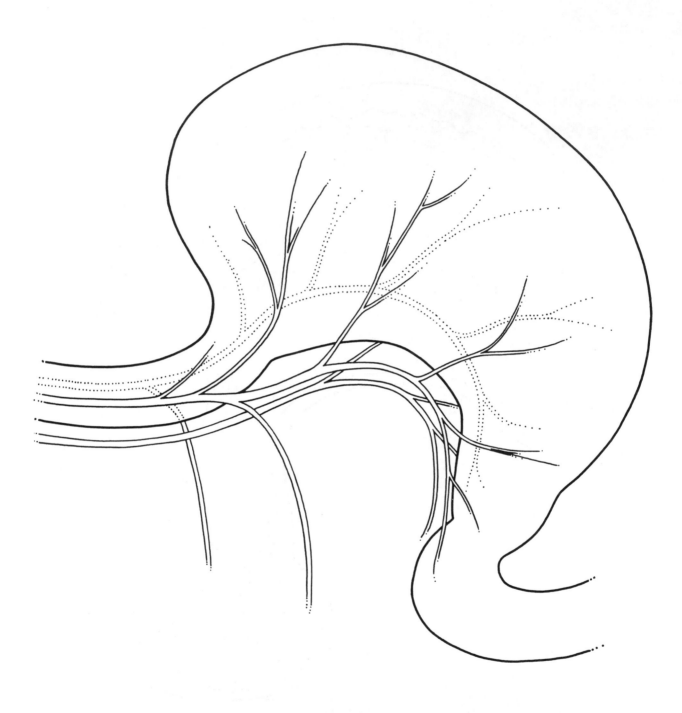

Fig. 4.7 Stomach - vagus nerve

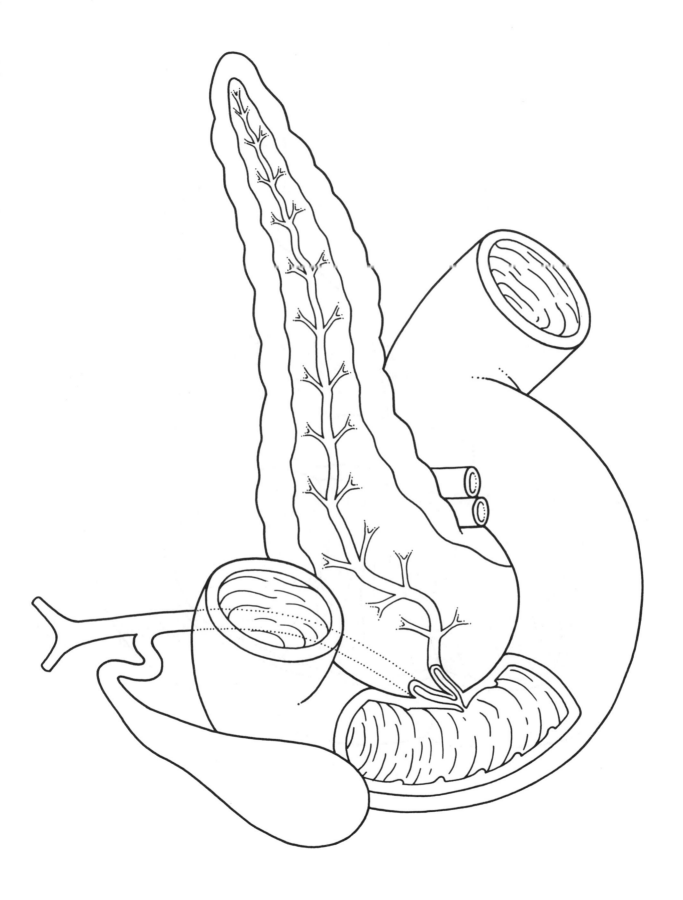

Fig. 4.8 Duodenum, Gallbladder, Pancreas

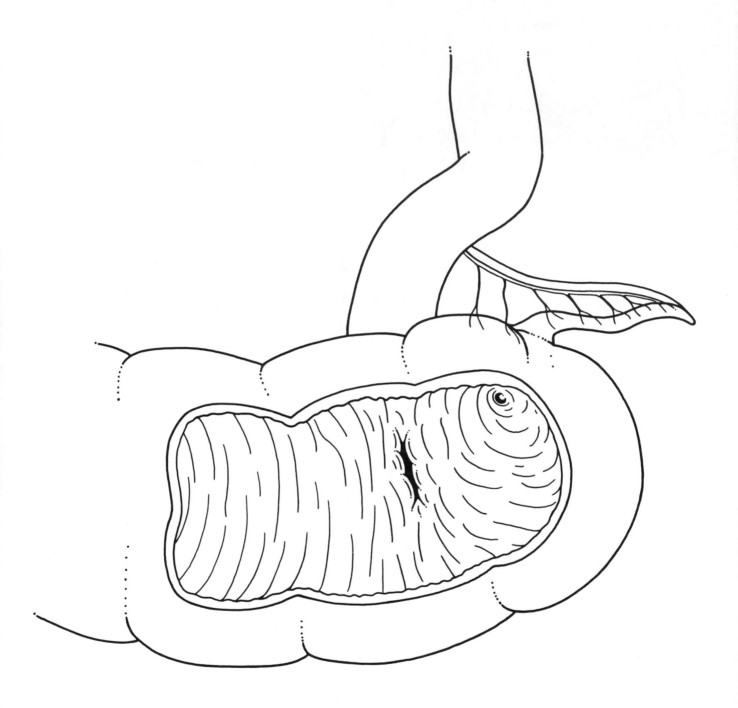

Fig. 4.9 Caecum, Appendix

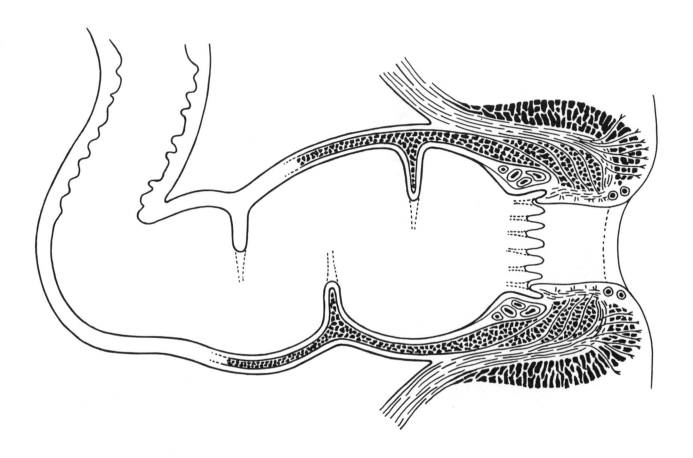

Fig. 4.10 Rectum, coronal section

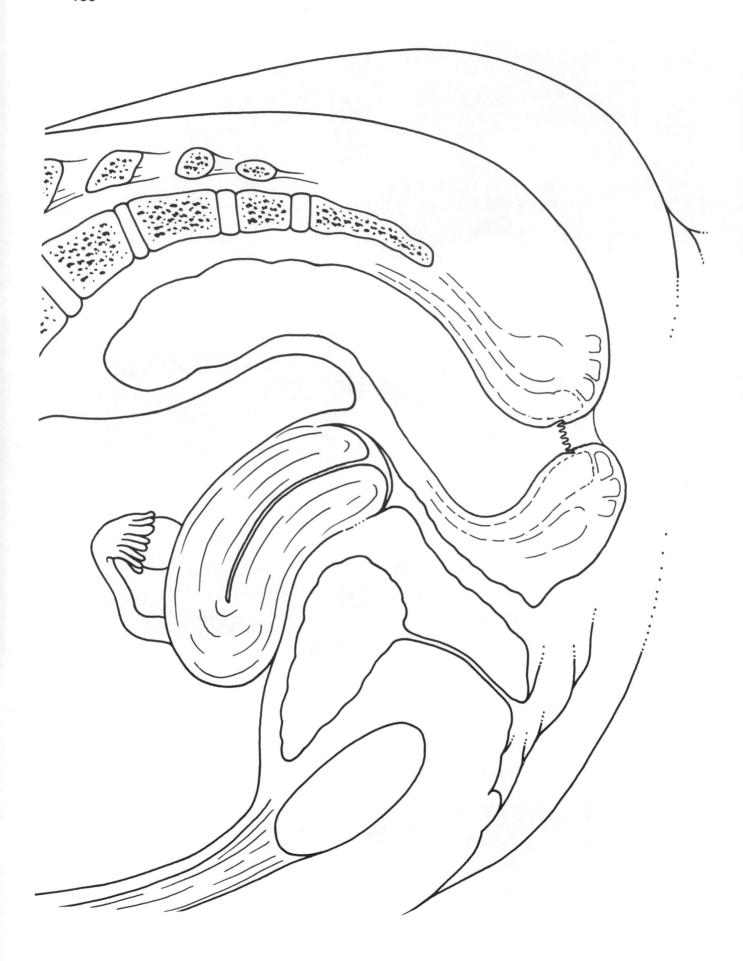

Fig. 4.11 Rectum, sagittal section

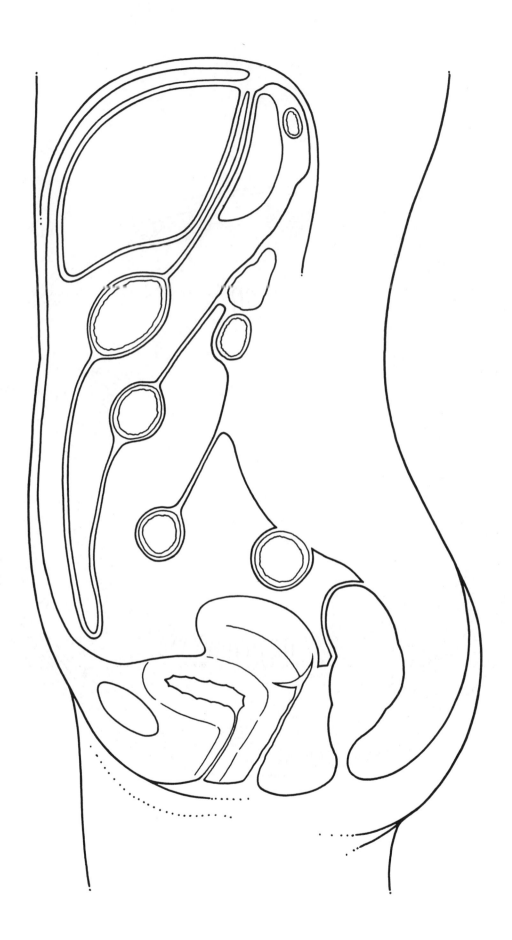

Fig. 4.12 Mesentery, peritoneal spaces

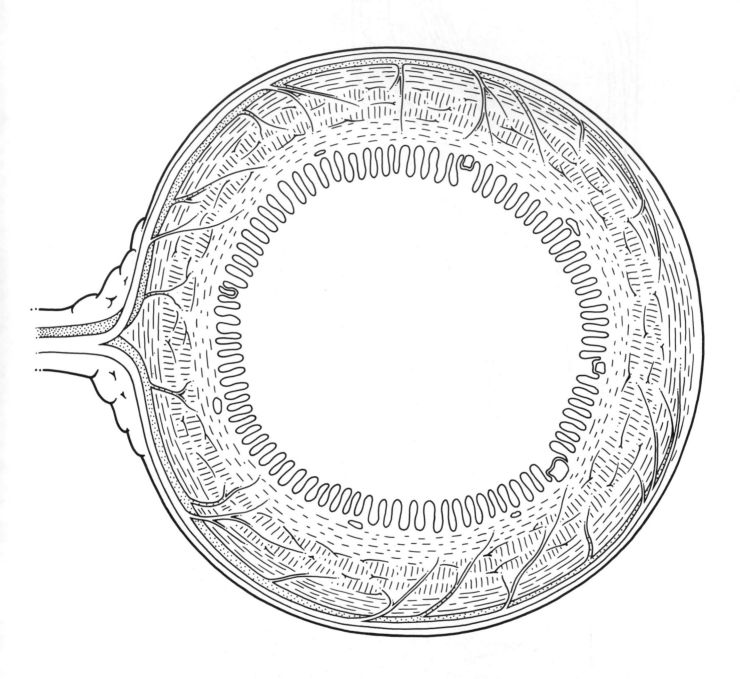

Fig. 4.13 Small bowel - section

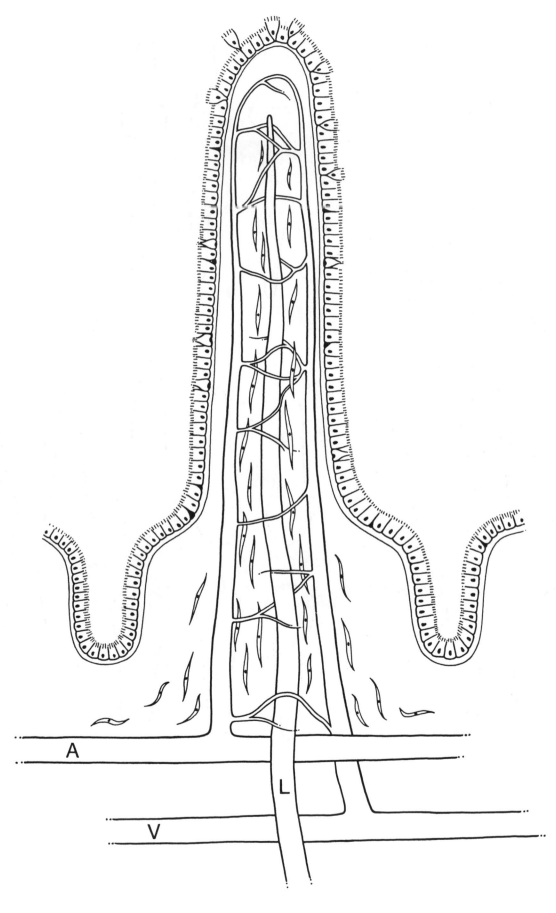

Fig. 4.14 Small bowel - villus

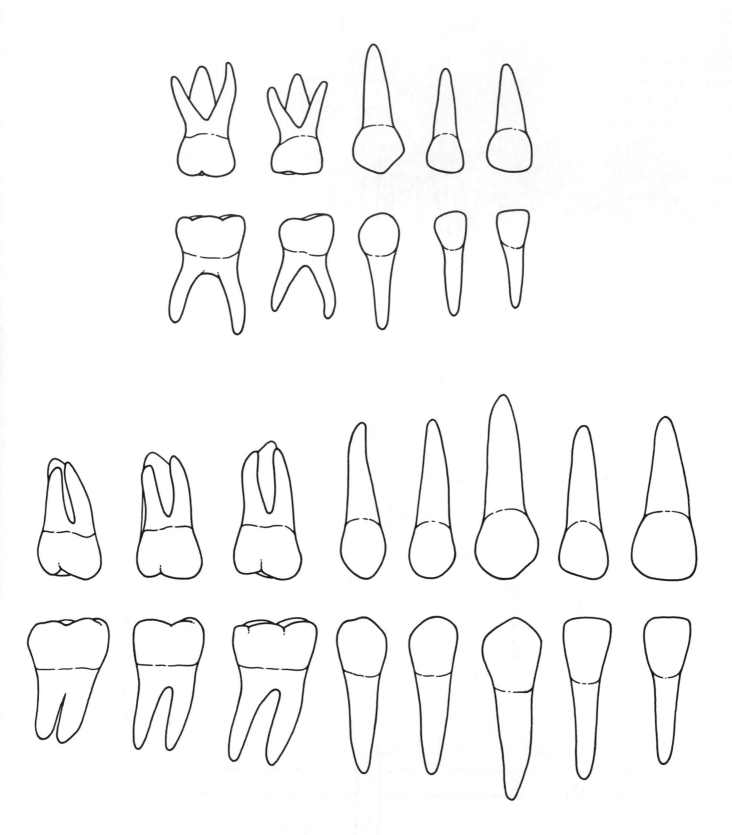

Fig. 4.15 Teeth, individual, deciduous and permanent

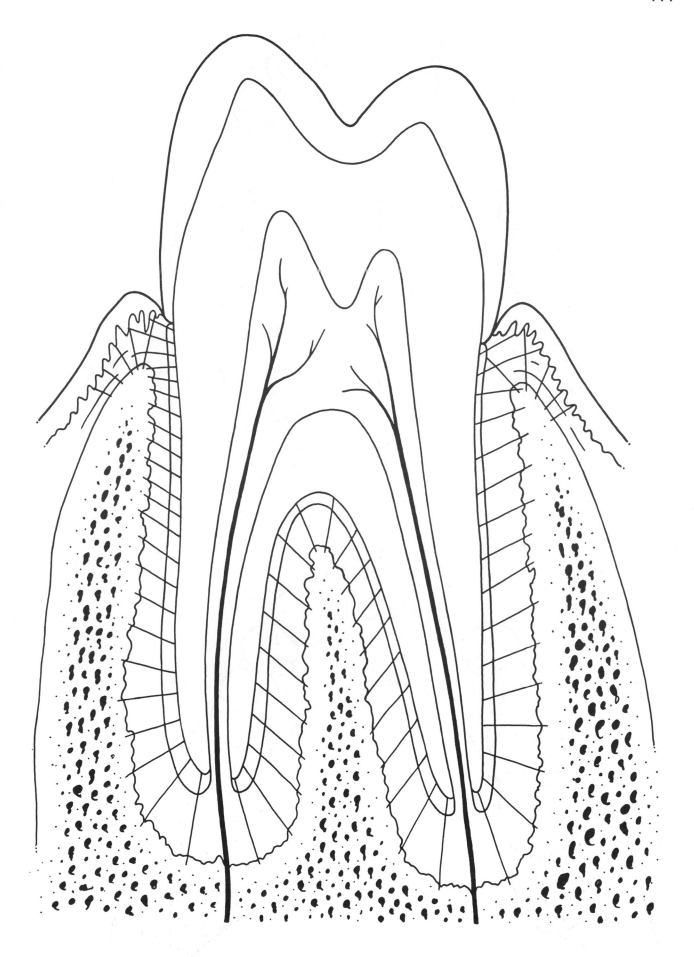

Fig. 4.16 Tooth - section

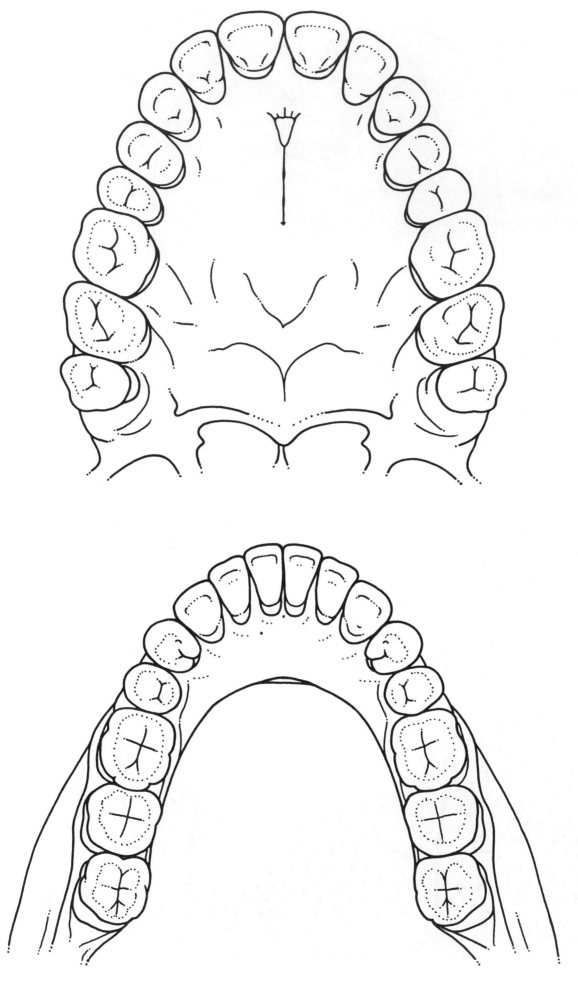

Fig. 4.17 Teeth in situ, upper jaw, lower jaw

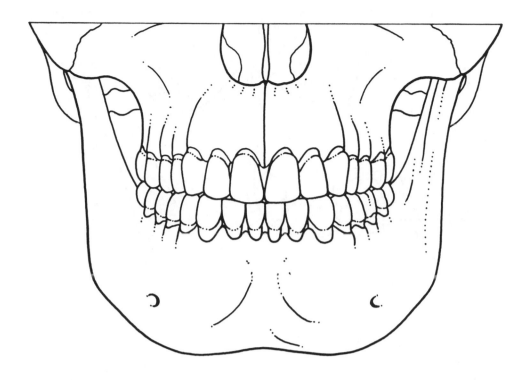

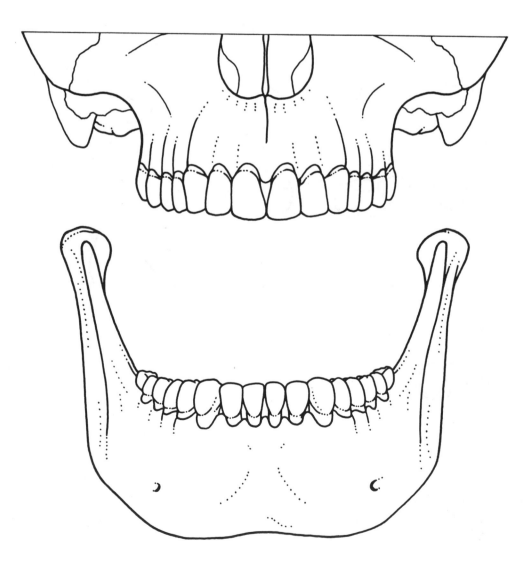

Fig. 4.18 Teeth in situ - anterior

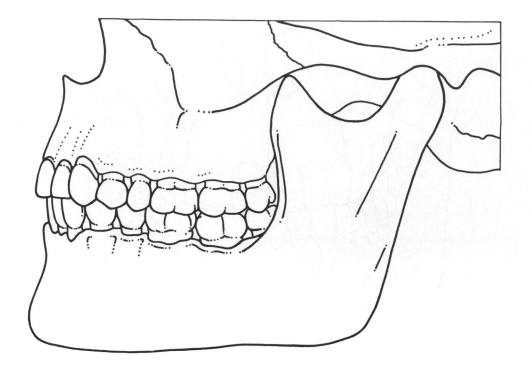

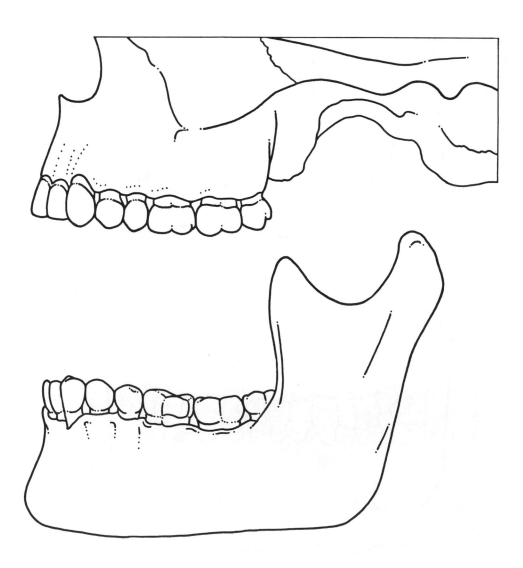

Fig. 4.19 Teeth in situ - left lateral

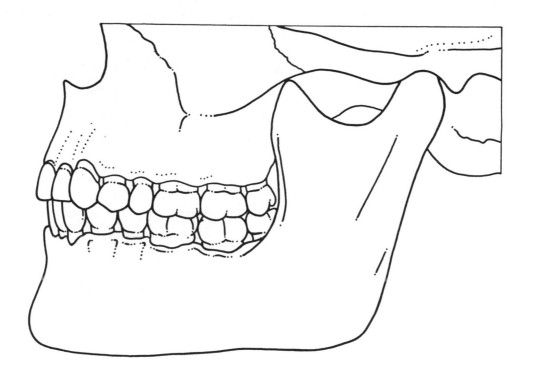

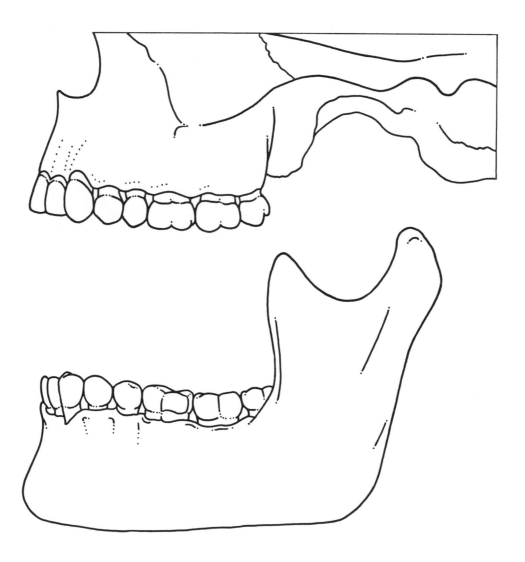

Fig. 4.20 Teeth in situ - right lateral

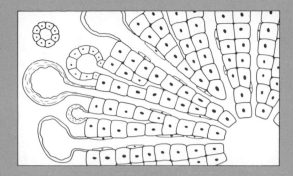

Section 5

Liver, Gallbladder, Pancreas and Spleen

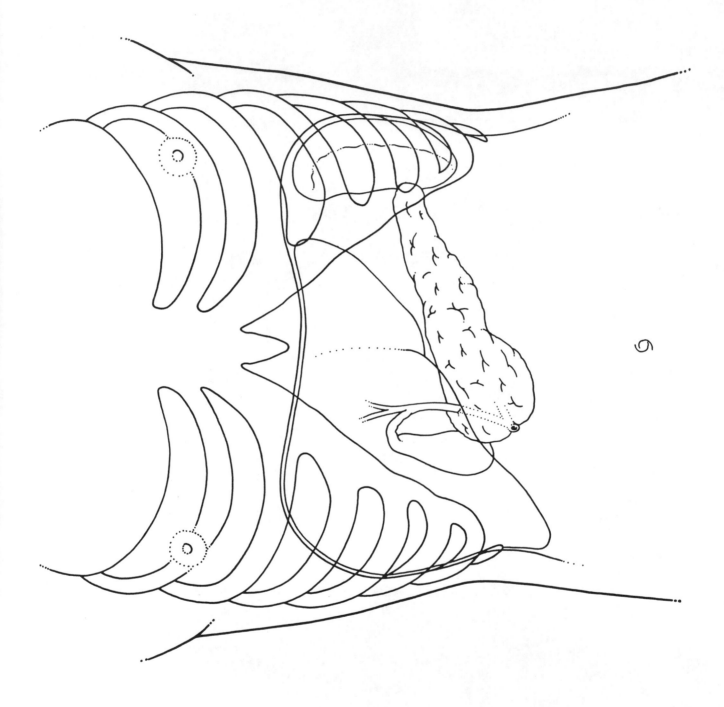

Fig. 5.1 Liver, Gallbladder, Pancreas, Spleen - position in body

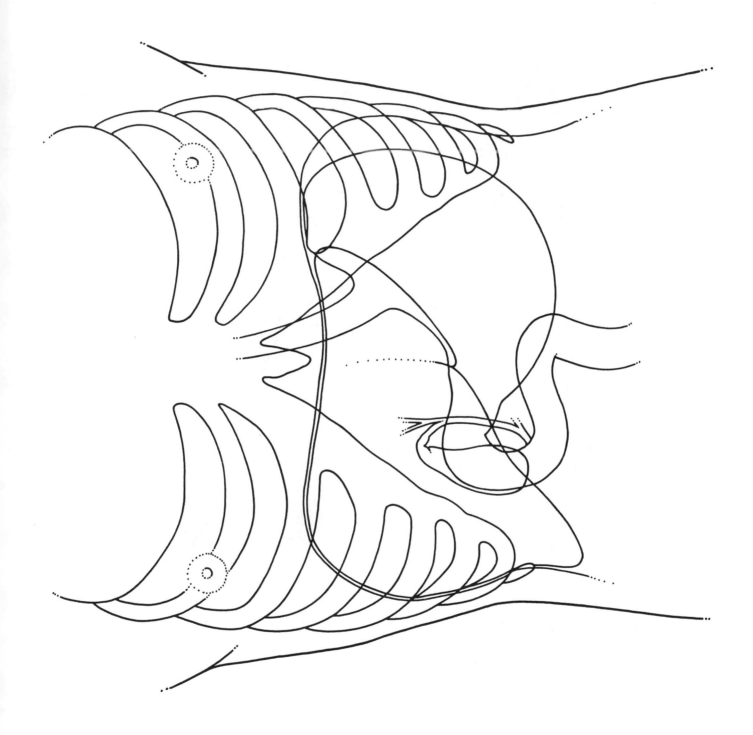

Fig. 5.2 Liver, Gallbladder, Stomach, Duodenum - position in body

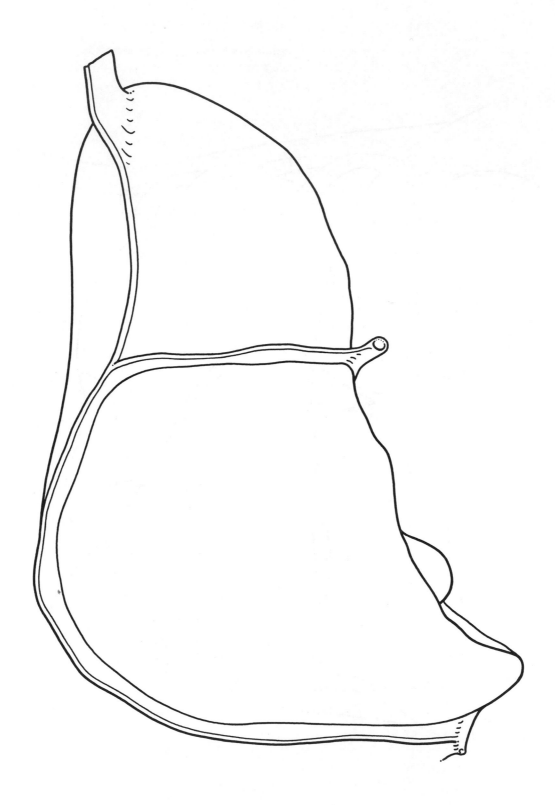

Fig. 5.3 Liver, AP

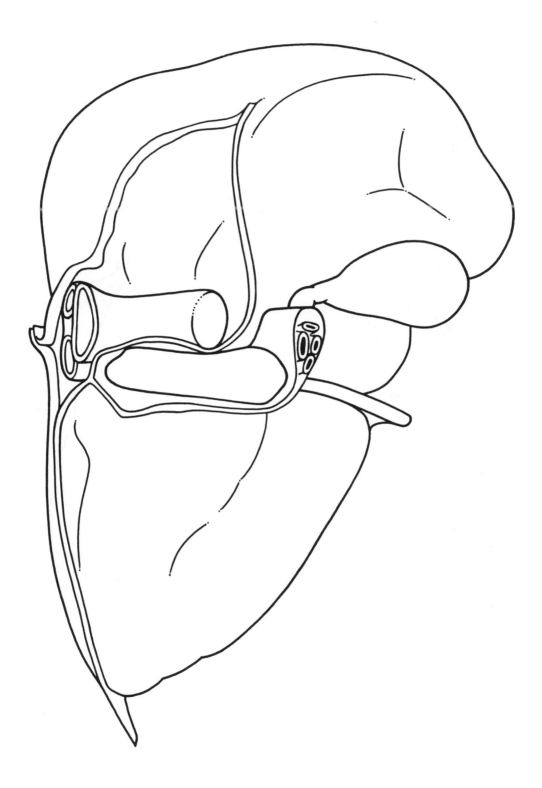

Fig. 5.4 Liver, PA

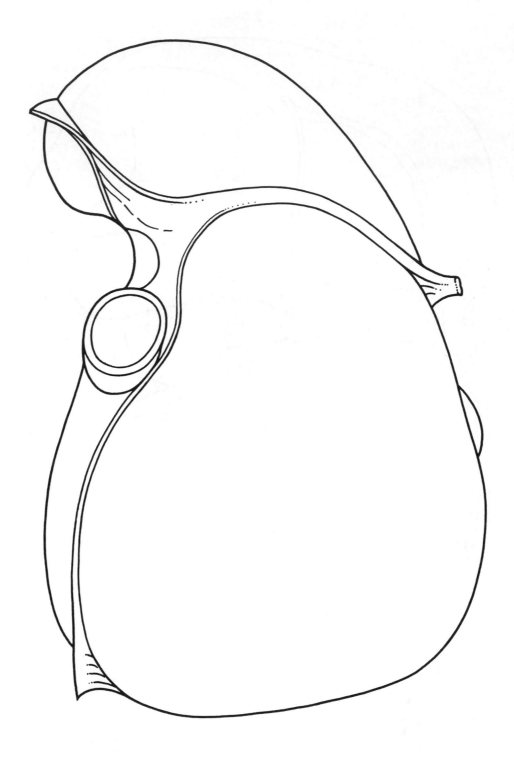

Fig. 5.5 Liver, superior

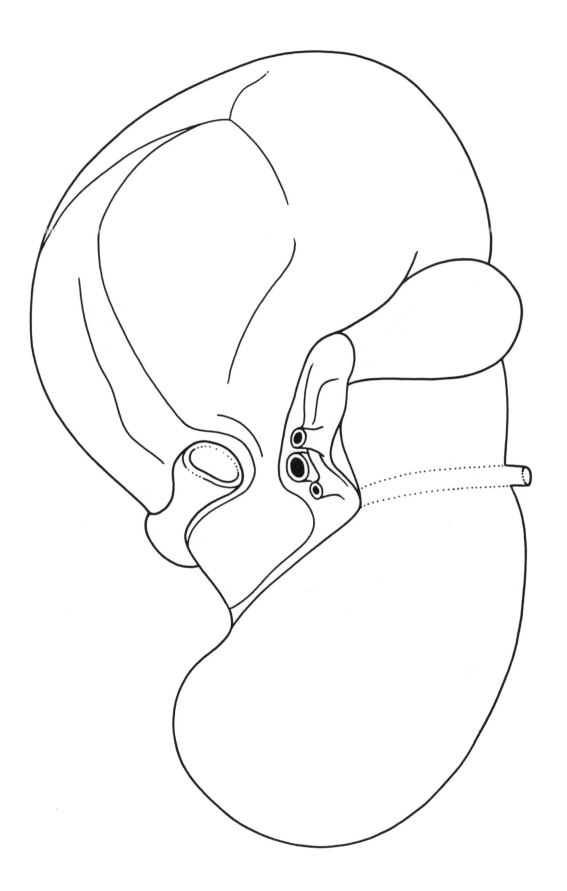

Fig. 5.6 Liver, inferior

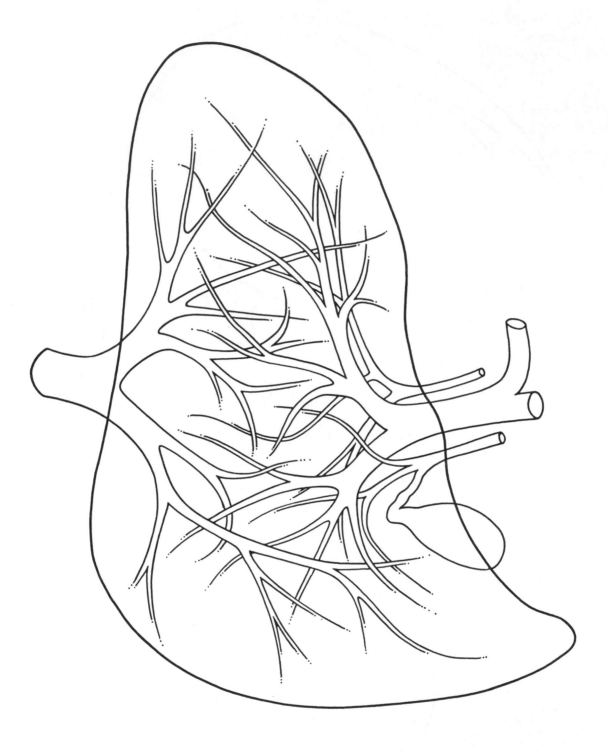

Fig. 5.7 Liver, anterior, arteries, veins, bile ducts

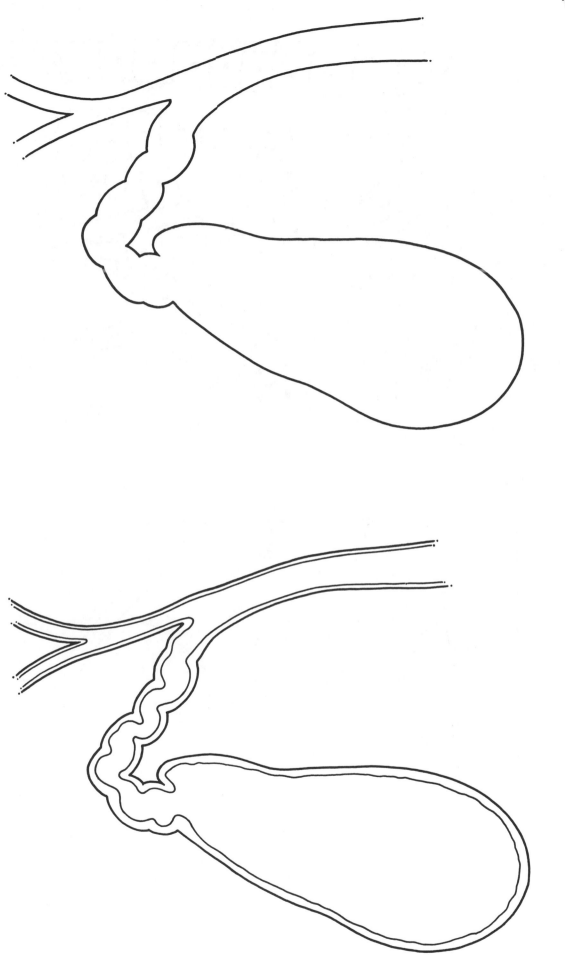

Fig. 5.8 Gallbladder and ducts - section

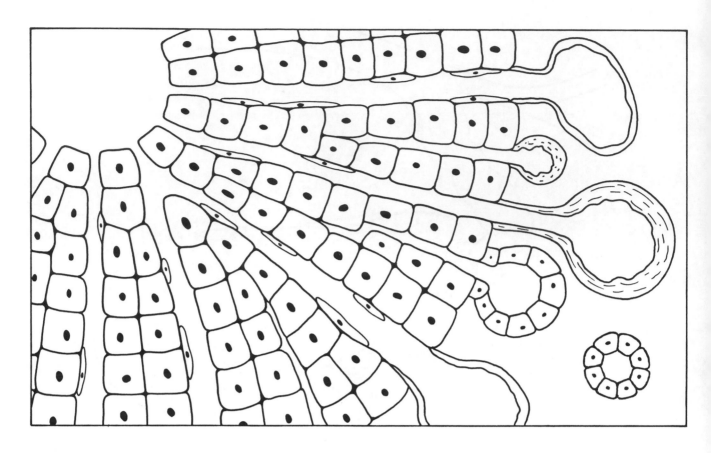

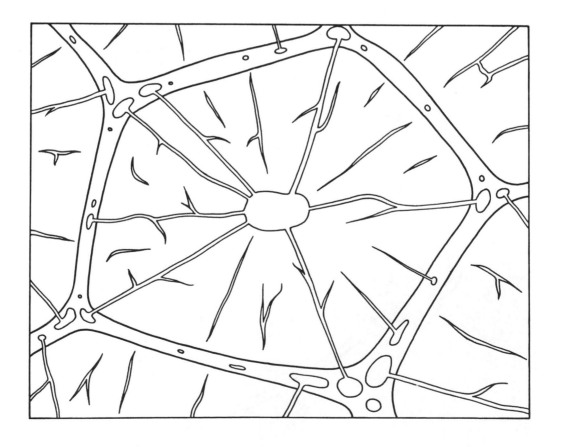

Fig. 5.9 Liver lobule - scheme, structure

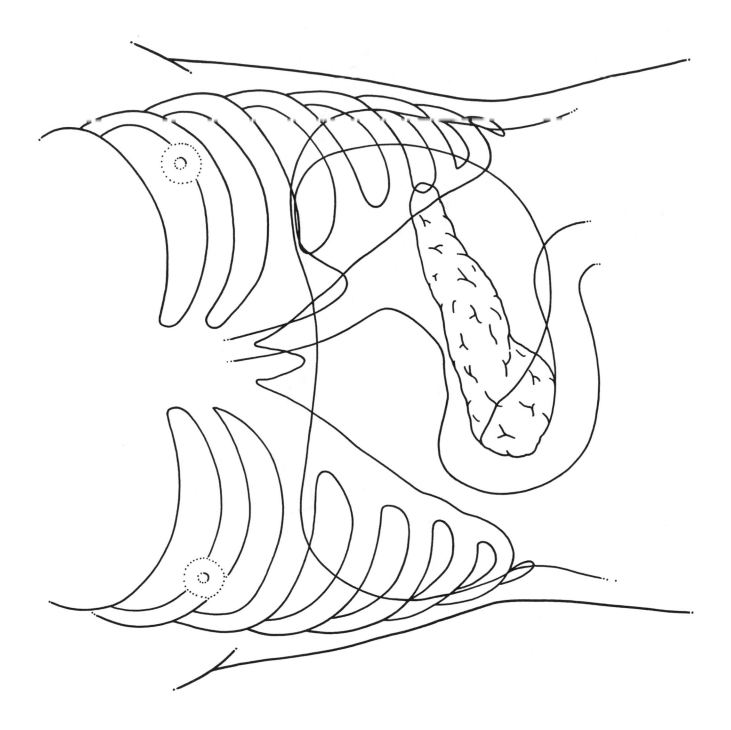

Fig. 5.10 Pancreas, stomach - position in body

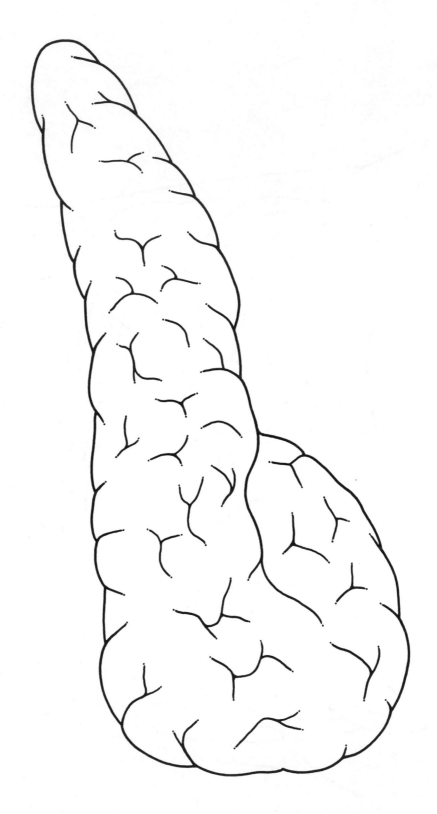

Fig. 5.11 Pancreas, AP, external surface

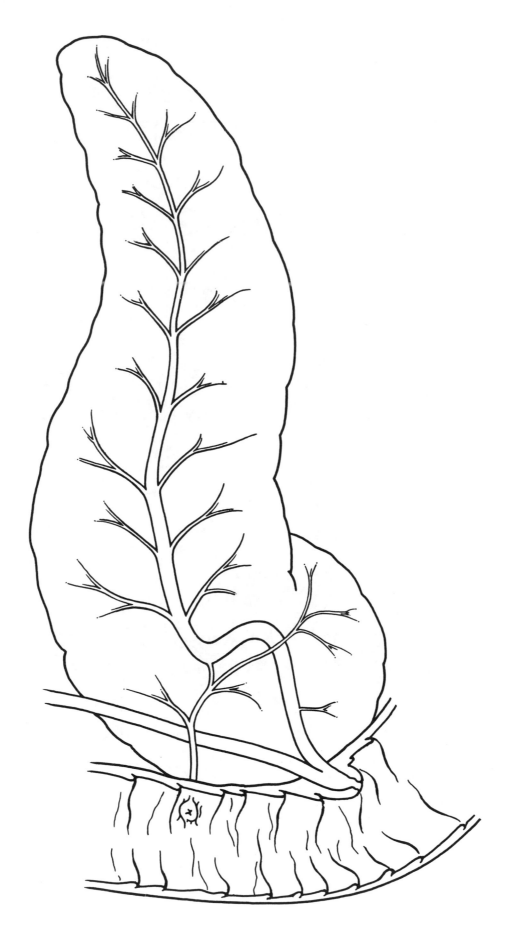

Fig. 5.12   Pancreas - Ducts, papilla

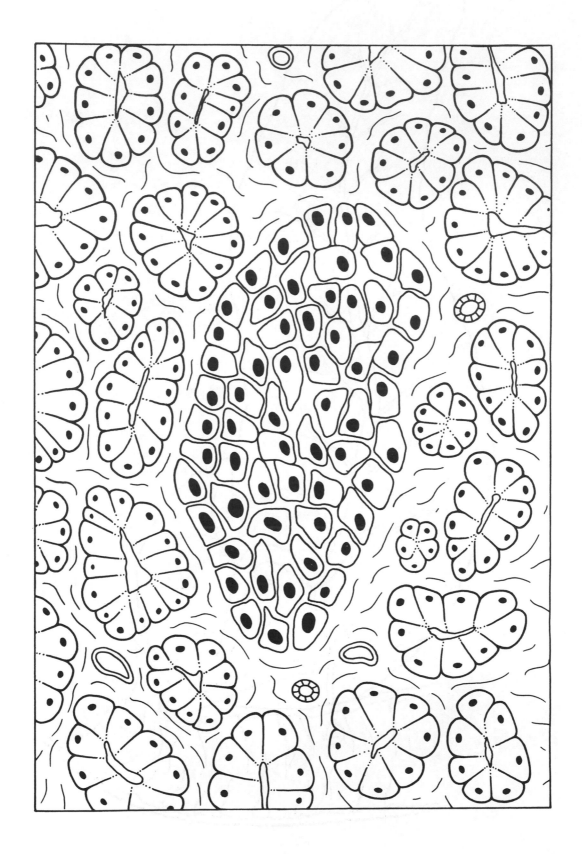

Fig. 5.13 Pancreas - Islets of Langerhans

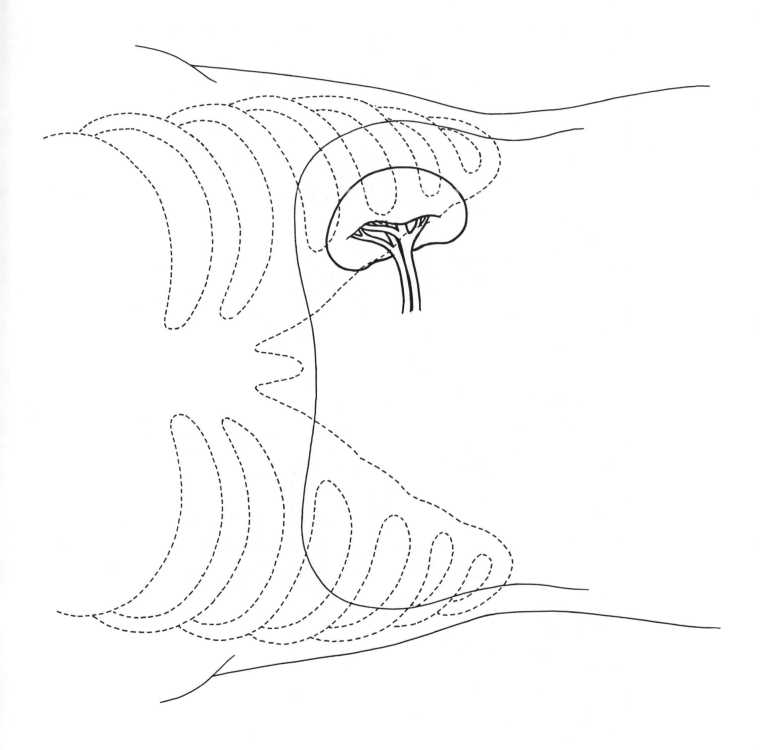

Fig. 5.14 Spleen - position in body, anterior

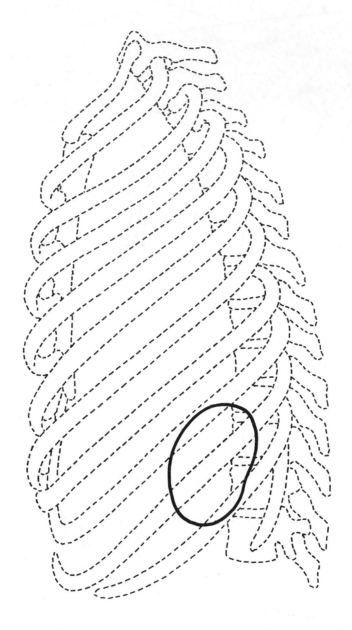

Fig. 5.15 Spleen - position in body, lateral

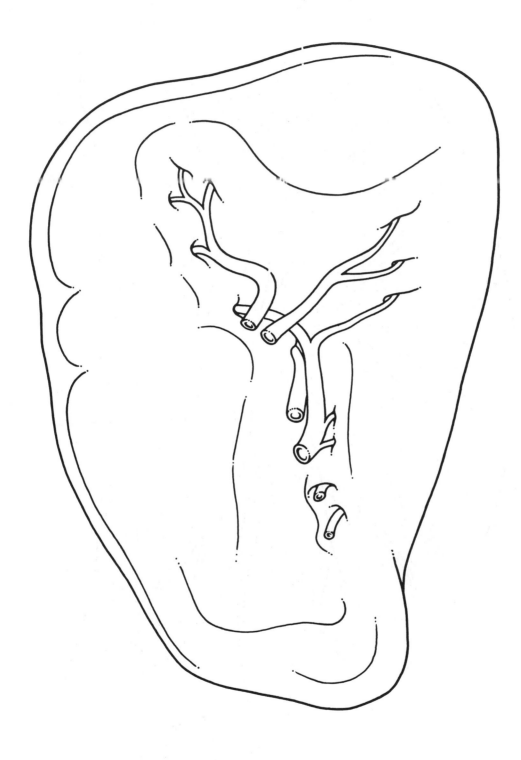

Fig. 5.16 Spleen - visceral view

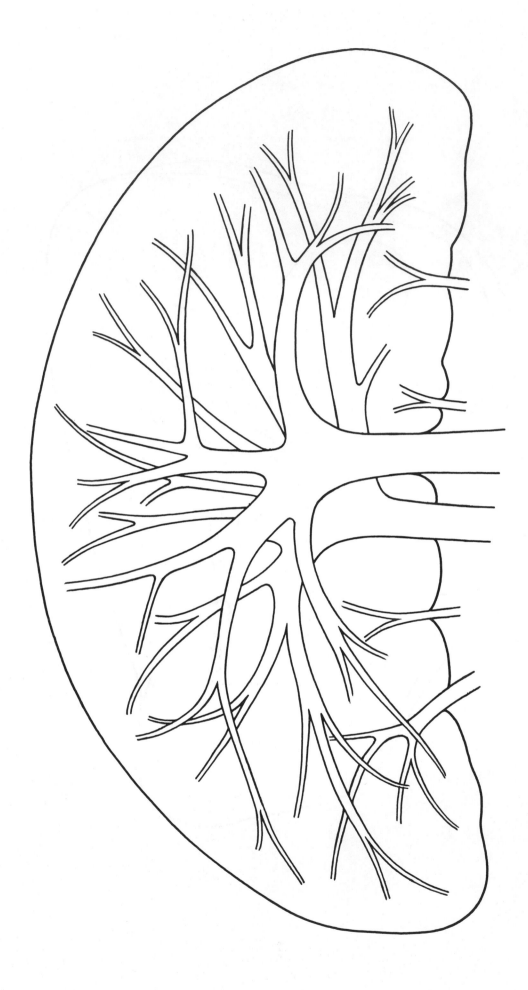

Fig. 5.17 Spleen - section

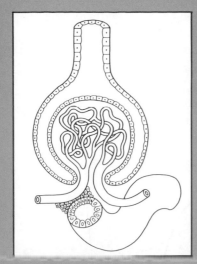

Section 6

Kidneys and Bladder

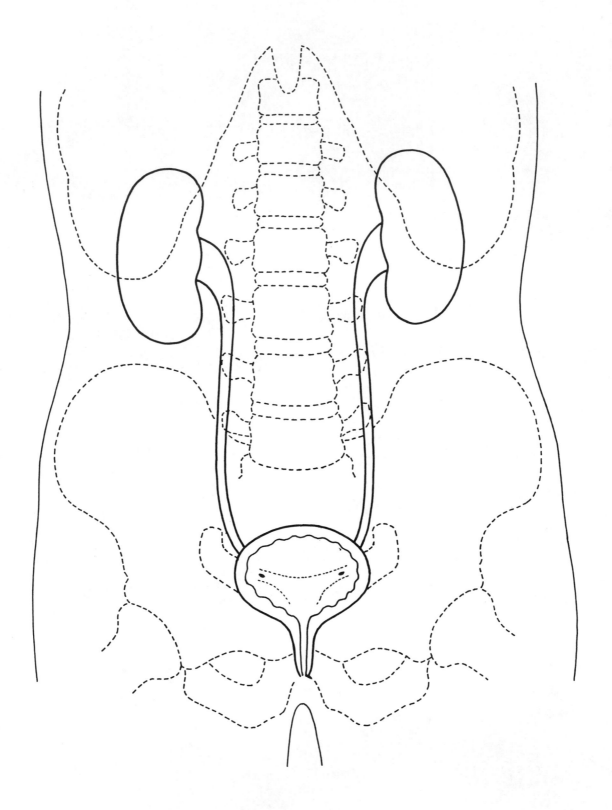

Fig. 6.1 Kidneys and bladder, position in body, AP

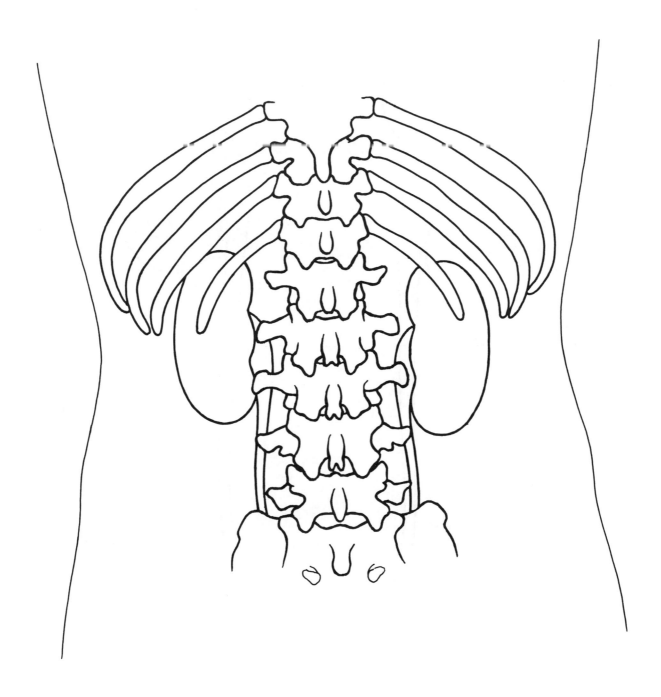

Fig. 6.2 Kidneys, position in body, PA

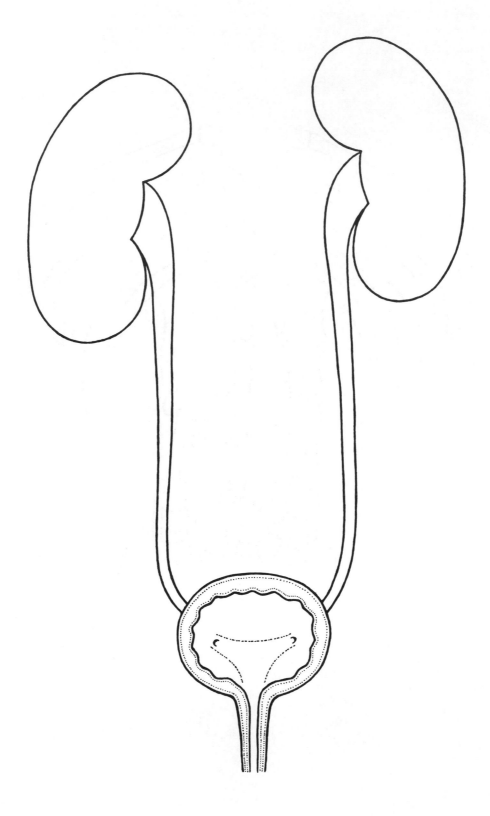

Fig. 6.3 Kidneys and bladder - scheme

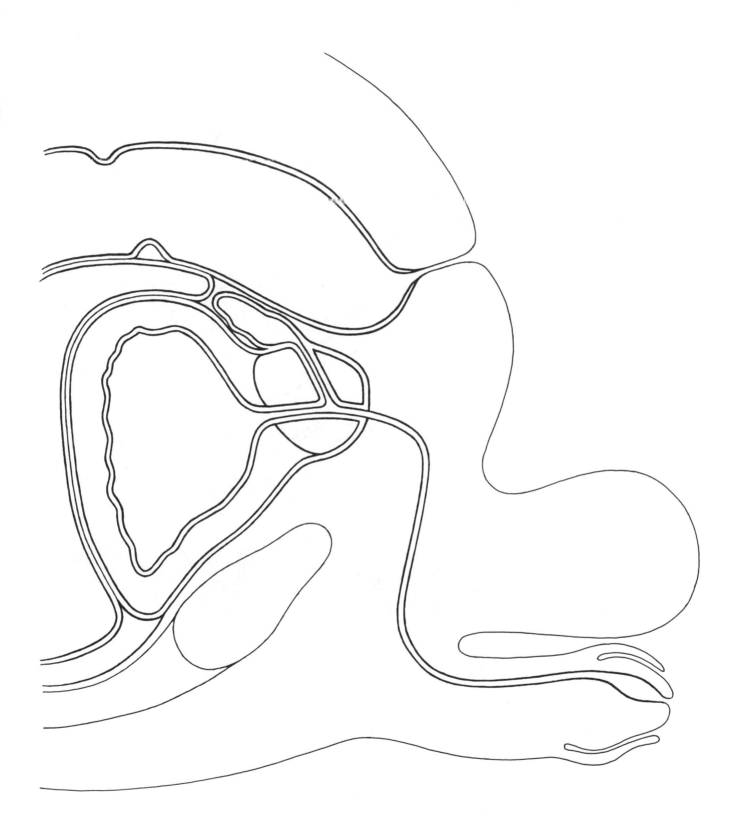

Fig. 6.4   Pelvic urinary organs, sagittal section - male

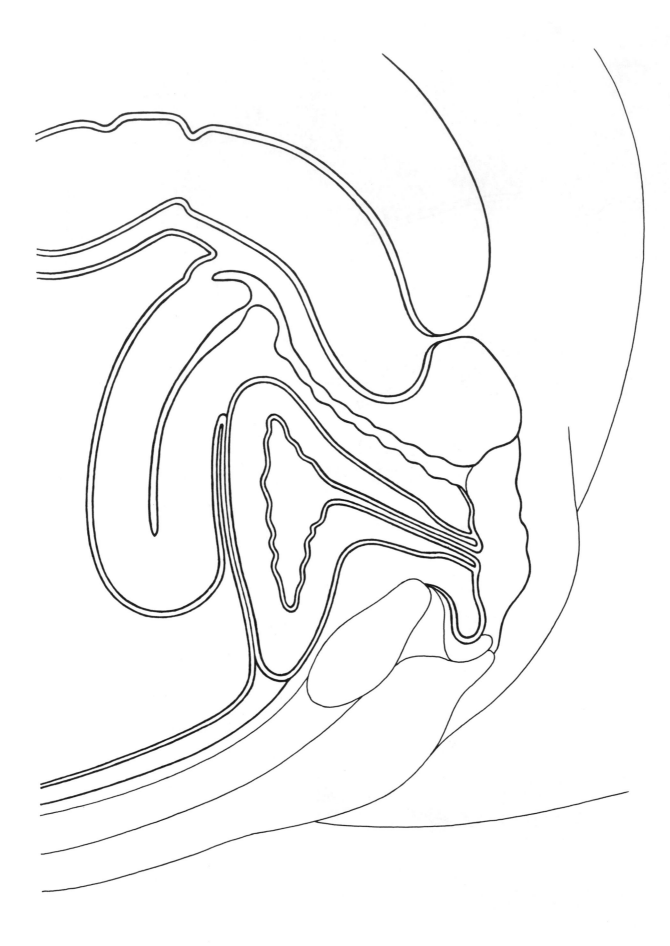

Fig. 6.5 Pelvic urinary organs, sagittal section - female

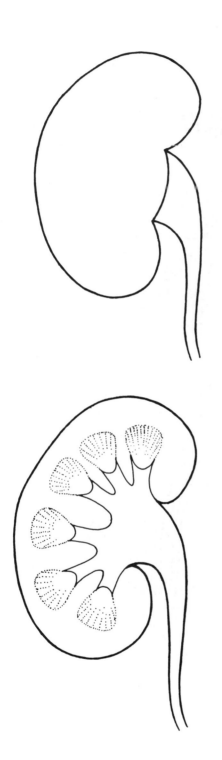
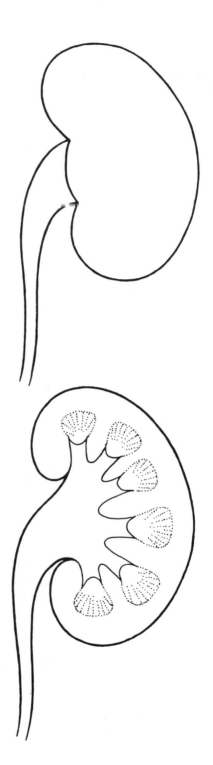

Fig. 6.6   Kidneys - outline, section

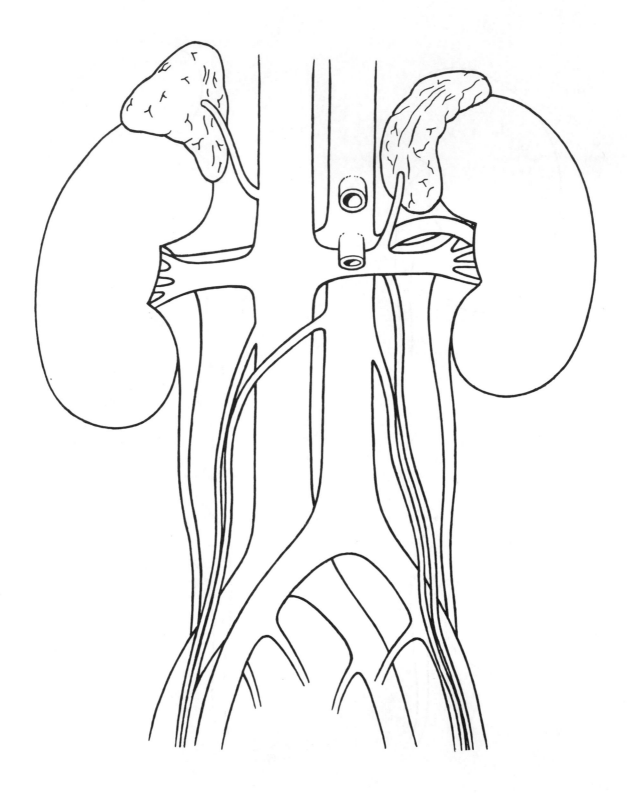

Fig. 6.7 Kidneys, adrenals - blood supply

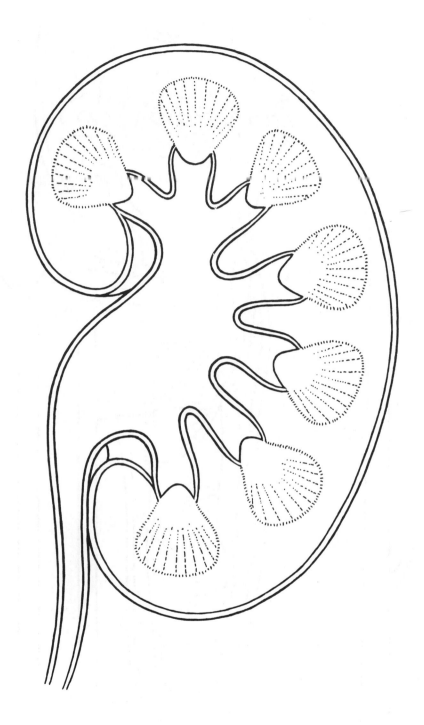

Fig. 6.8 Kidney - section

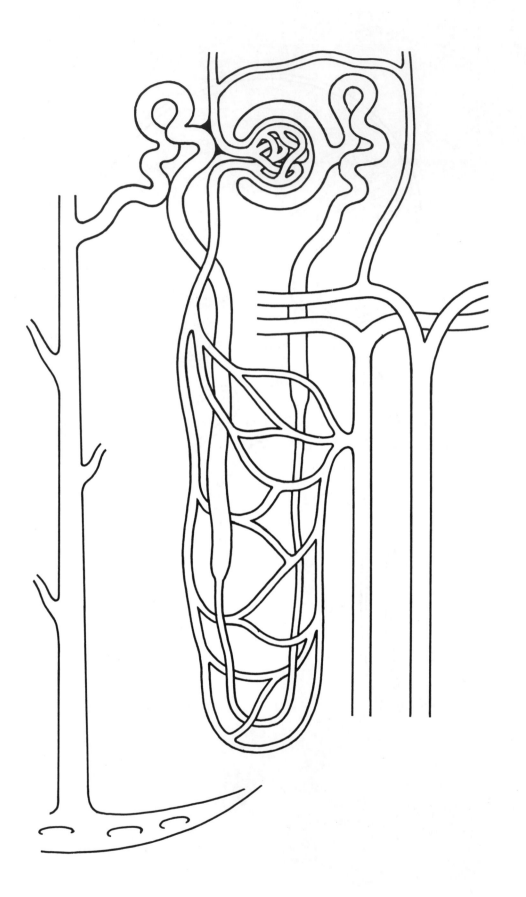

Fig. 6.9 Nephron

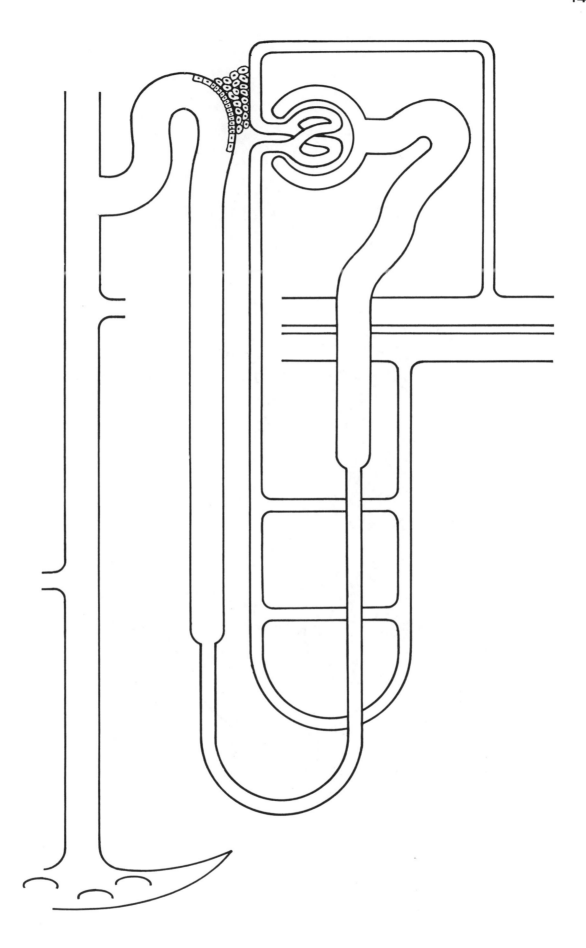

Fig. 6.10 Nephron - scheme

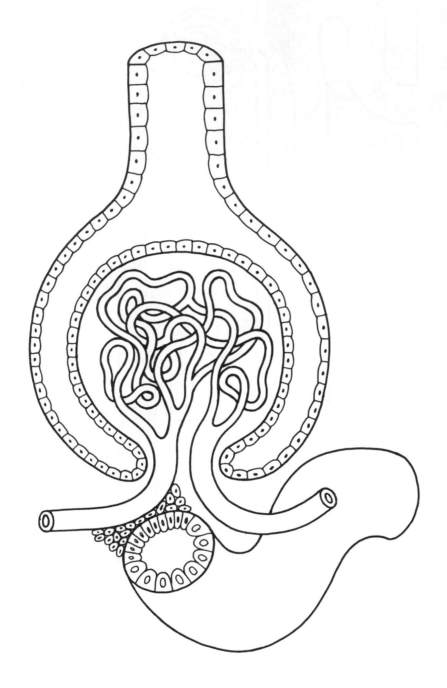

Fig. 6.11 Glomerulus

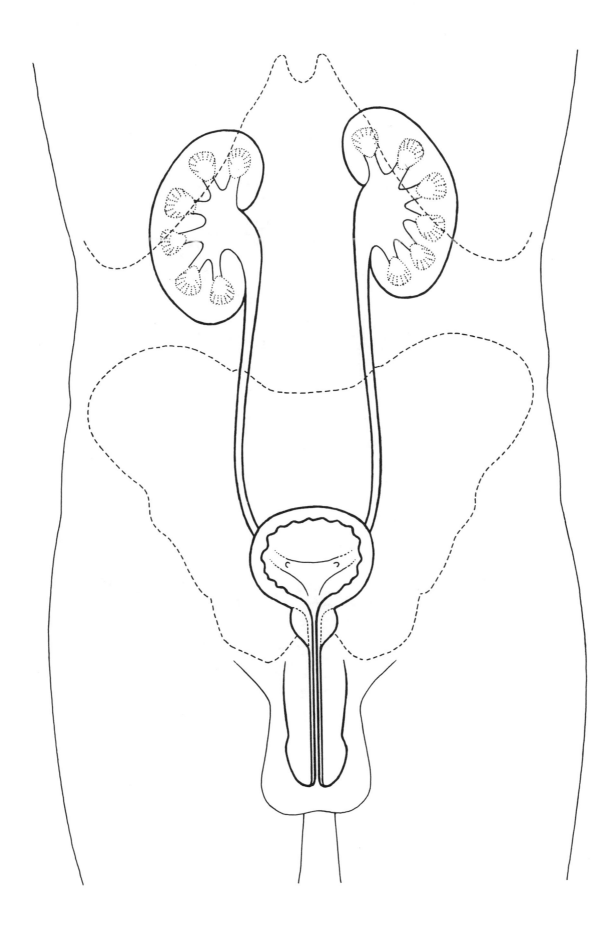

Fig. 6.12 Bladder, coronal section - male

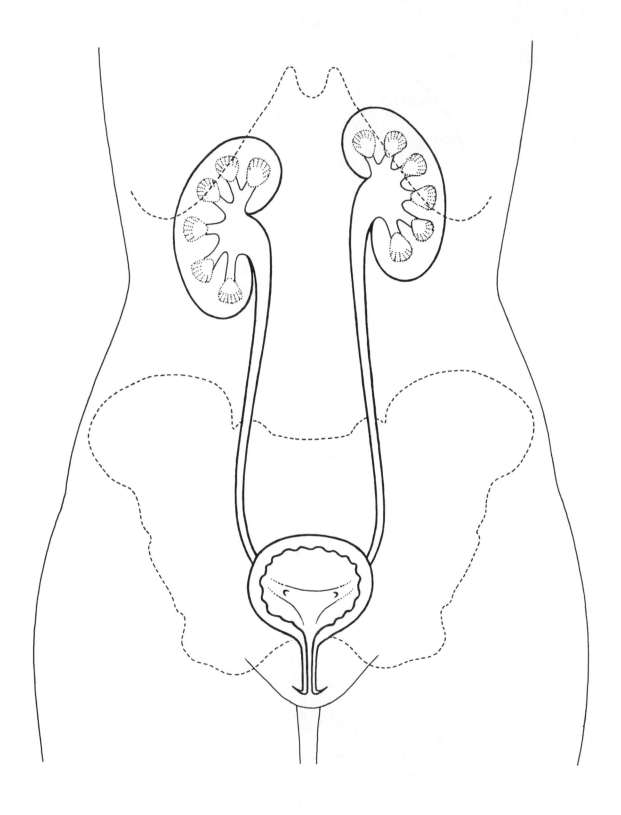

Fig. 6.13 Bladder, coronal section - female

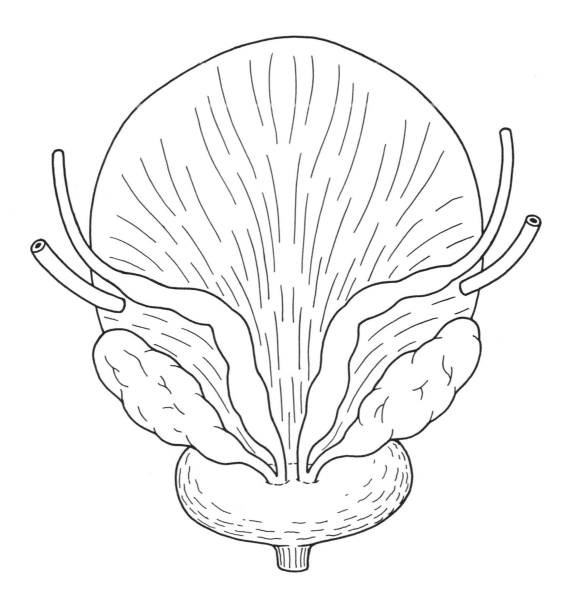

Fig. 6.14 Bladder, PA - male

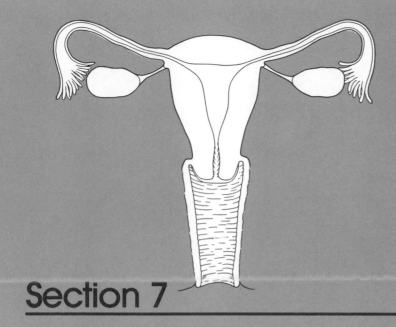

Section 7

Female Genital Tract

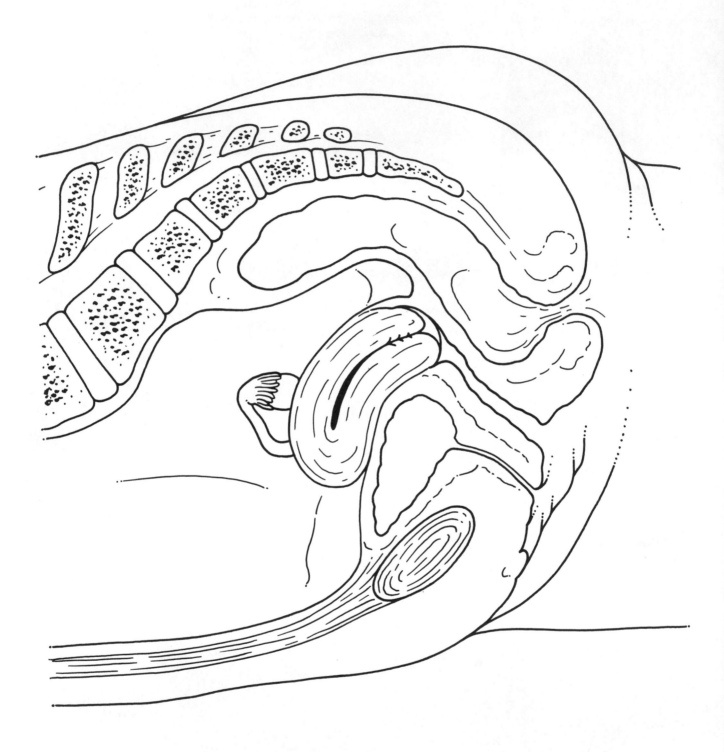

Fig. 7.1 Pelvic organs, sagittal section

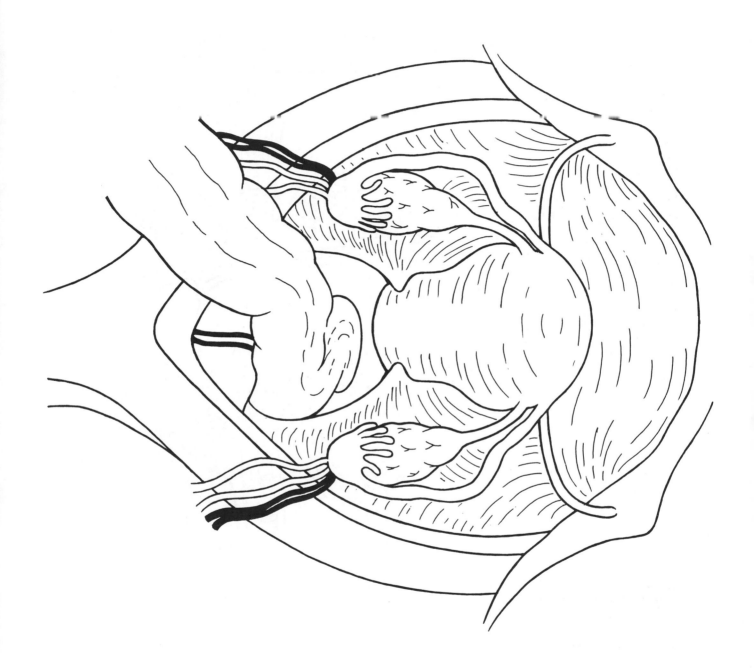

Fig. 7.2 Pelvic organs, superior

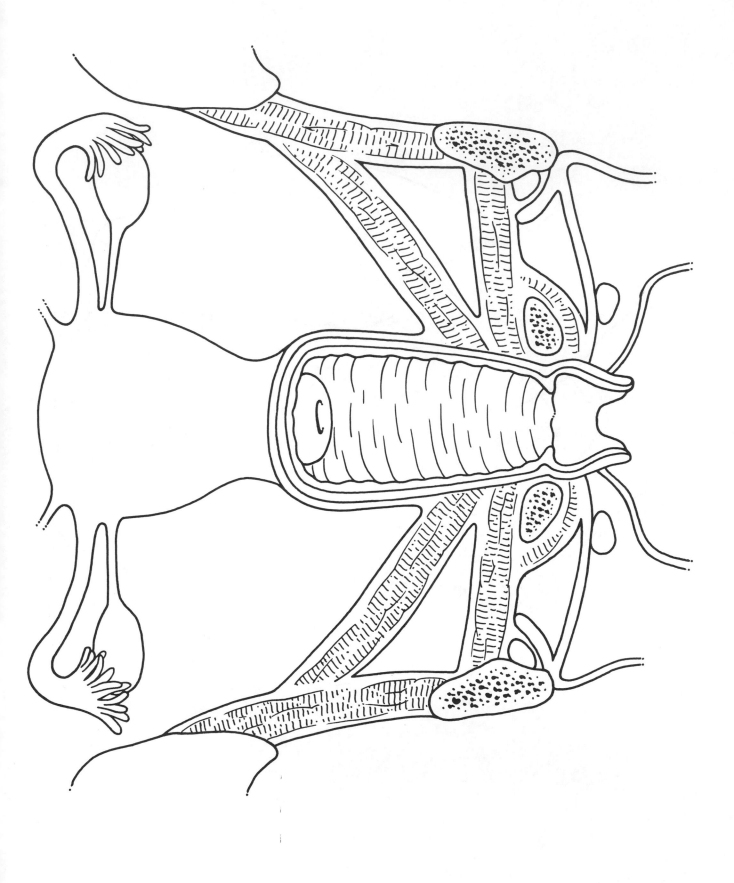

Fig. 7.3 Pelvic floor and organs, coronal section

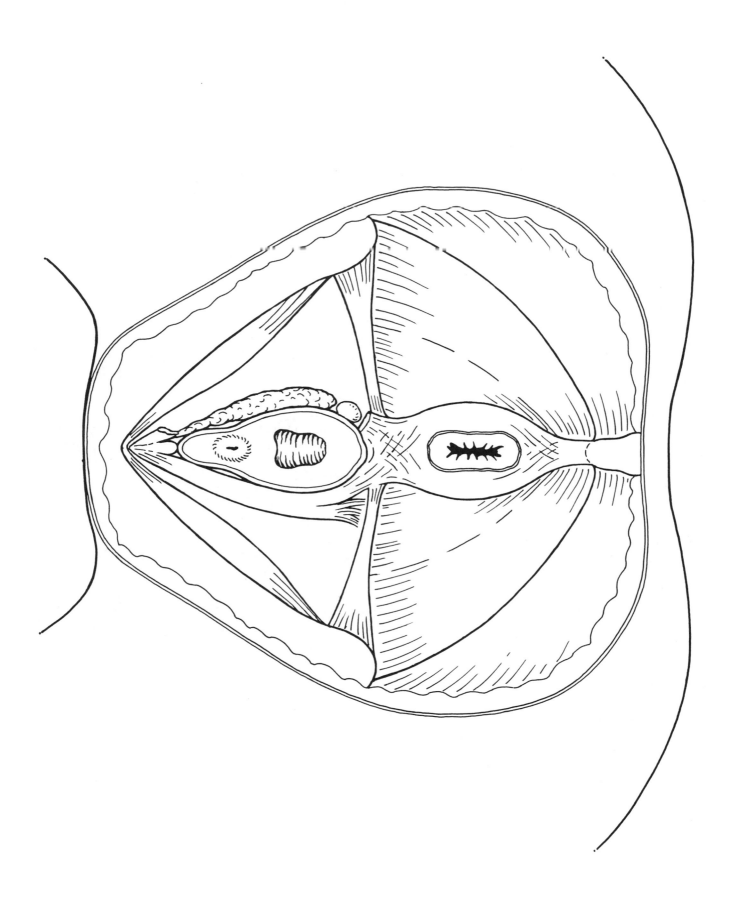

Fig. 7.4 Perineum, structure

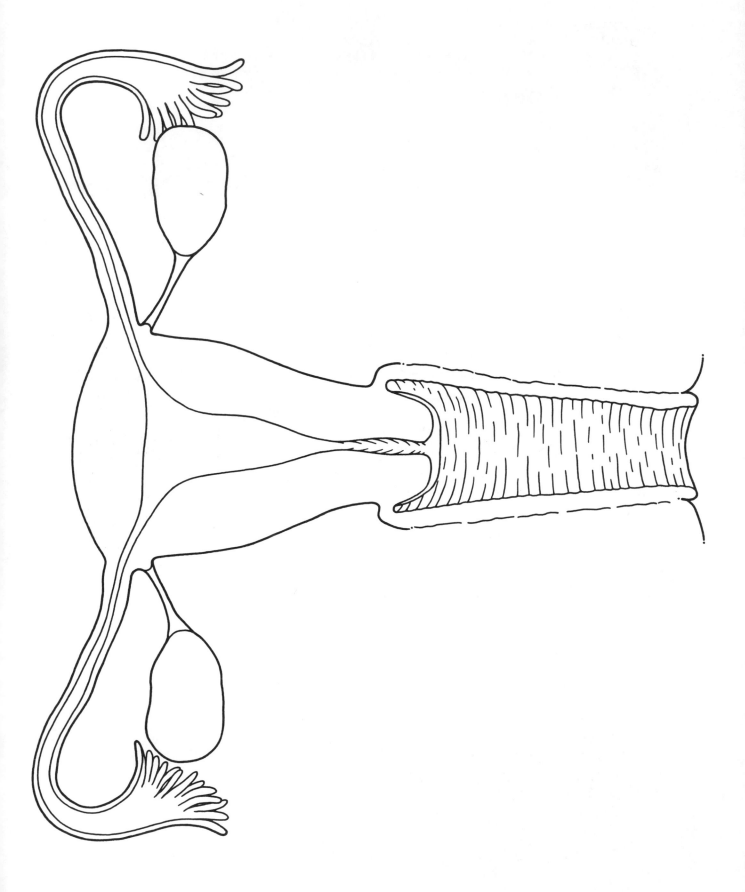

Fig. 7.5 Uterus, fallopian tubes, ovaries, vagina, coronal section

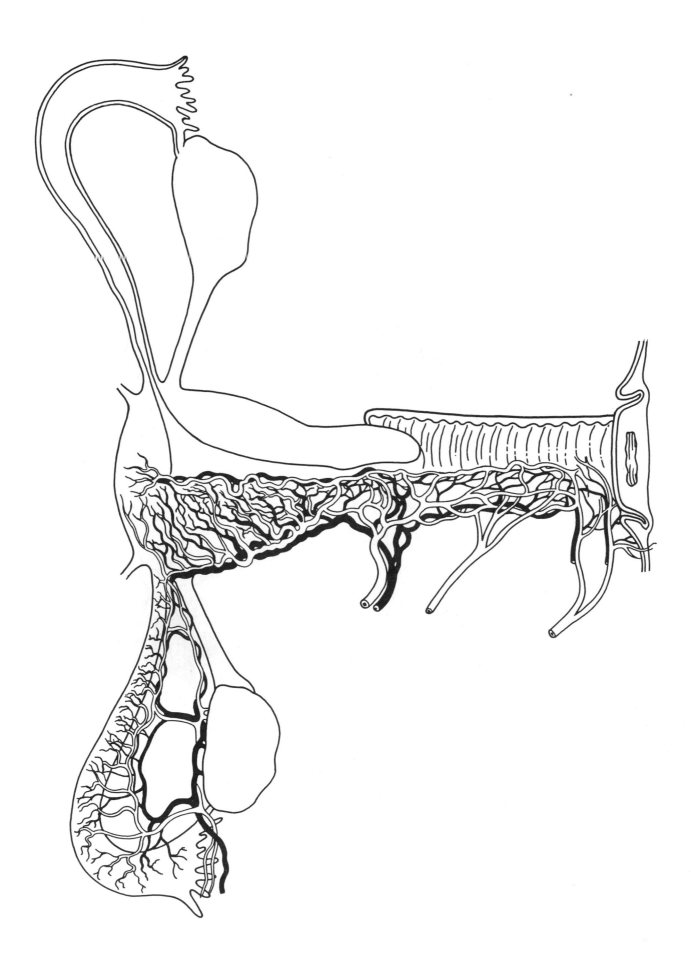

Fig. 7.6 Uterus, fallopian tubes, ovaries, vagina, blood supply

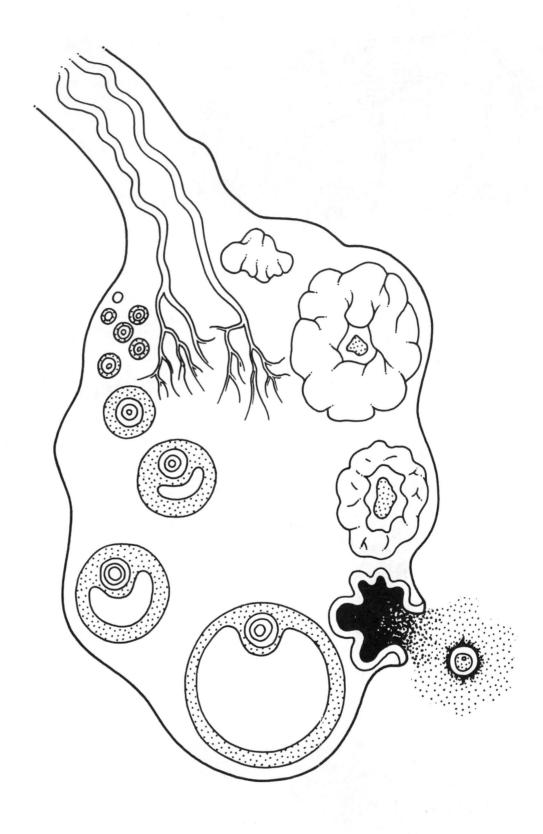

Fig. 7.7   Ovary, graafian follicle development

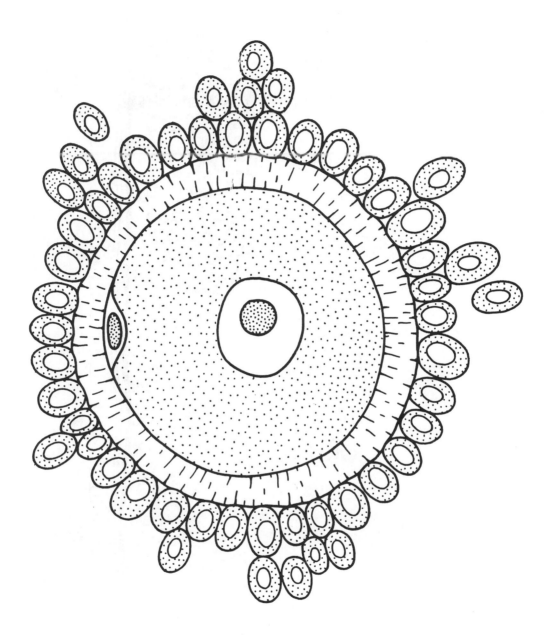

Fig. 7.8 Ovum

160

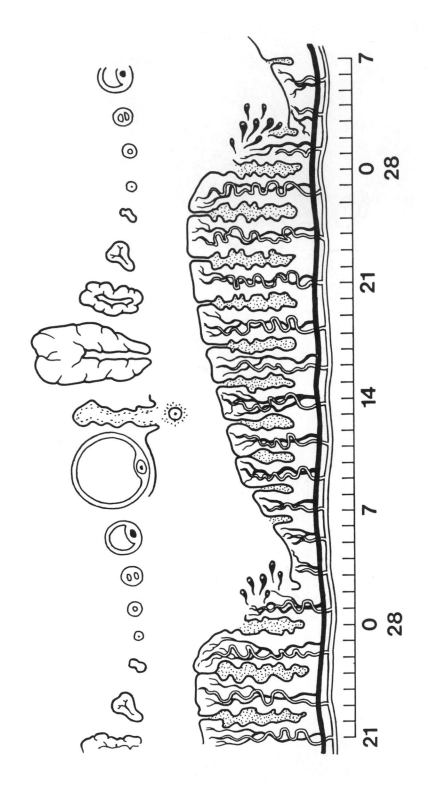

Fig. 7.9 Menstrual cycle

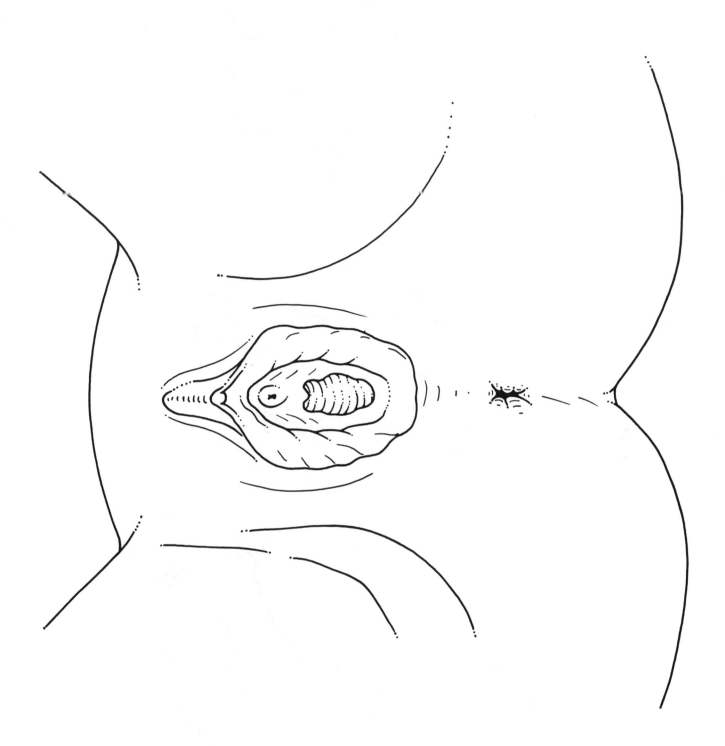

Fig. 7.10 External genitalia

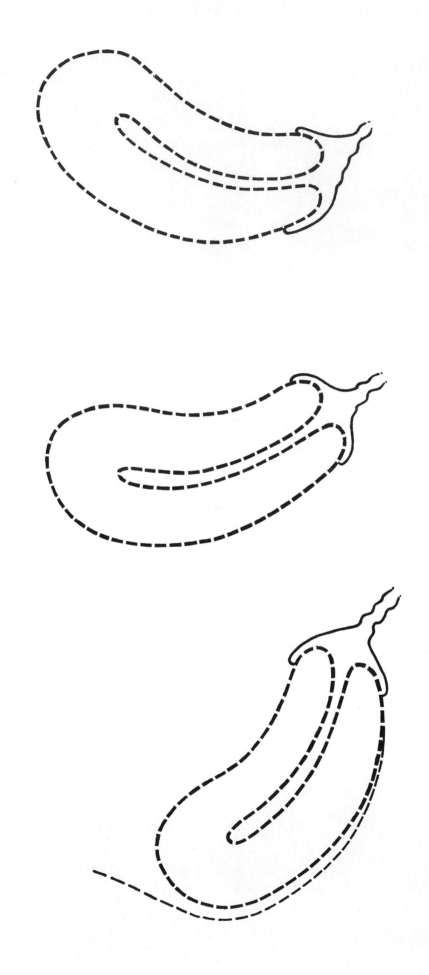

Fig. 7.11 Uterus, retroversion 1st, 2nd and 3rd degree

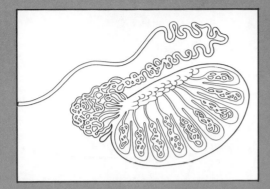

Section 8

Male Genital Tract

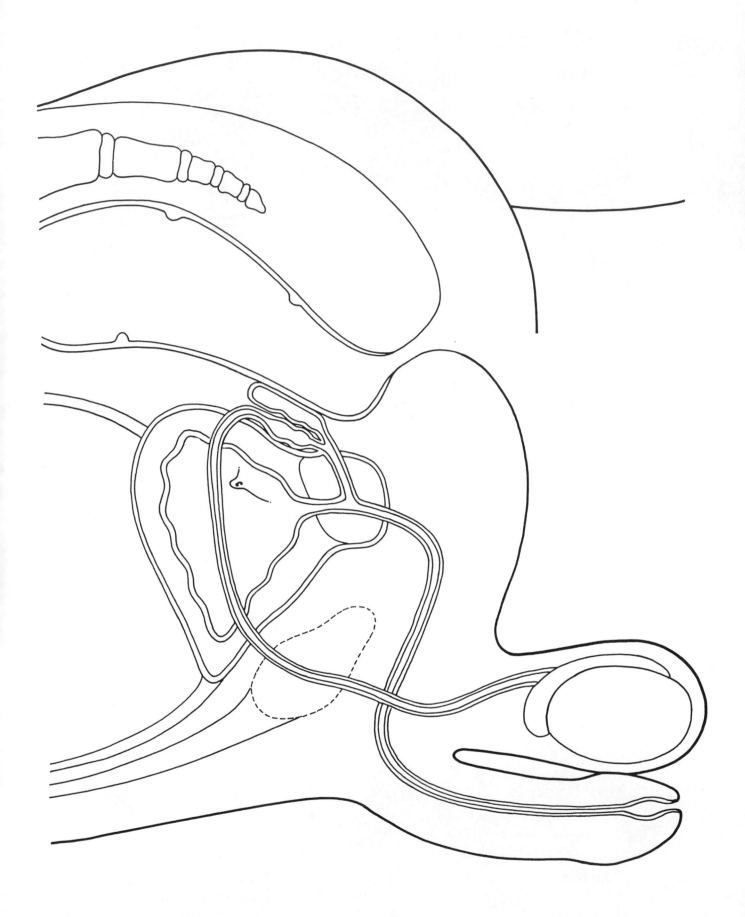

Fig. 8.1 Pelvic organs, sagittal section

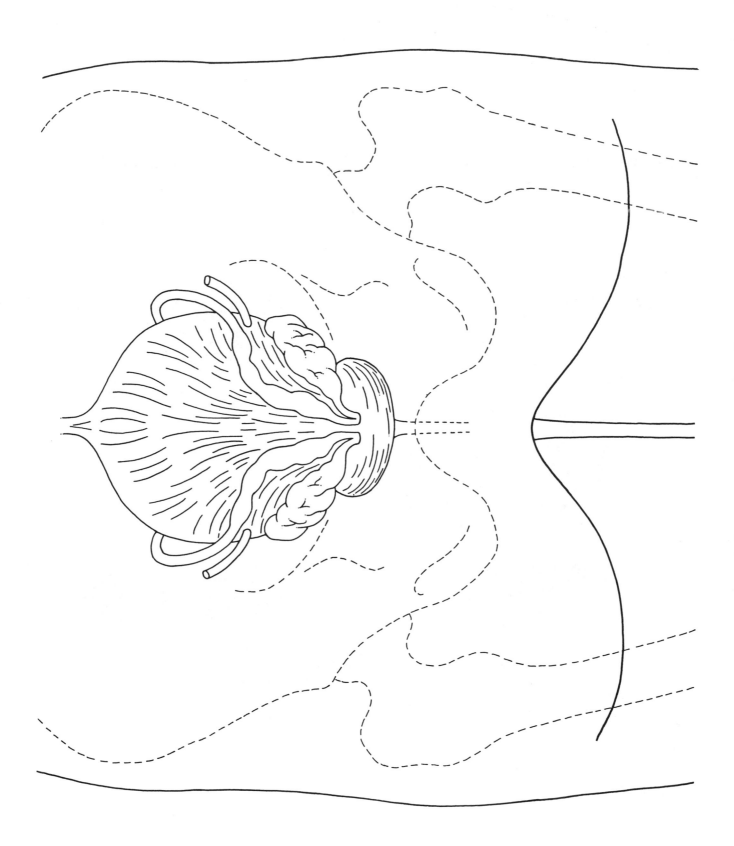

Fig. 8.2 Pelvic organs, posterior

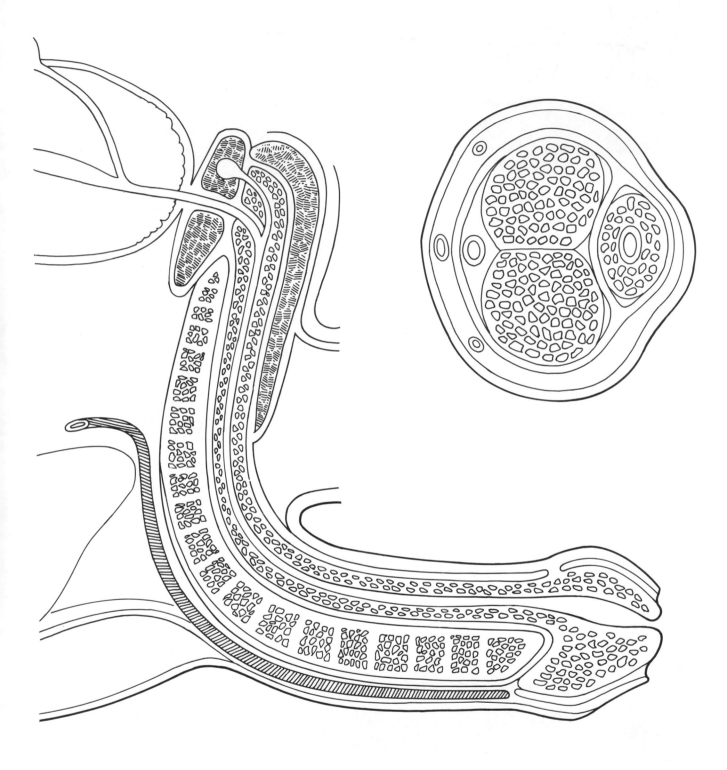

Fig. 8.3 Penis, longitudinal and transverse sections

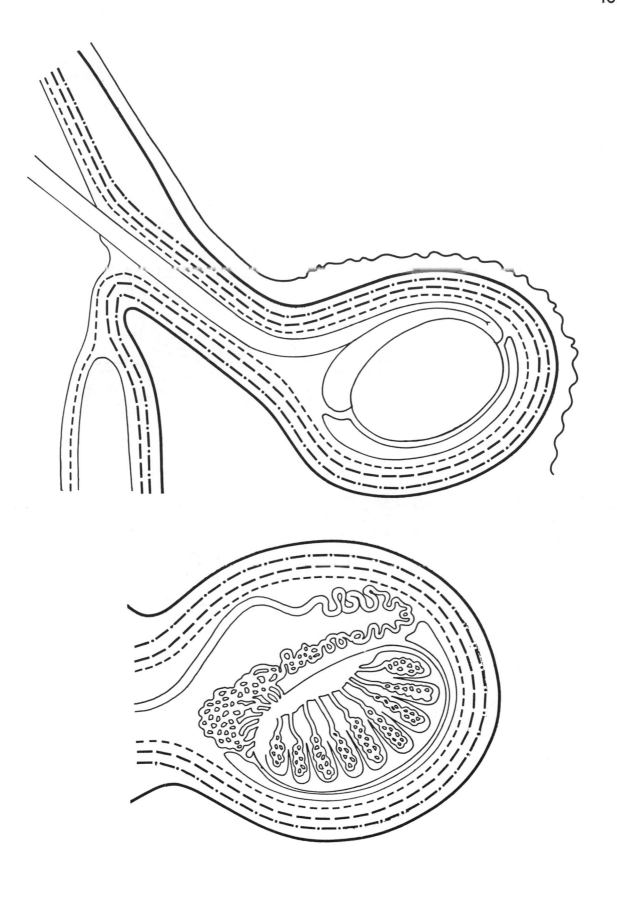

Fig. 8.4 Scrotum and testes - scheme

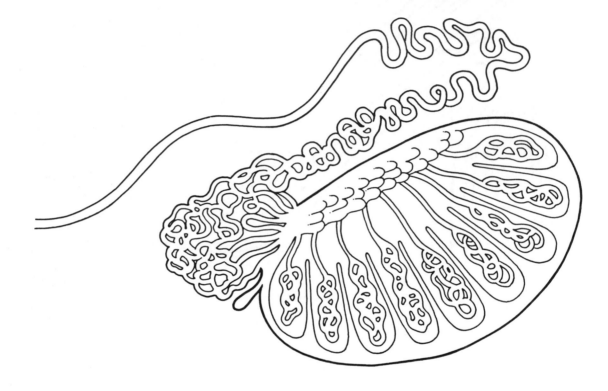

Fig. 8.5 Testis and epididymis, vertical section

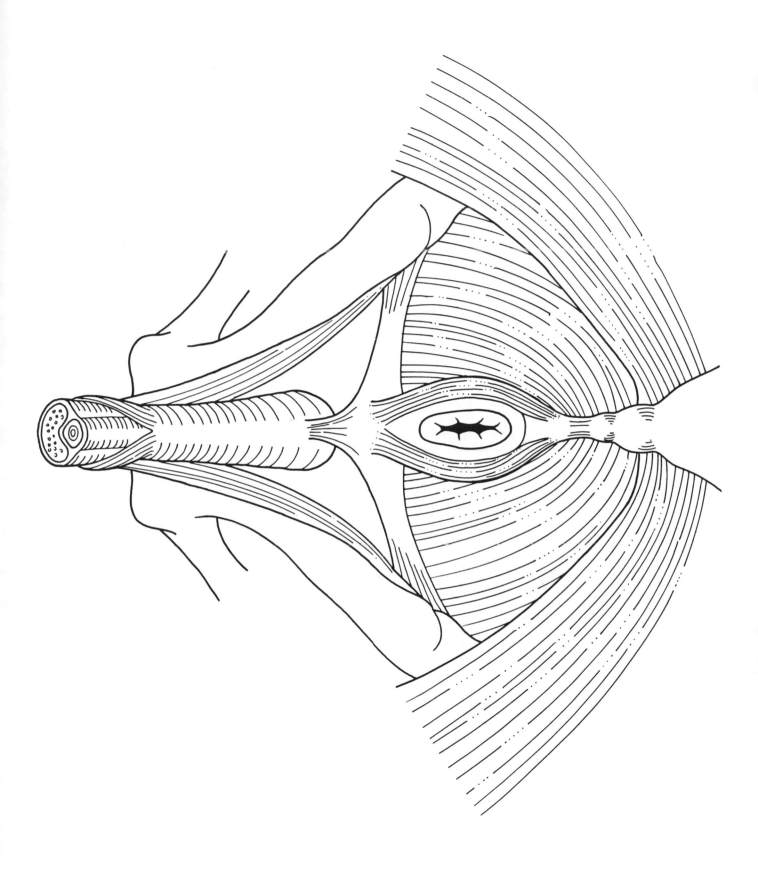

Fig. 8.6 Perineum, structure

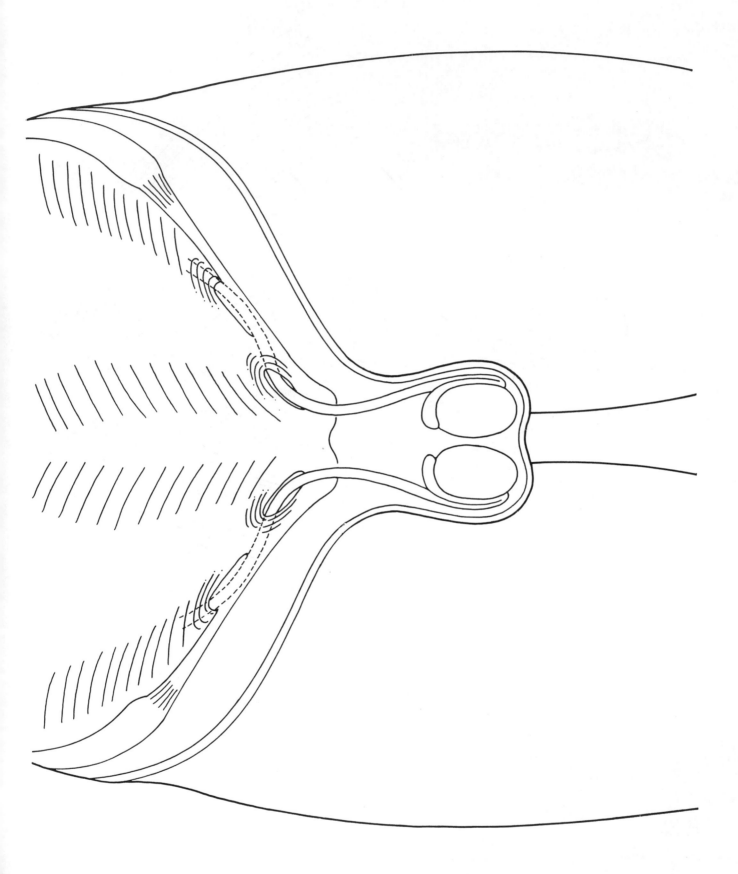

Fig. 8.7 Inguinal canal, scheme

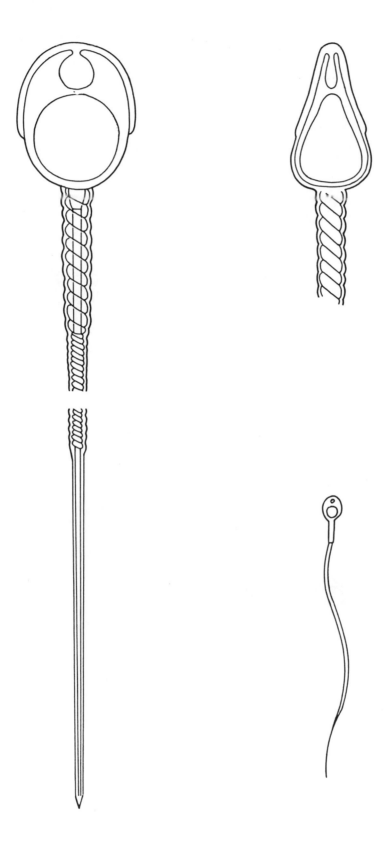

Fig. 8.8 Sperm

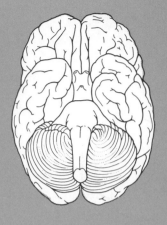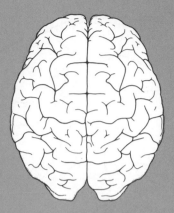

Section 9

Brain and Nervous System

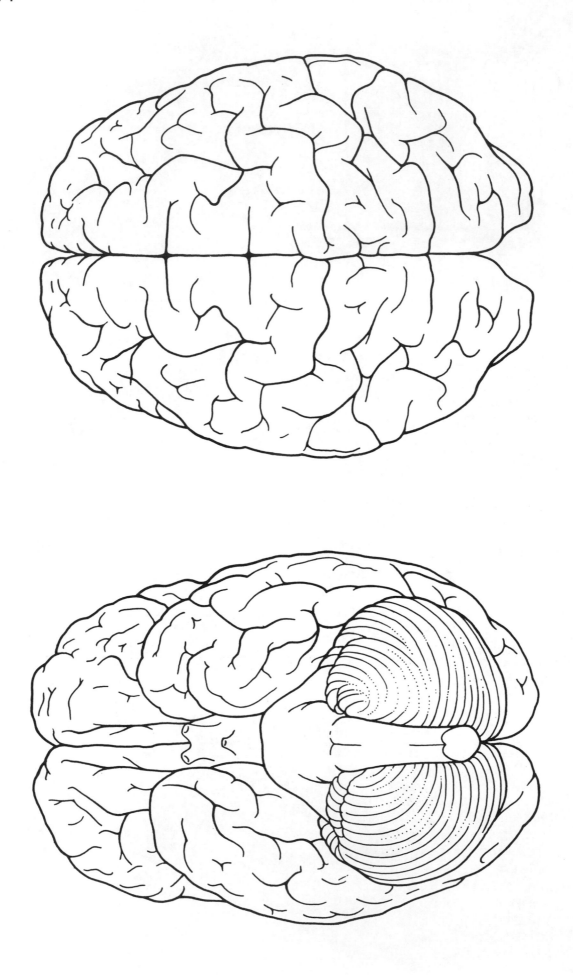

Fig. 9.1 Brain, superior, inferior

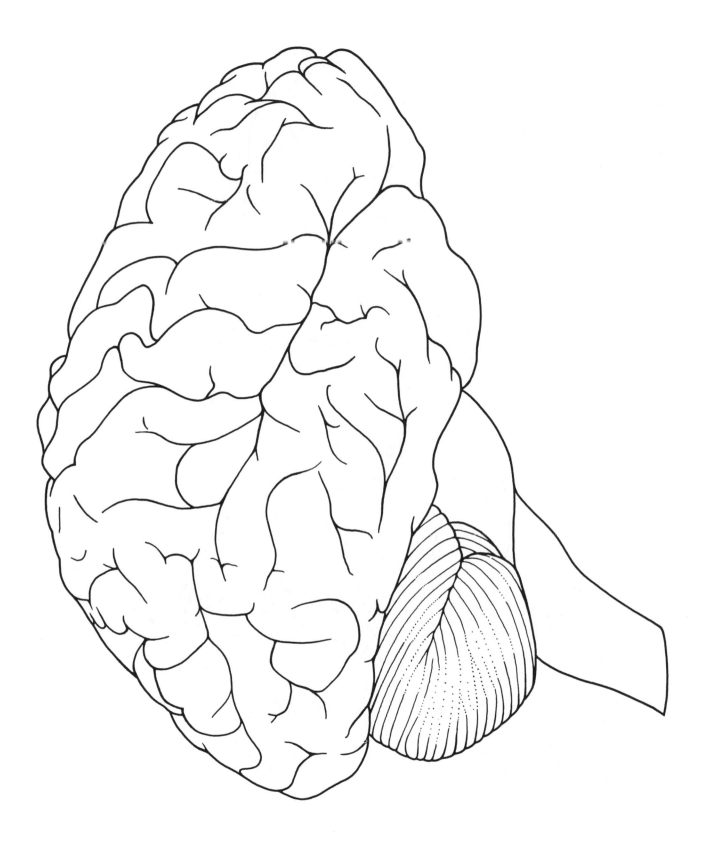

Fig. 9.2 Brain, lateral

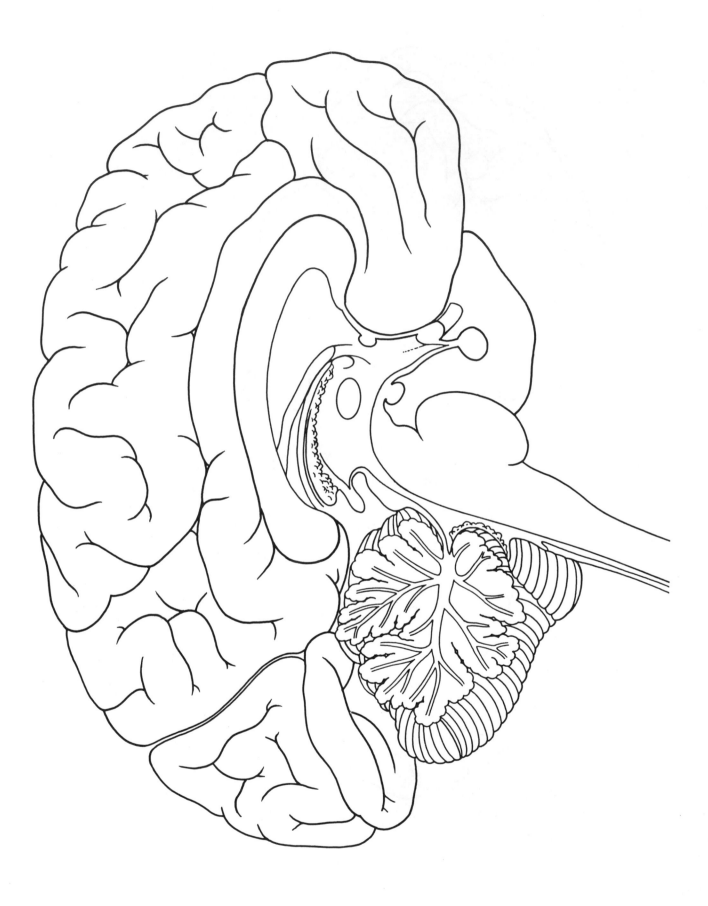

Fig. 9.3 Brain, sagittal section

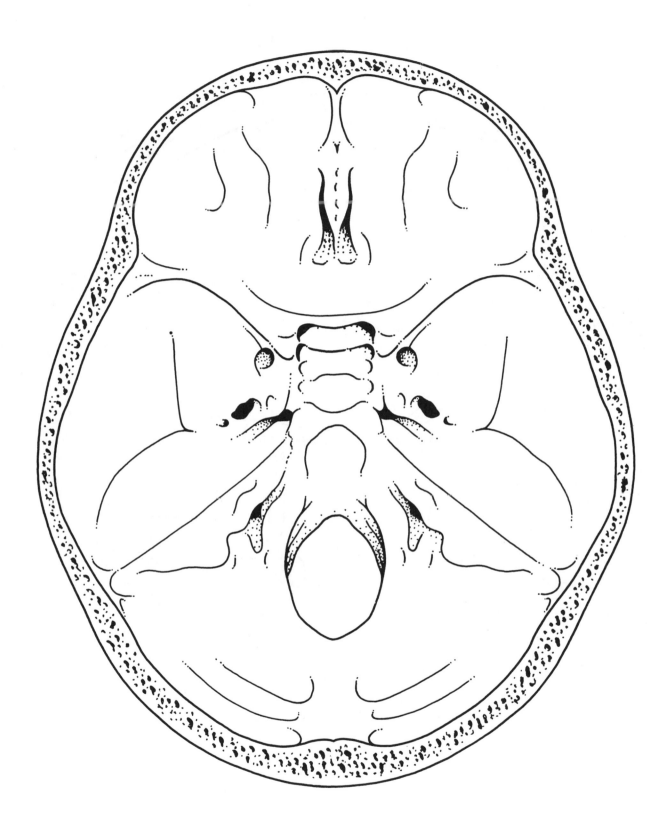

Fig. 9.4 Skull, interior of base

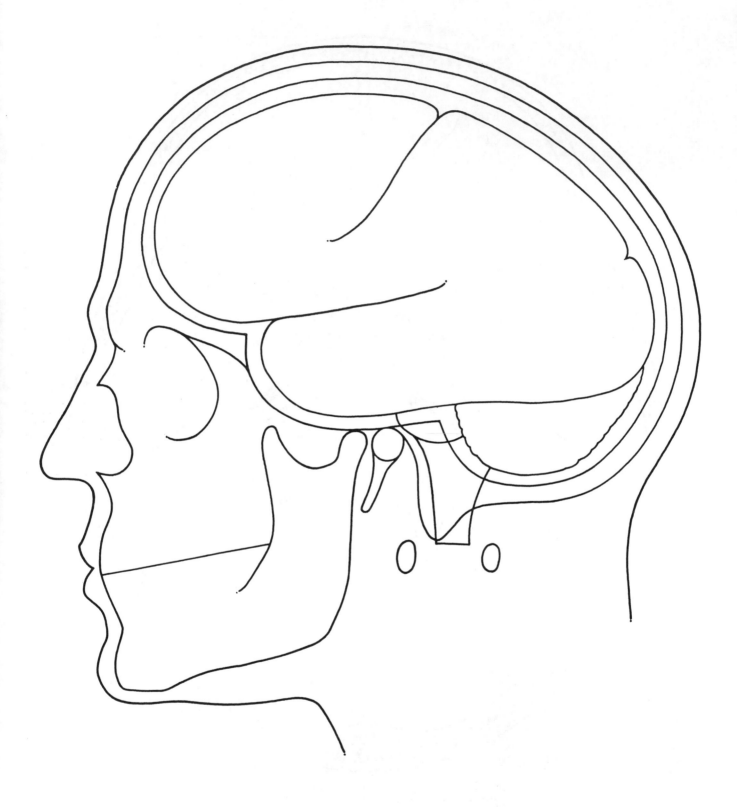

Fig. 9.5 Brain - relationship to skull

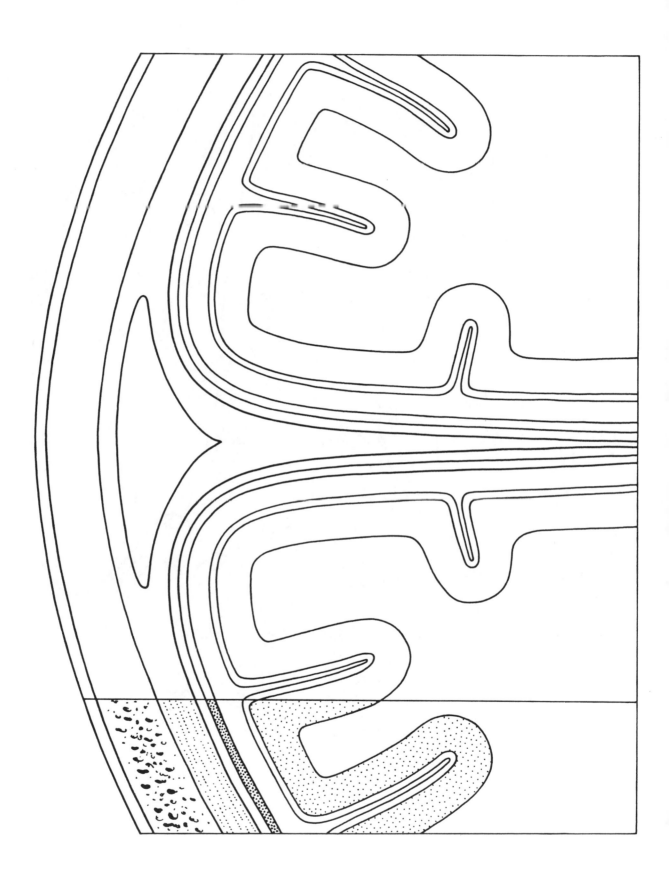

Fig. 9.6 Brain, meninges

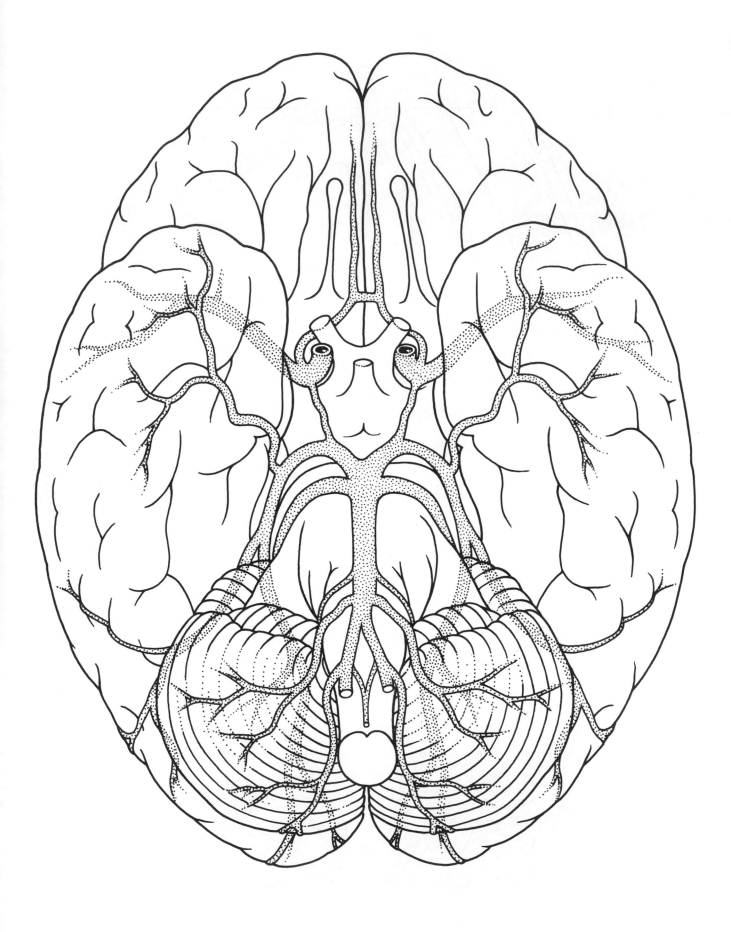

Fig. 9.7 Brain, inferior, arteries

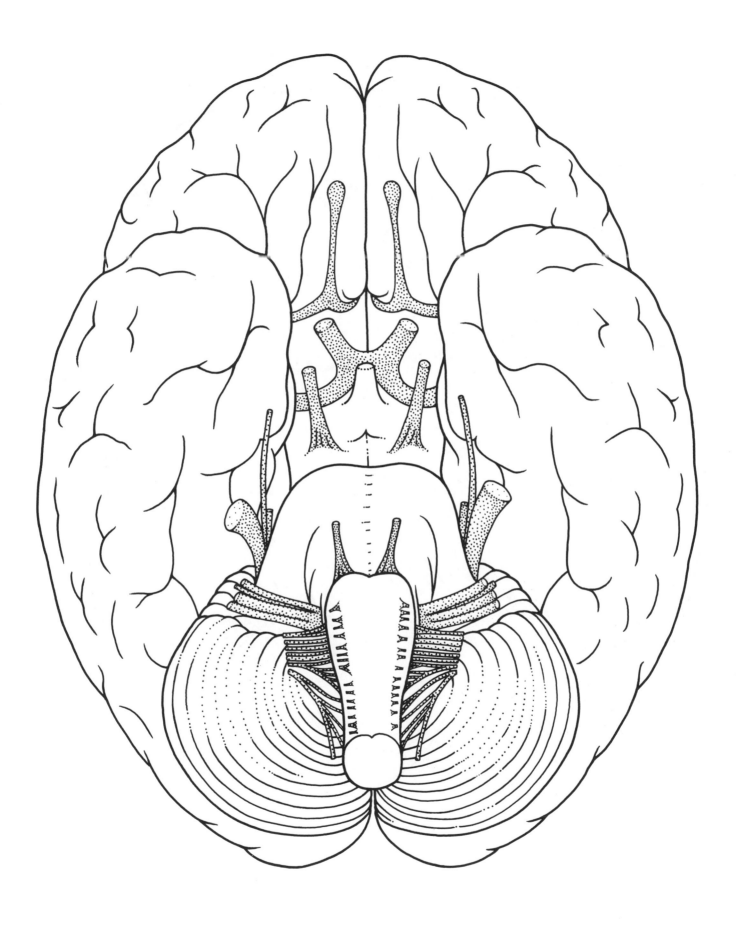

Fig. 9.8 Brain, inferior, cranial nerves

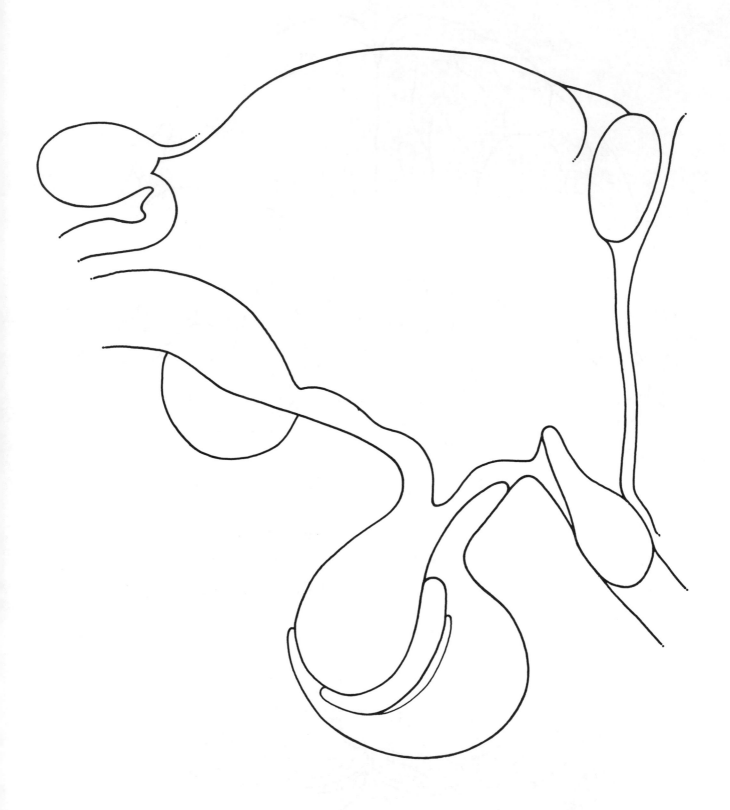

Fig. 9.9 Pineal body, pituitary section

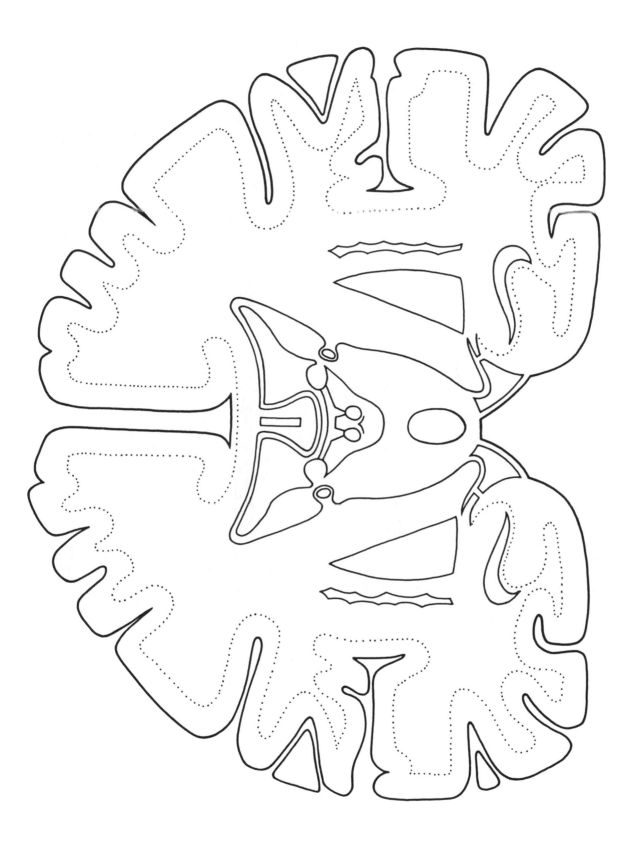

Fig. 9.10 Brain - coronal section, (diencephalon)

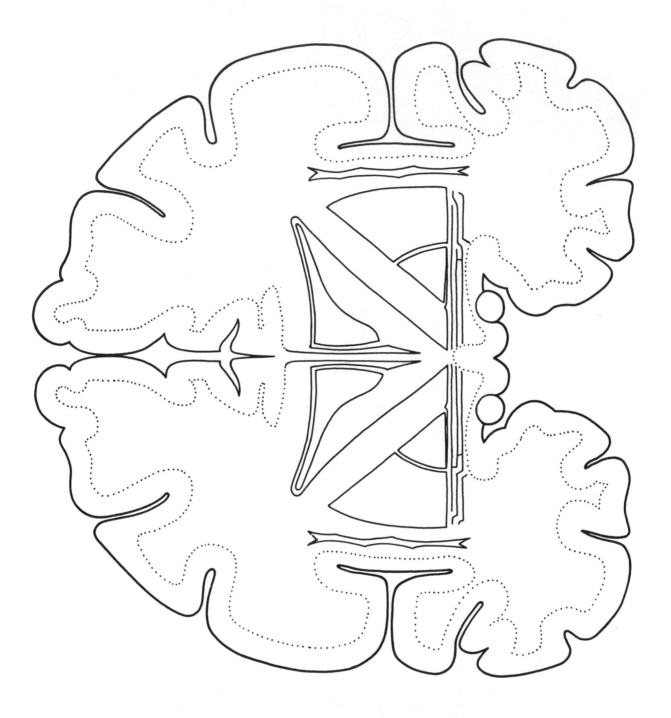

Fig. 9.11 Brain - coronal section, (anterior commisure)

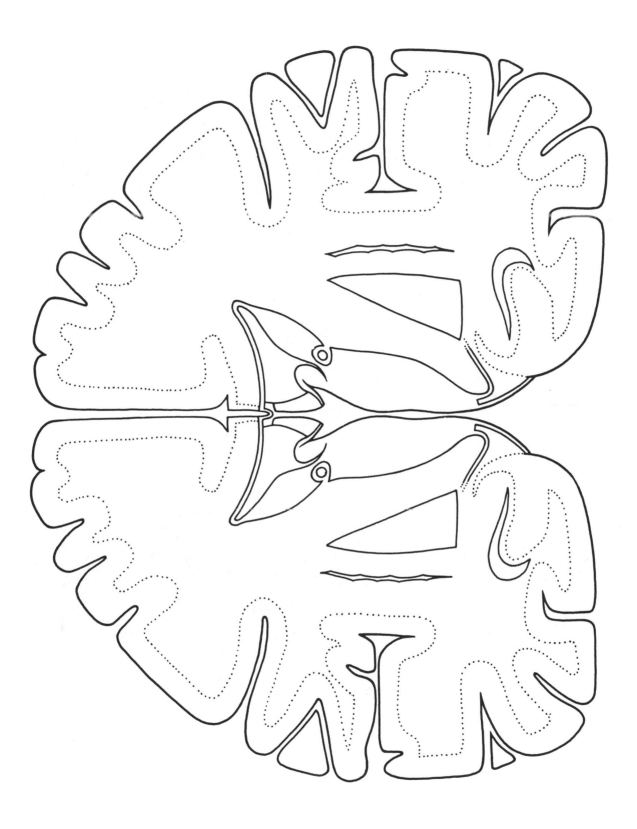

Fig. 9.12 Brain - coronal section, (mamillary body)

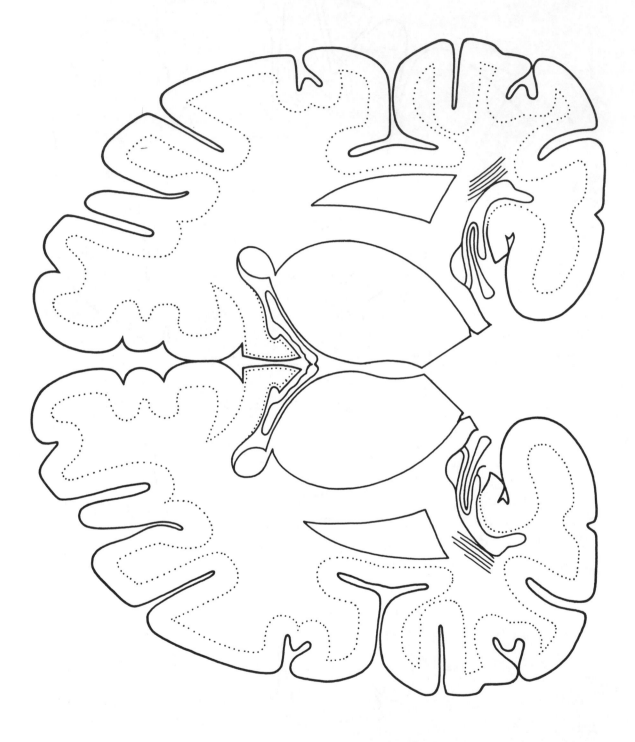

Fig. 9.13 Brain - coronal section, (crus cerebri)

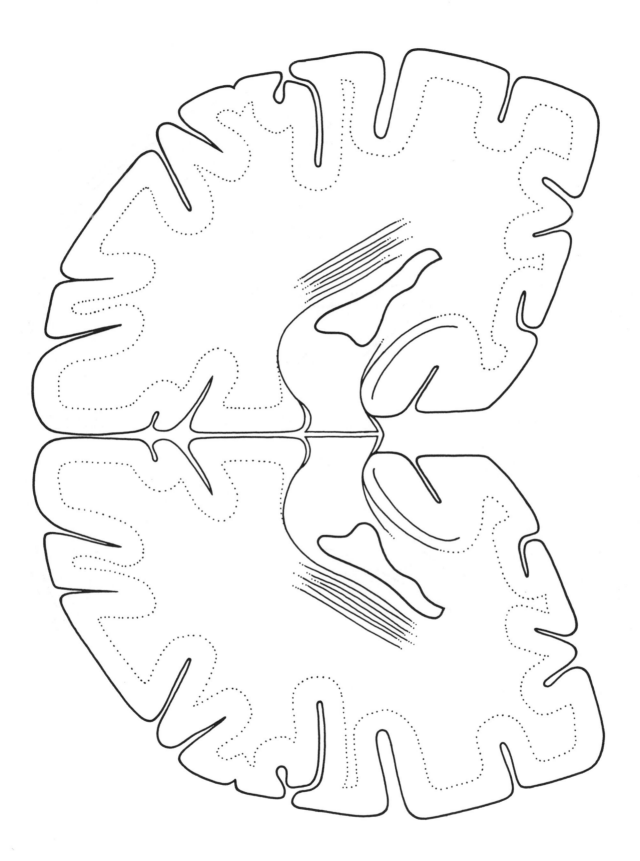

Fig. 9.14   Brain - coronal section, (splenium, corpus callosum)

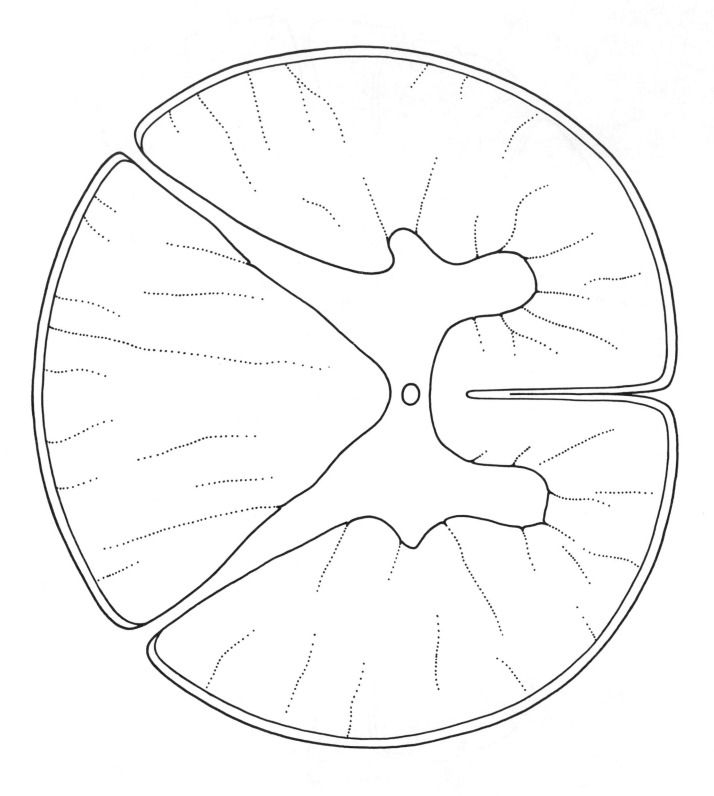

Fig. 9.15 Spinal cord, slice

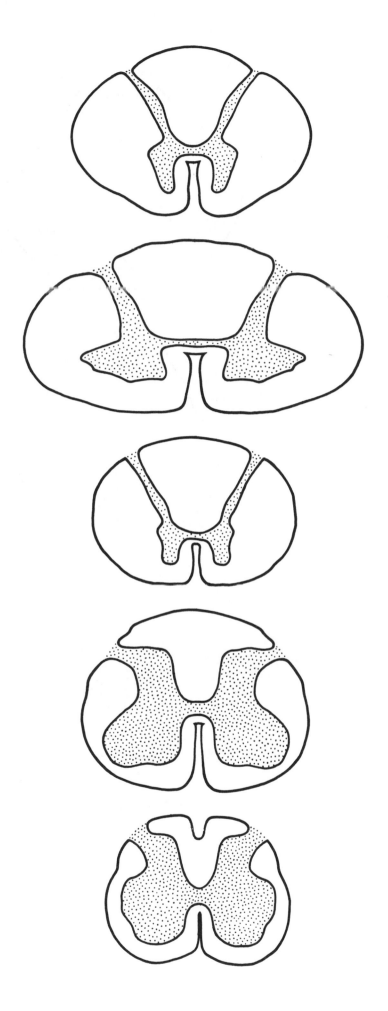

Fig. 9.16 Spinal cord - sections at various levels

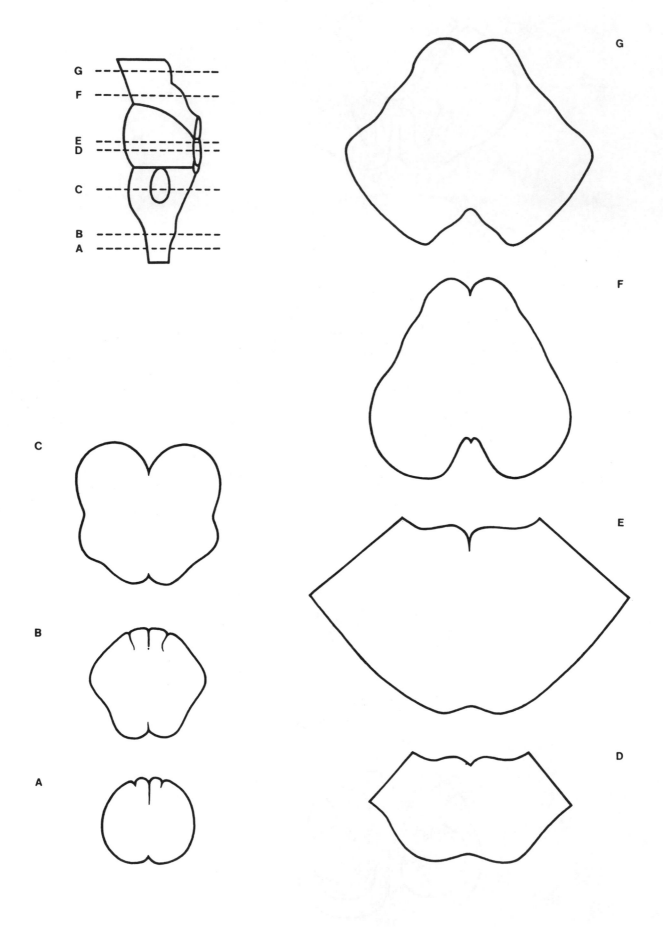

Fig. 9.17 Brain stem - sections at various levels

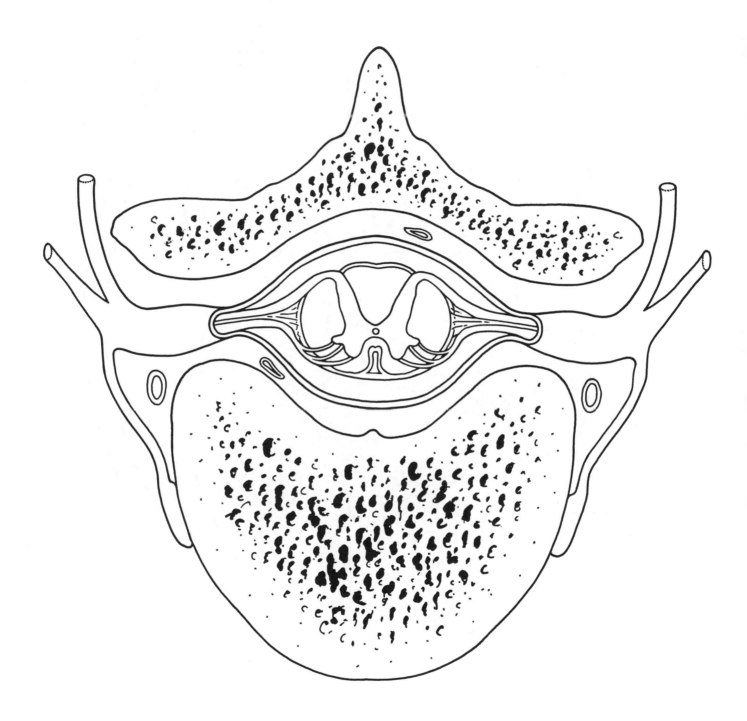

Fig. 9.18 Spinal cord in vertebra

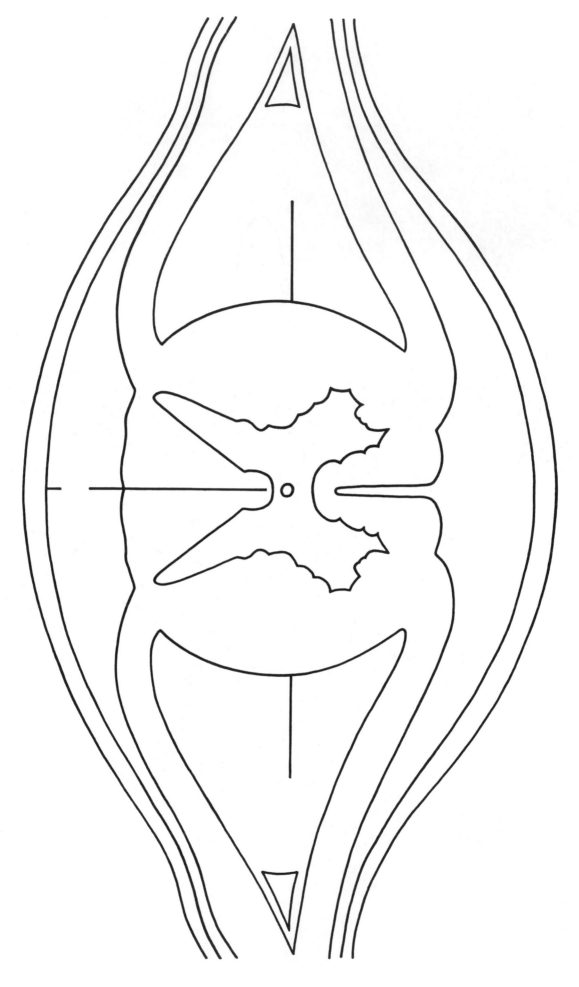

Fig. 9.19 Spinal cord - horizontal section

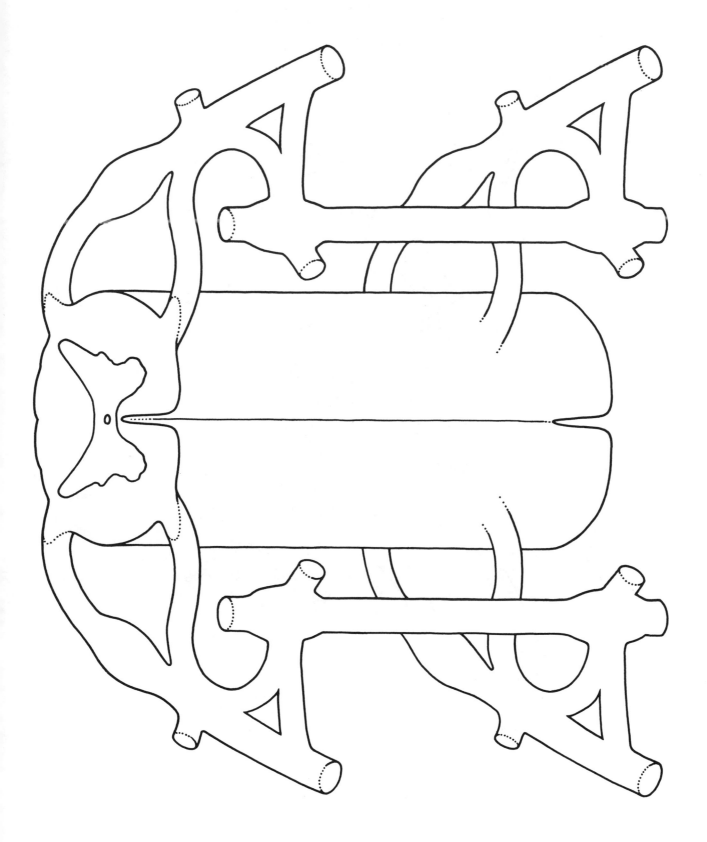

Fig. 9.20 Spinal cord and nerves - scheme

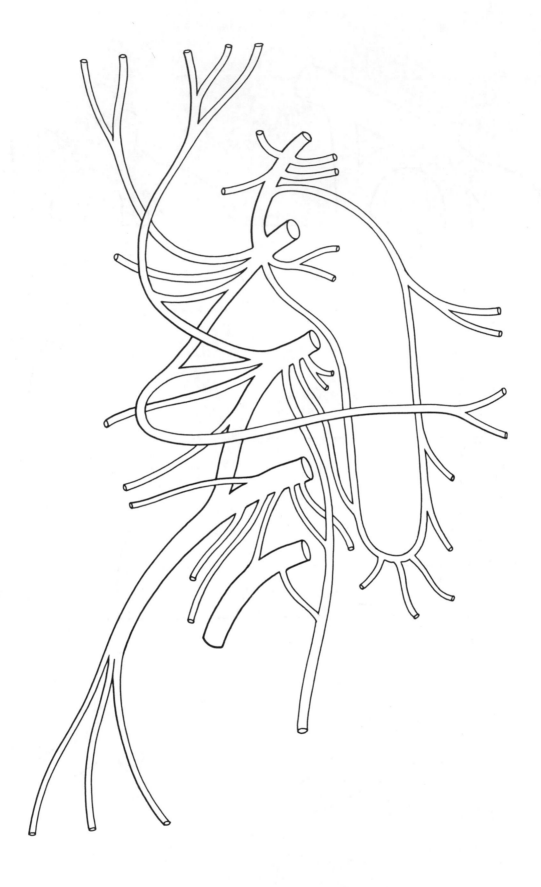

Fig. 9.21 Cervical plexus

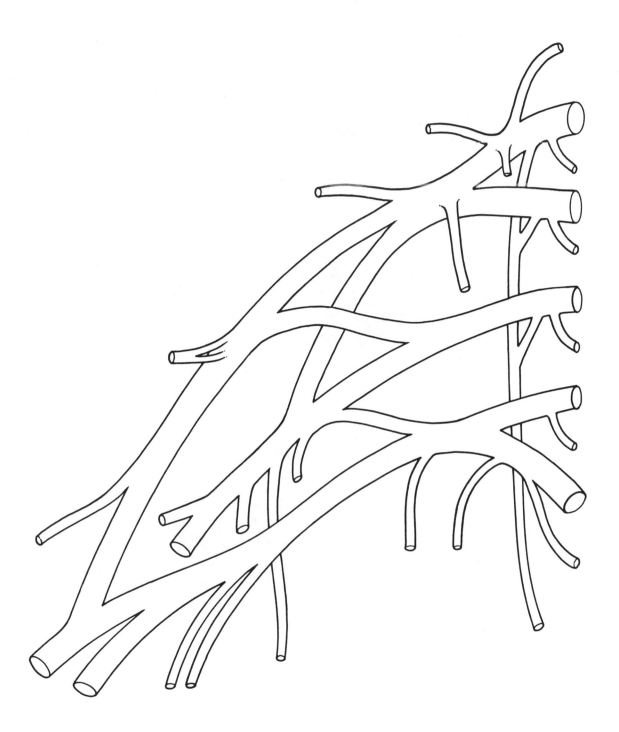

Fig. 9.22 Brachial plexus

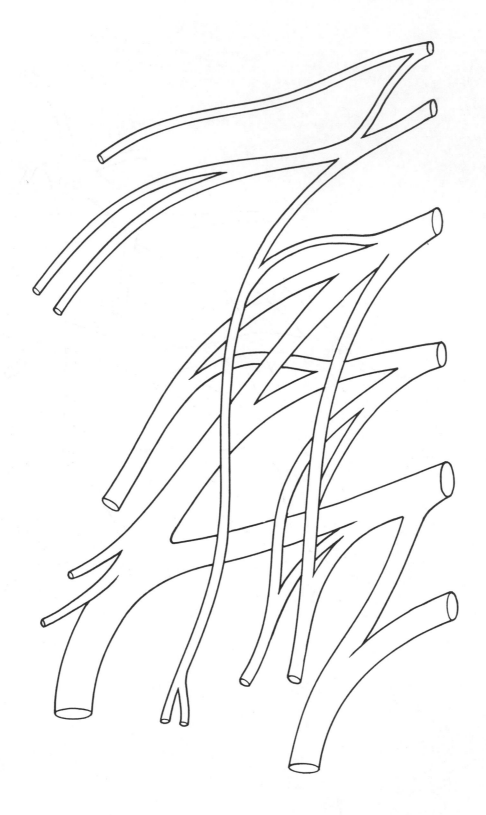

Fig. 9.23 Lumbar plexus

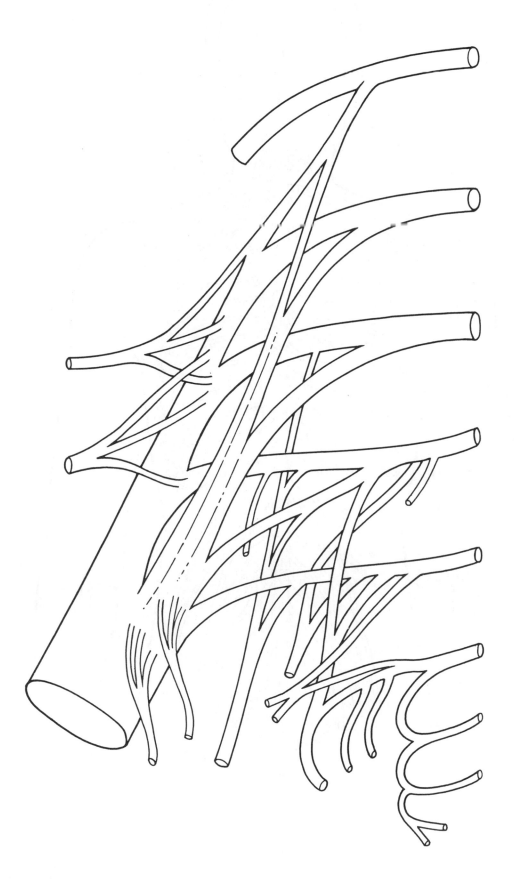

Fig. 9.24 Sacral, coccygeal plexus

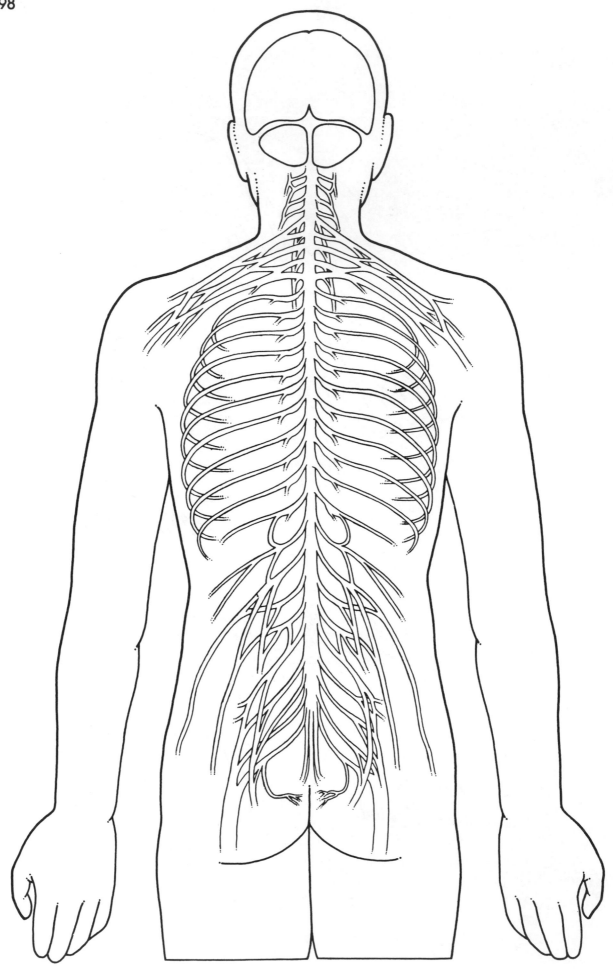

Fig. 9.25 Spinal nerves

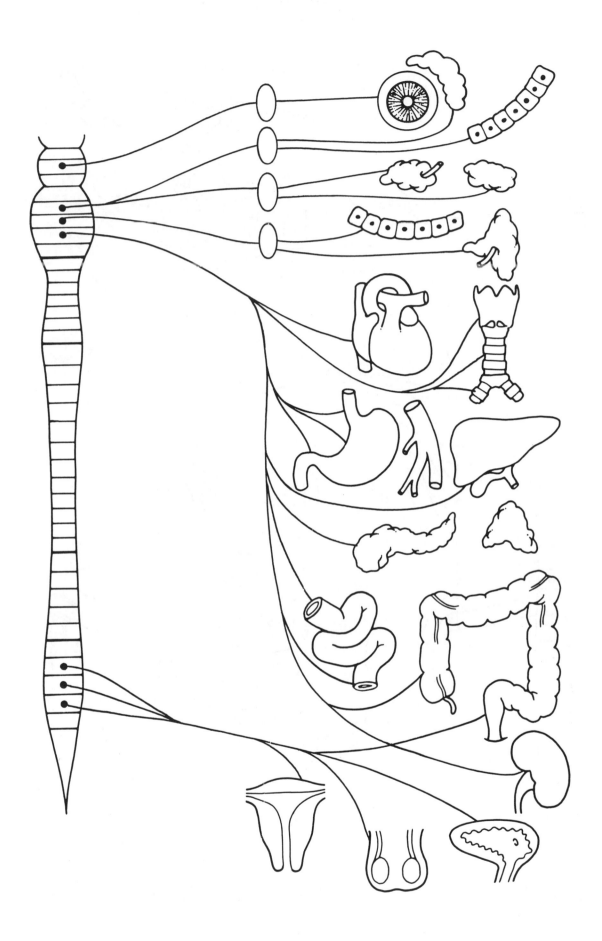

Fig. 9.26 Parasympathetic system - scheme

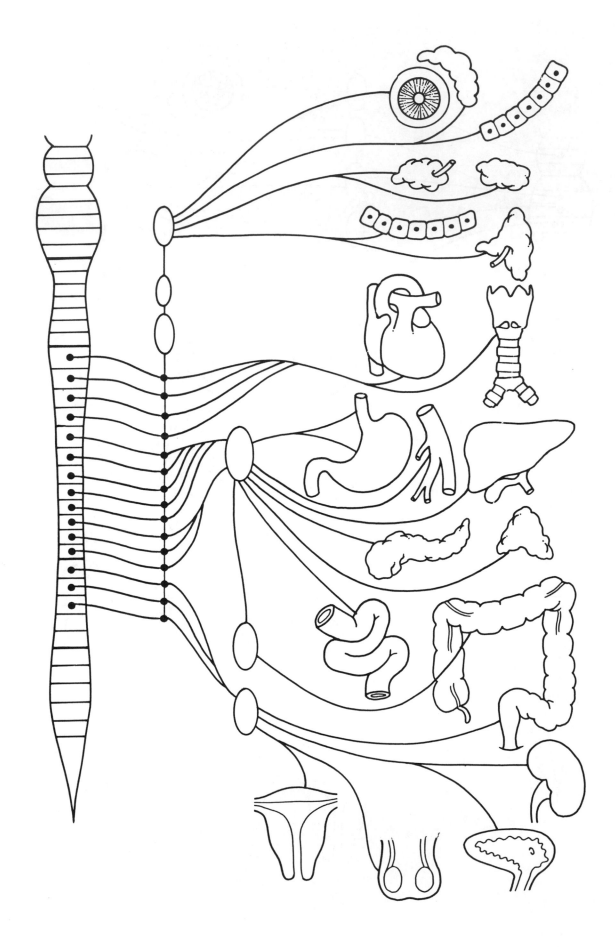

Fig. 9.27 Autonomic system - scheme

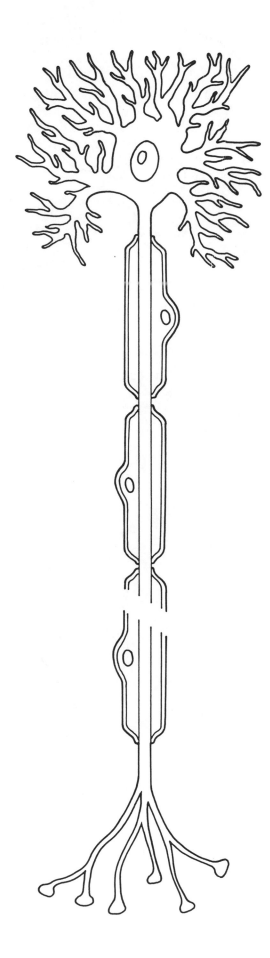

Fig. 9.28 Motor neuron

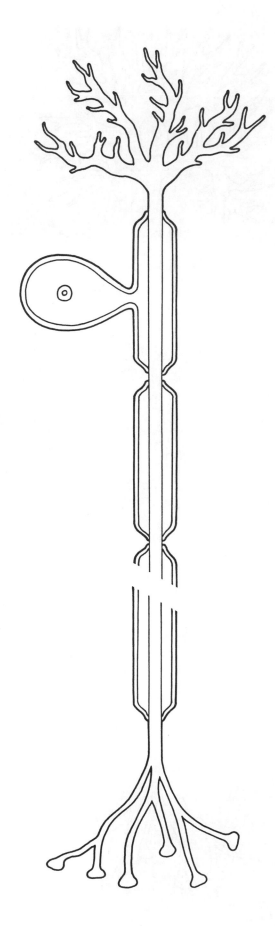

Fig. 9.29 Sensory neuron

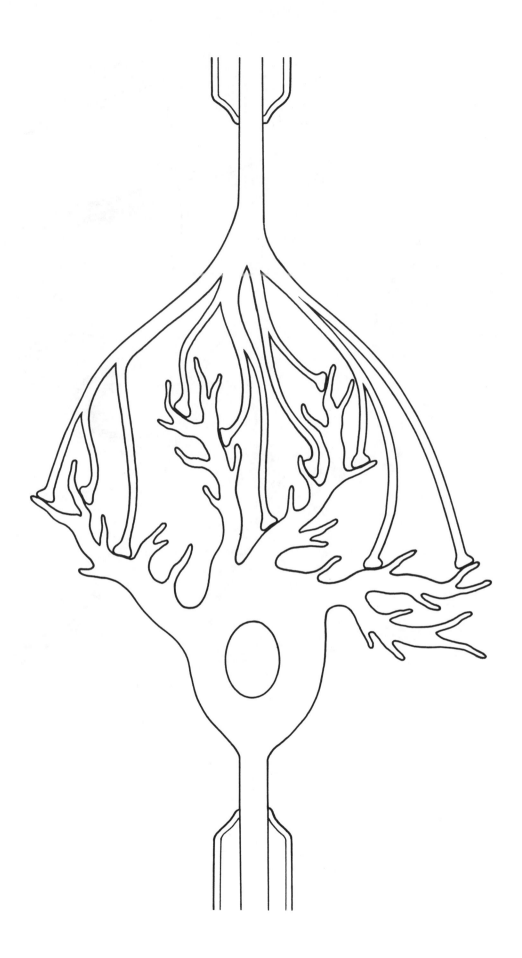

Fig. 9.30 Synapse

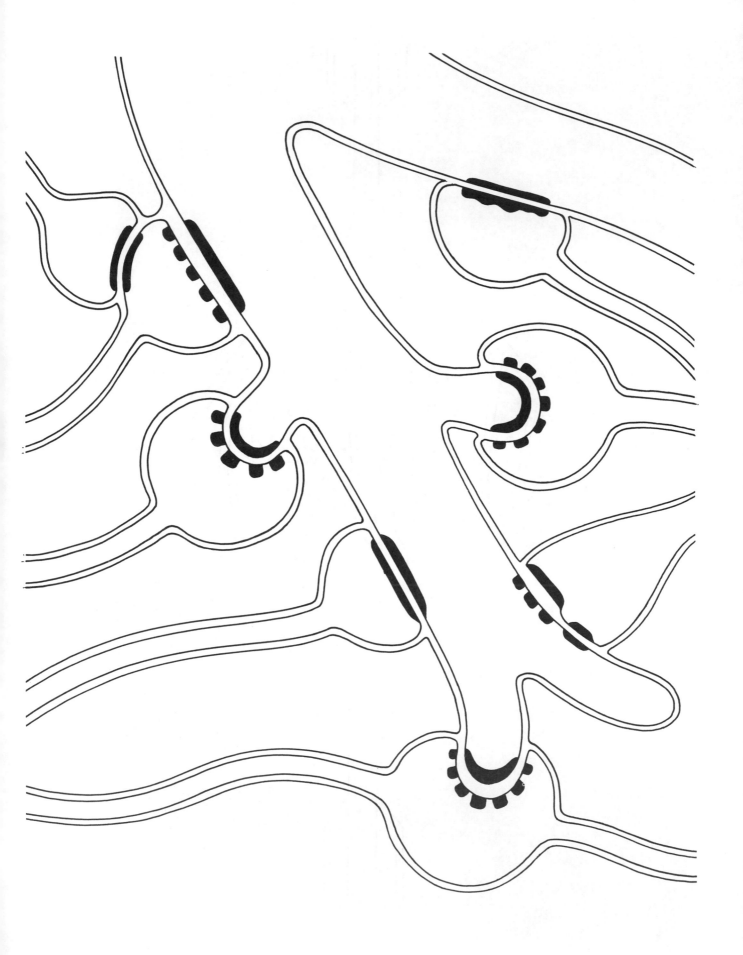

Fig. 9.31 Synaptic junctions

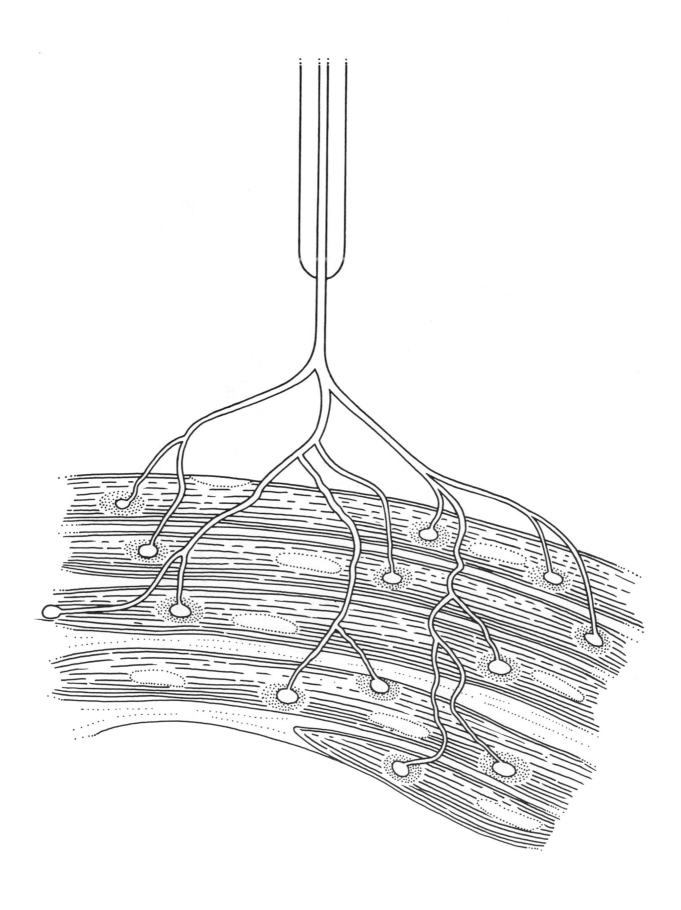

Fig. 9.32 Motor nerve ending

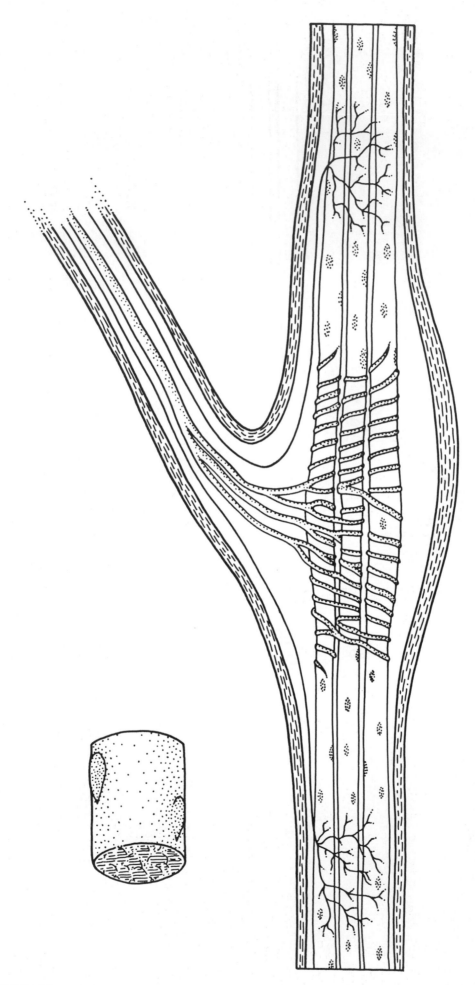

Fig. 9.33 Neuromuscular junction

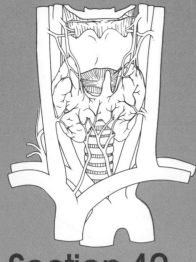

Section 10

Endocrine and Ductless Glands

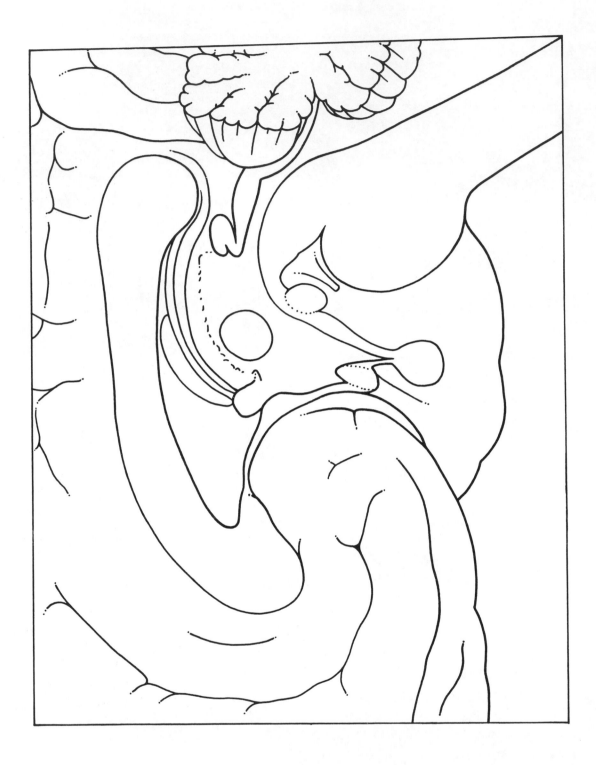

Fig. 10.1 Pituitary - location in brain

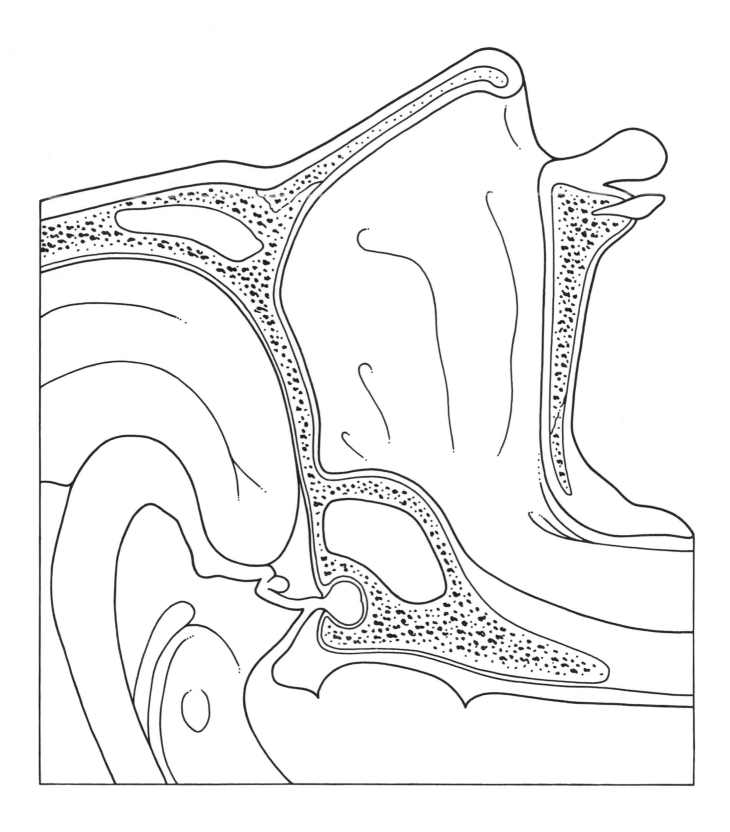

Fig. 10.2 Pituitary in fossa

210

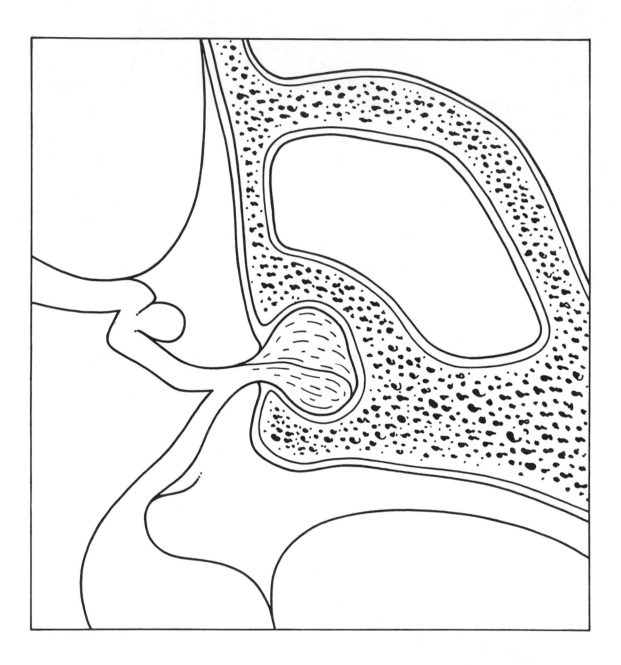

Fig. 10.3 Pituitary in fossa

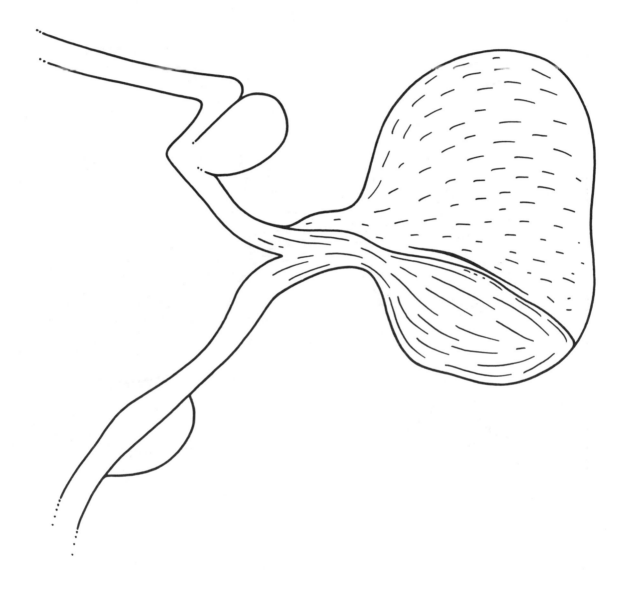

Fig. 10.4 Pituitary - section

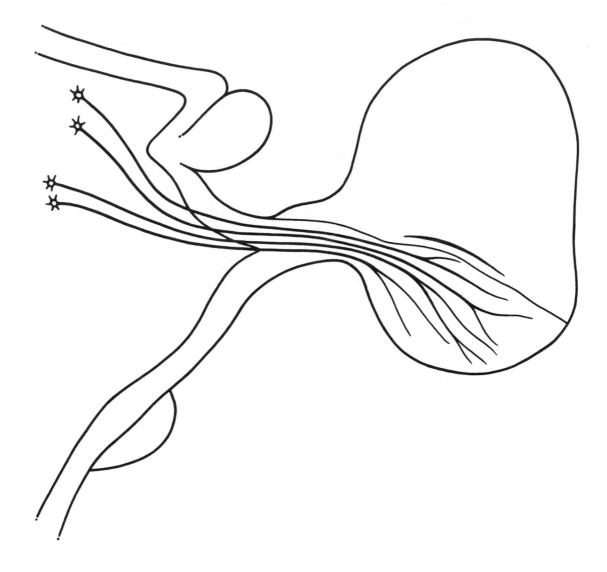

Fig. 10.5 Pituitary - section, nerves

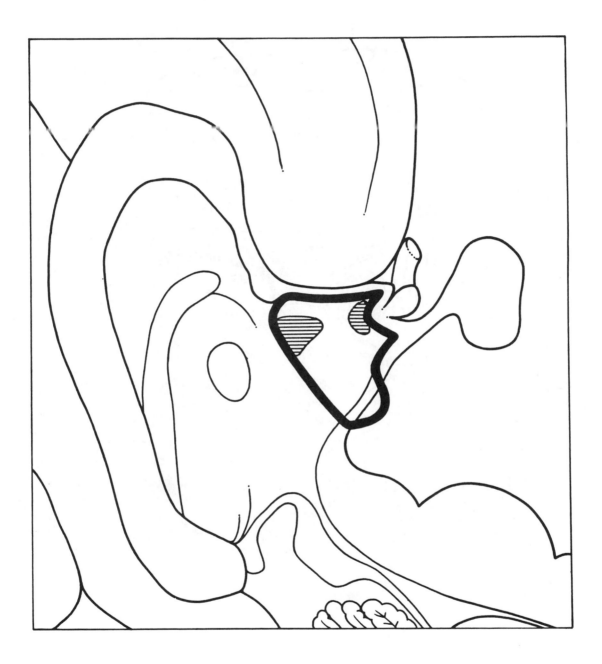

Fig. 10.6 Hypothalamus - median sagittal section

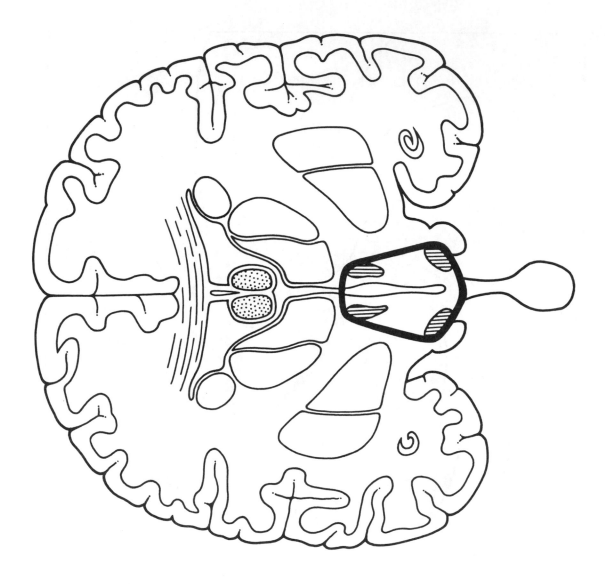

Fig. 10.7 Hypothalamus - coronal section

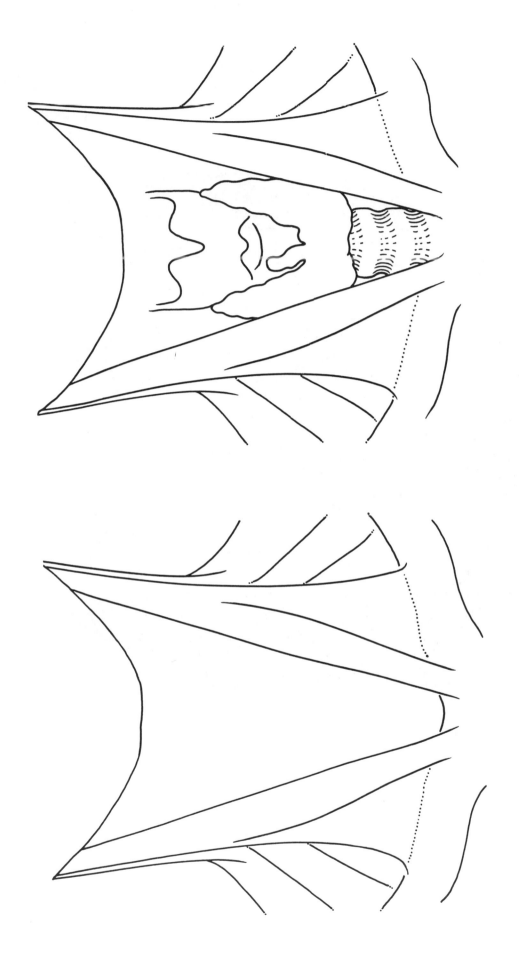

Fig. 10.8 Thyroid , position in neck

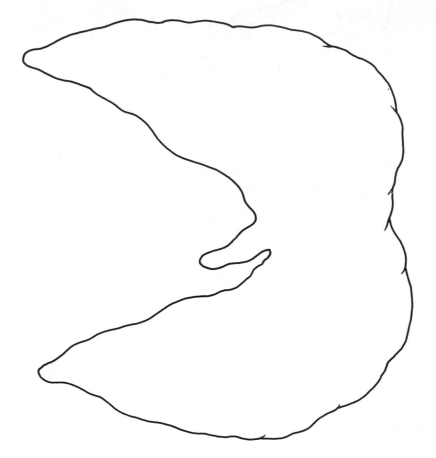

Fig. 10.9 Thyroid - outline

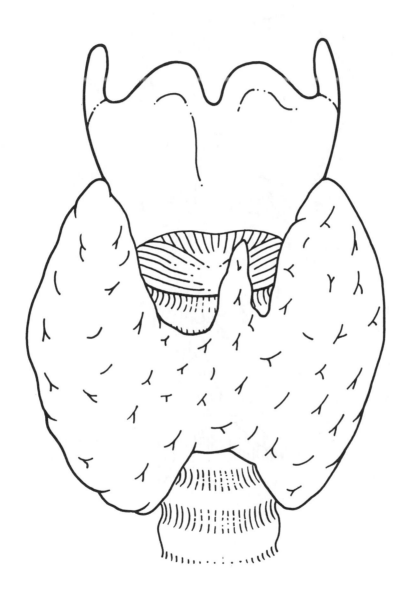

Fig. 10.10 Thyroid, trachea, AP

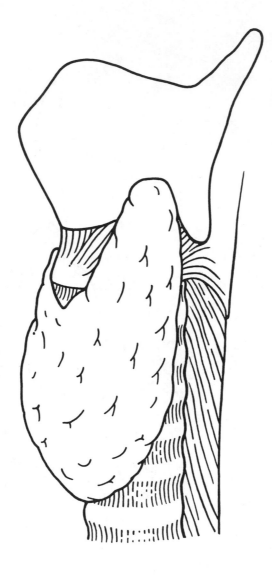

Fig. 10.11 Thyroid, trachea, lateral

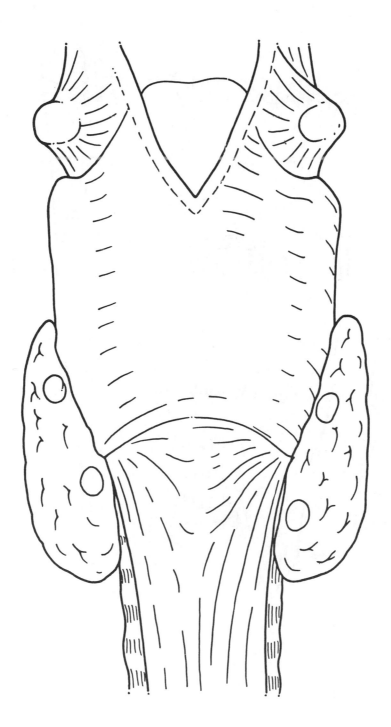

Fig. 10.12 Thyroid, parathyroids, trachea, PA

220

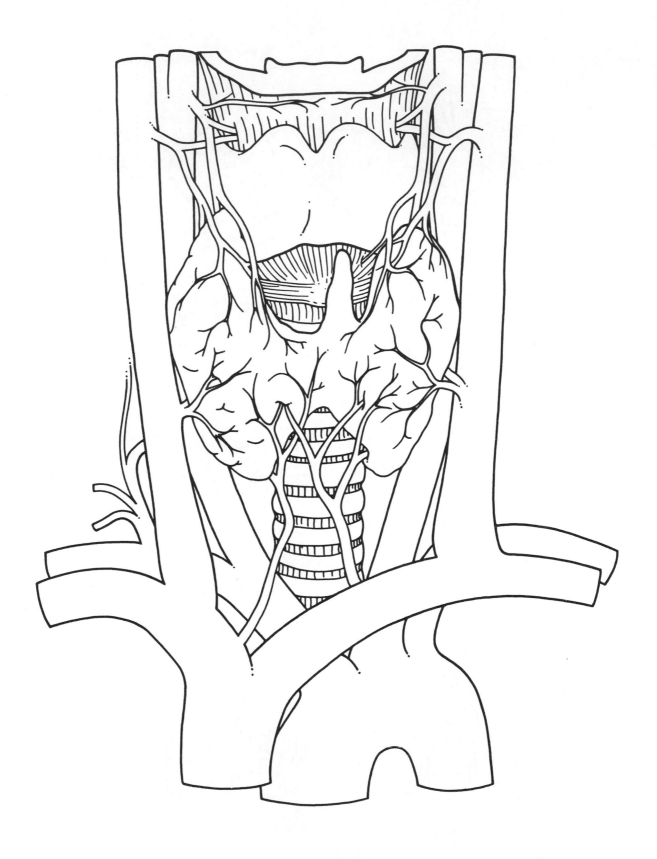

Fig. 10.13 Thyroid, trachea - blood supply, AP

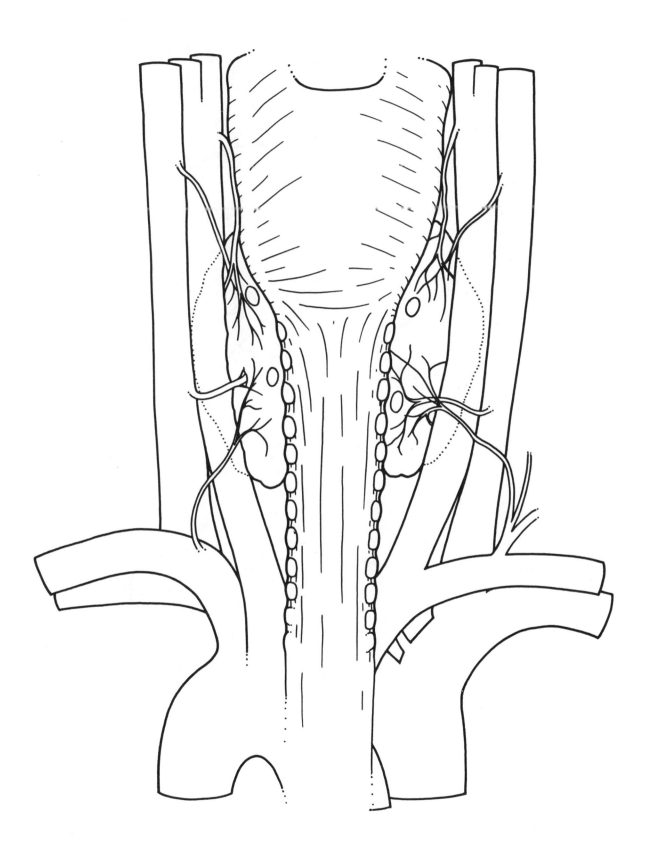

Fig. 10.14 Thyroid, parathyroids, trachea - blood supply, PA

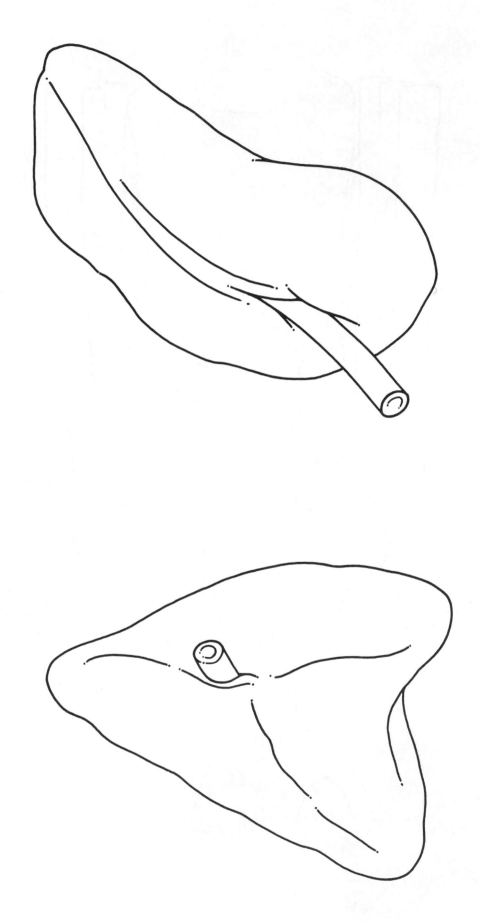

Fig. 10.15 Adrenal glands - outline

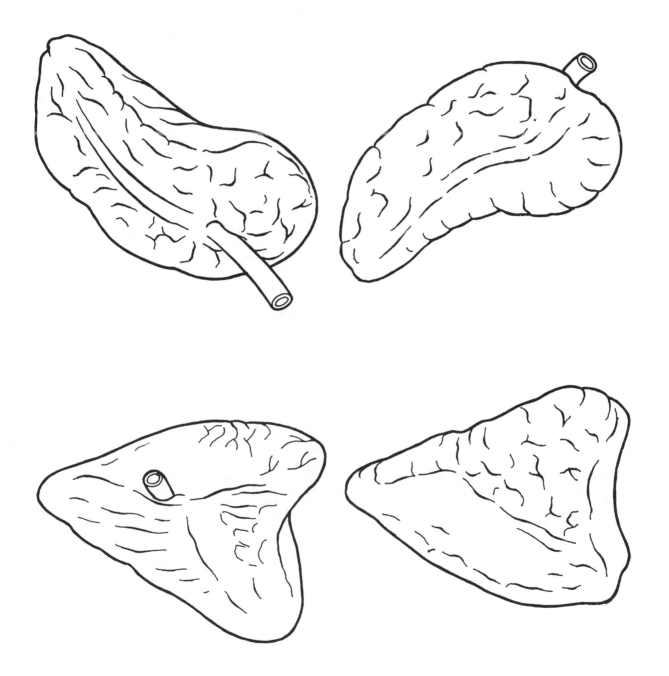

Fig. 10.16 Adrenal glands, AP. PA

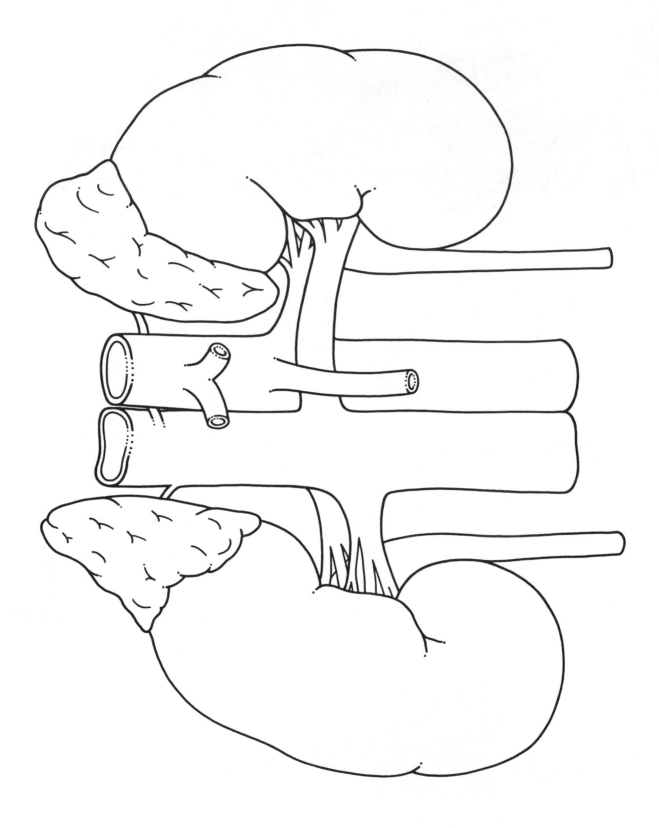

Fig. 10.17   Adrenal glands, kidney, AP

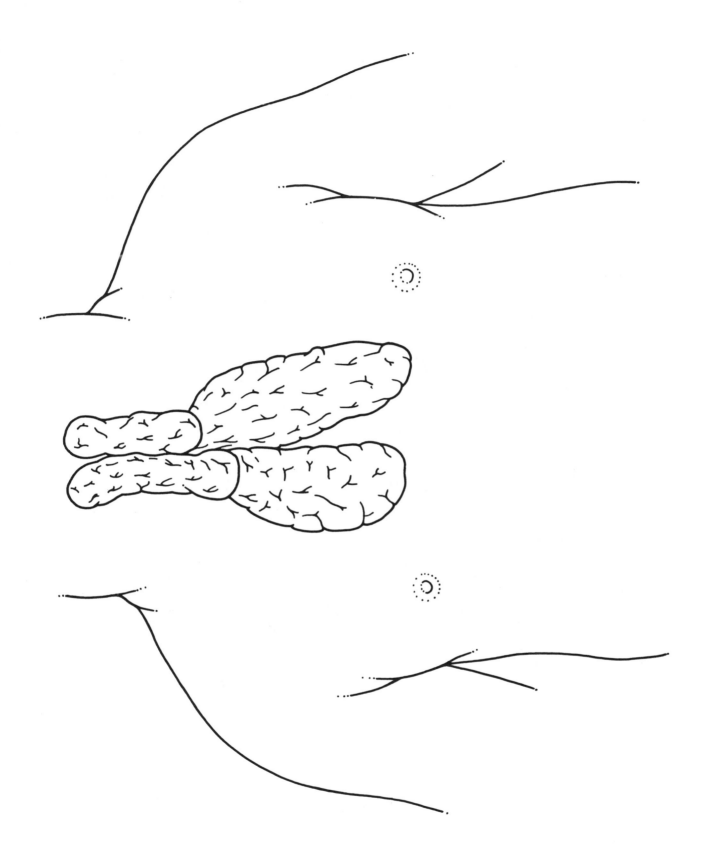

Fig. 10.18 Thymus gland - infant, AP

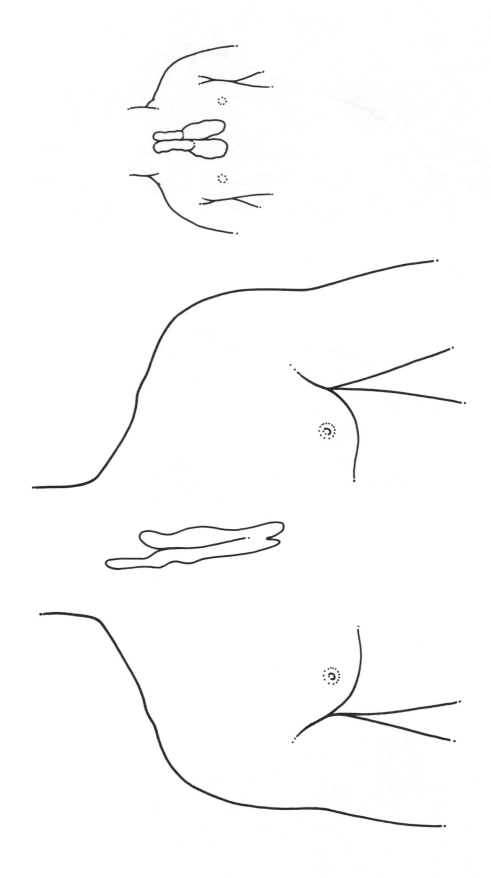

Fig. 10.19 Thymus gland - adult, infant, AP

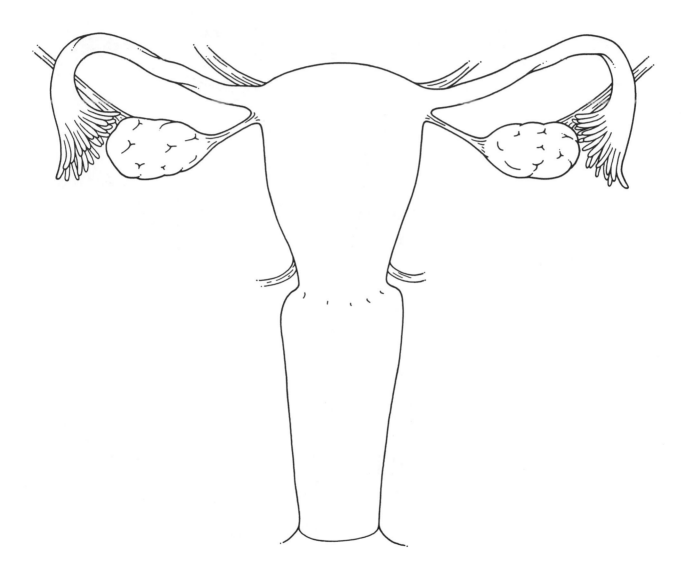

Fig. 10.20 Ovaries, fallopian tubes, uterus, vagina, AP

228

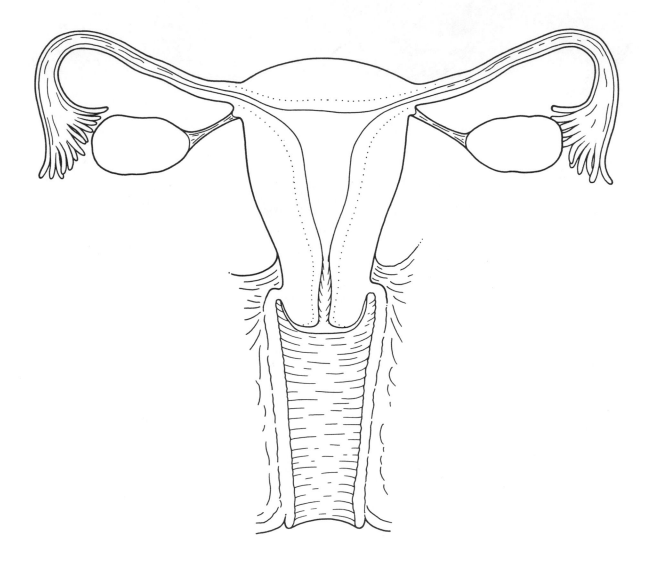

Fig. 10.21 Ovaries, fallopian tubes, uterus, vagina - section

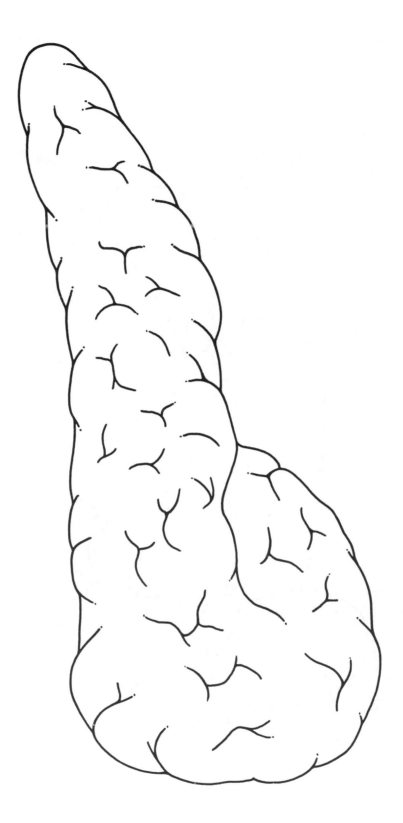

Fig. 10.22 Pancreas, AP

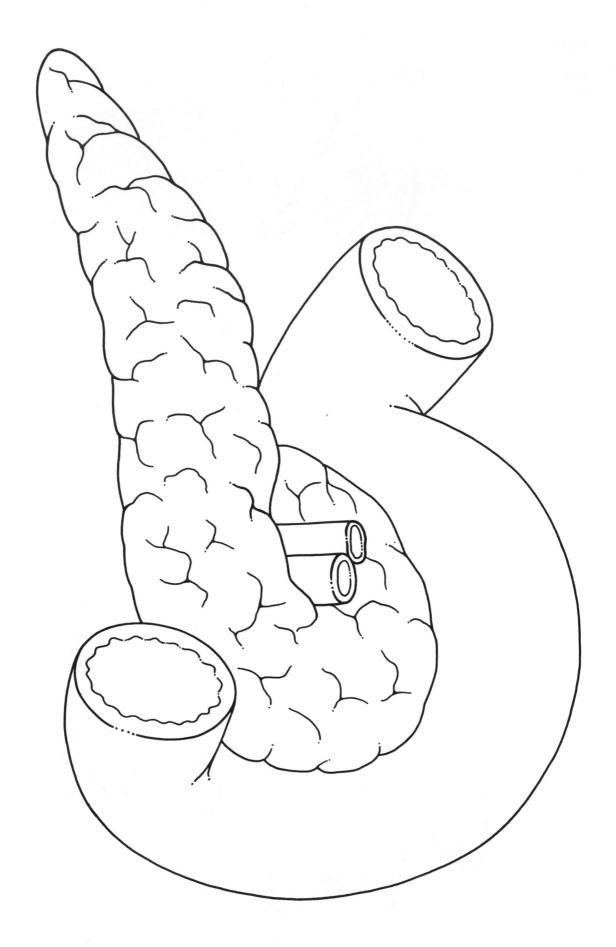

Fig. 10.23 Pancreas, duodenum, AP

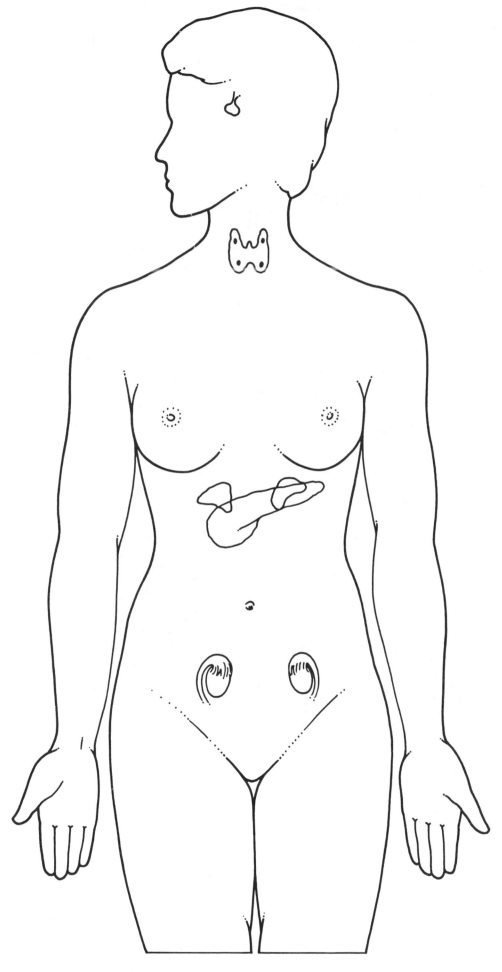

Fig. 10.24 Endocrine glands - female, AP

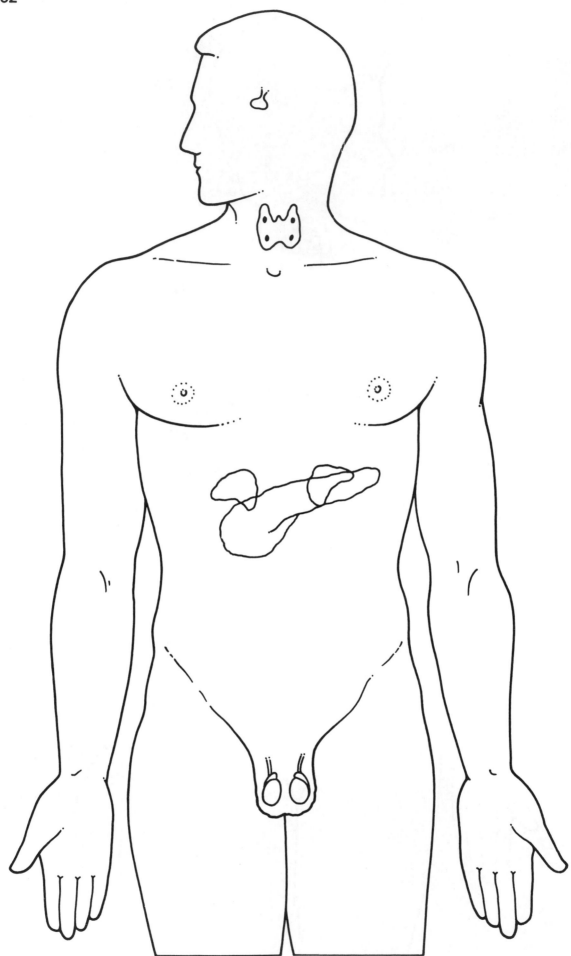

Fig. 10.25 Endocrine glands - male, AP

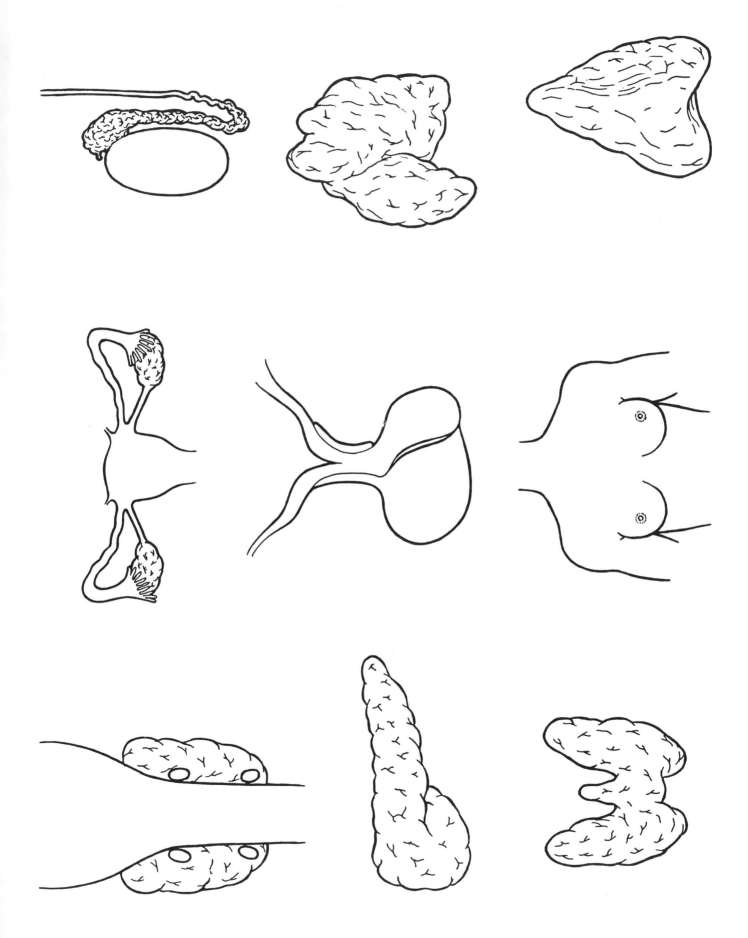

Fig. 10.26 Endocrine - miscellaneous

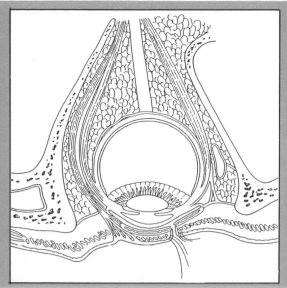

Section 11

Eye, Ear, Nose, Throat

236

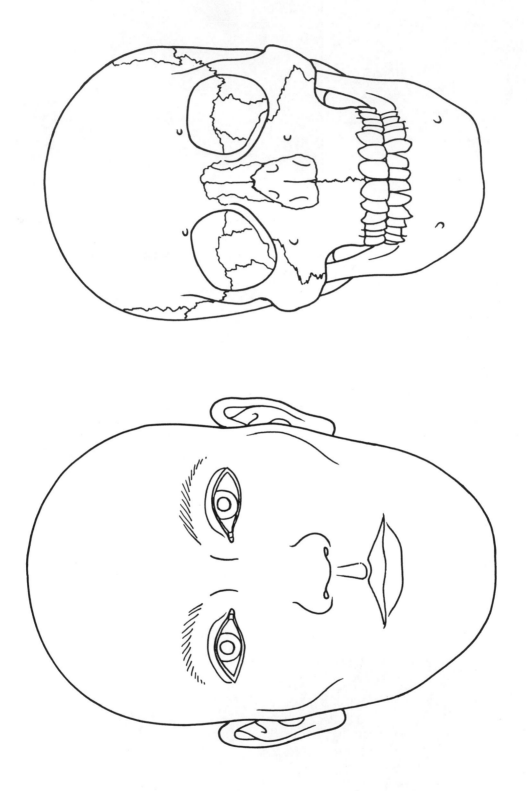

Fig. 11.1 Head, skull, AP

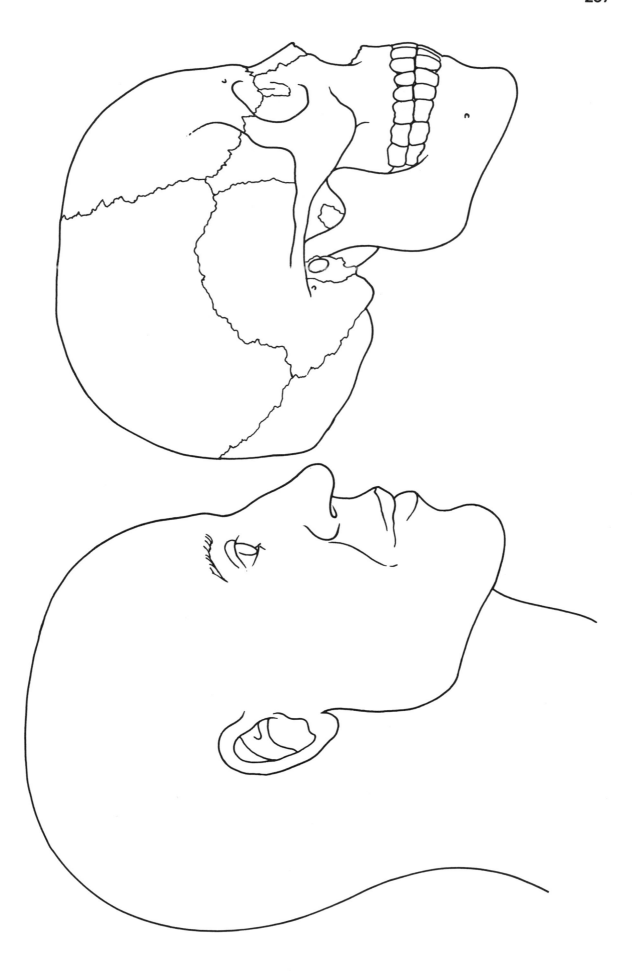

Fig. 11.2 Head, skull, lateral

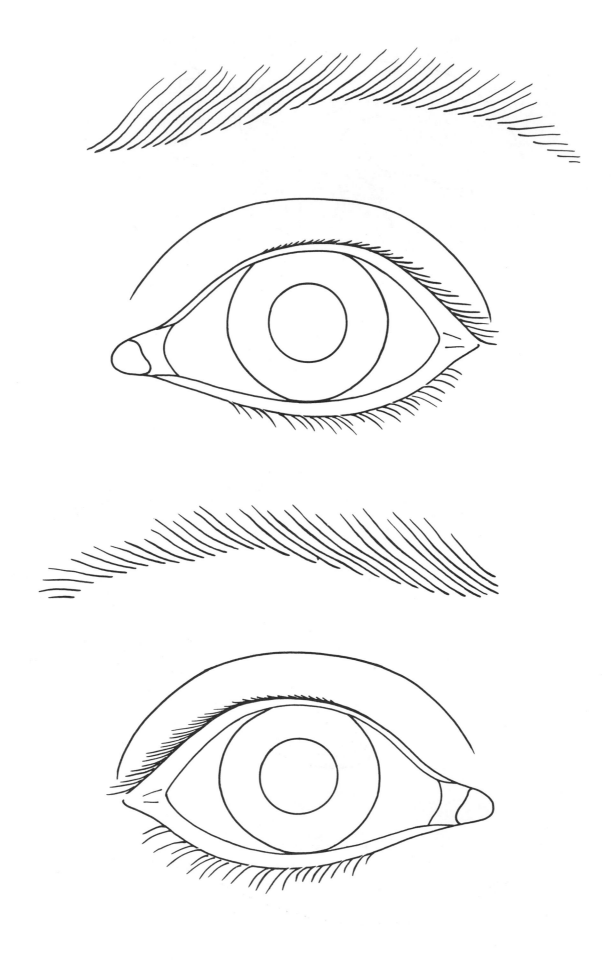

Fig. 11.3 Eye - external

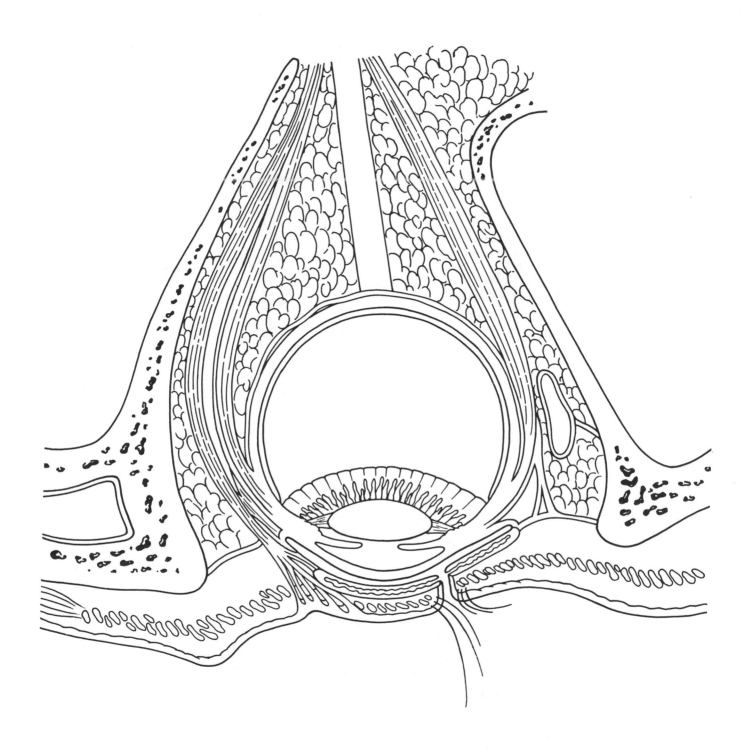

Fig. 11.4 Eye - in situ

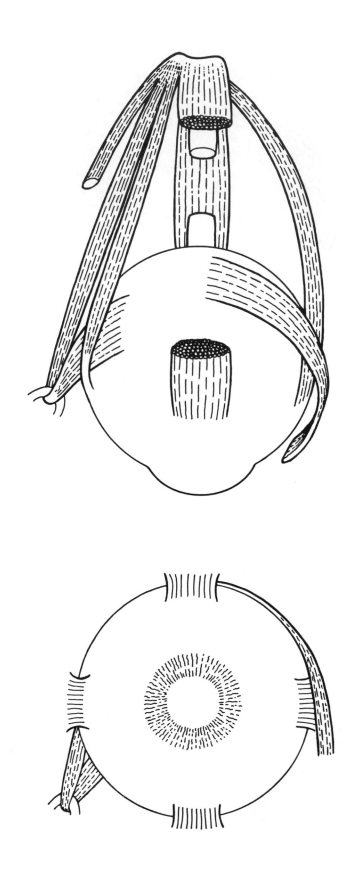

Fig. 11.5 Eye - extrinsic muscles, AP/lateral

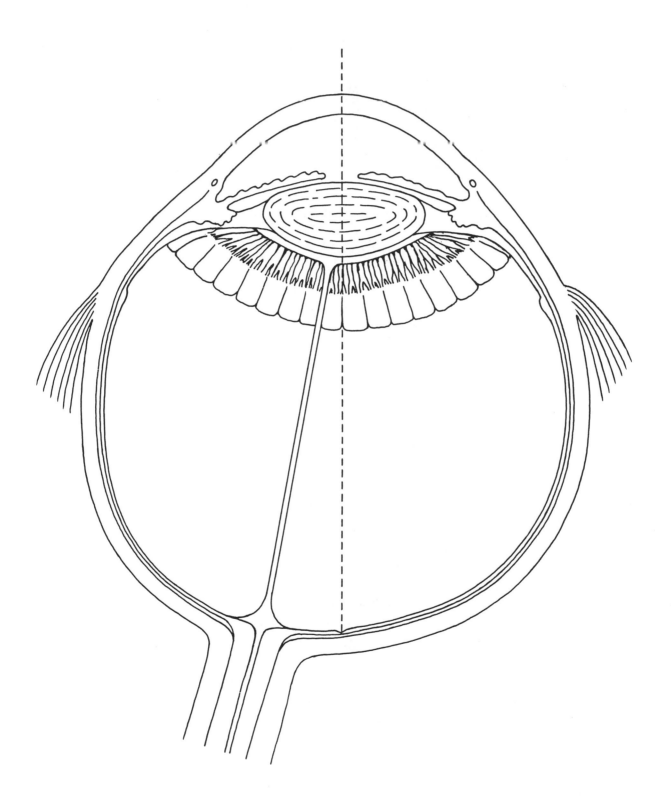

Fig. 11.6 Eye - section

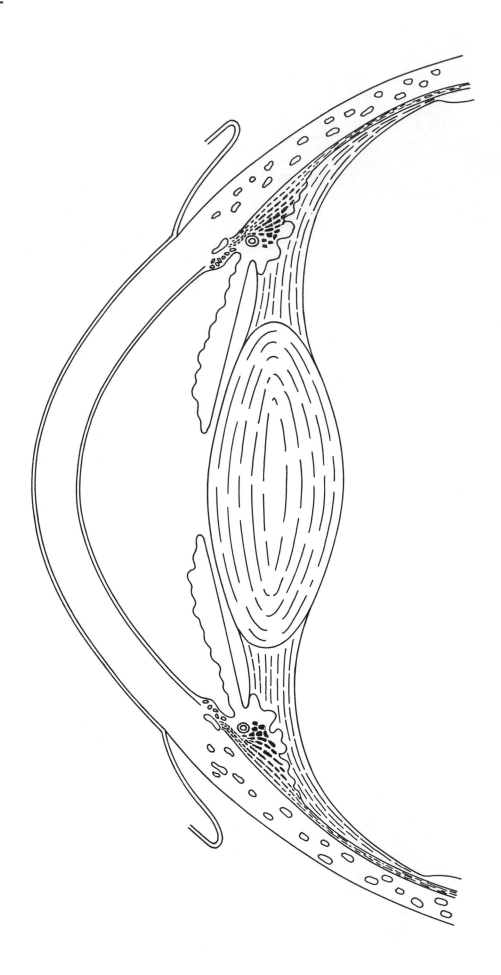

Fig. 11.7 Cornea, iris, lens - section

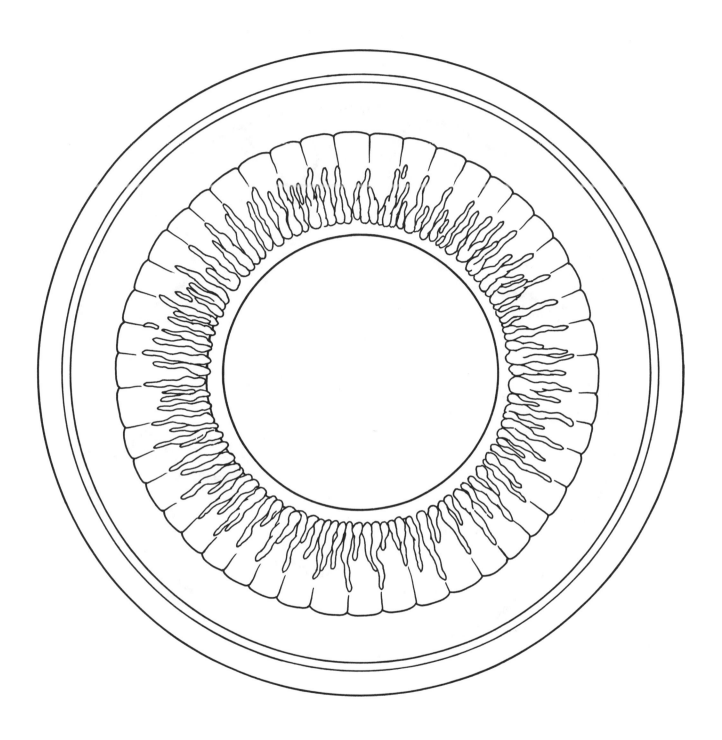

Fig. 11.8 Eye - interior of anterior half

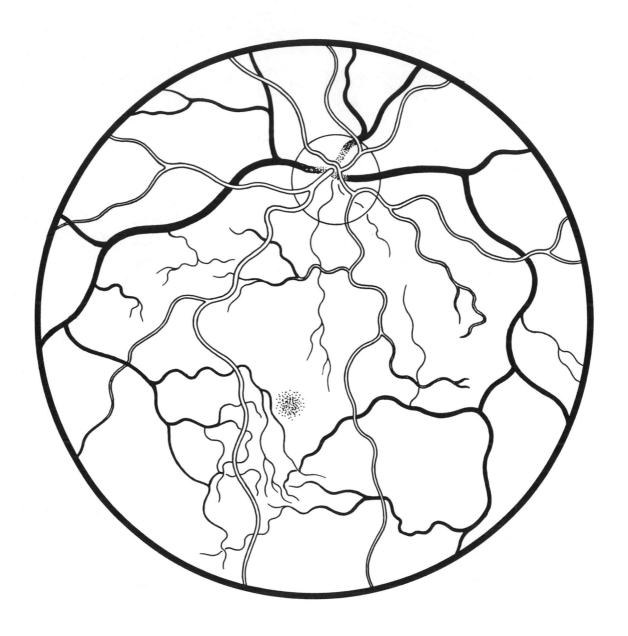

Fig. 11.9 Retina

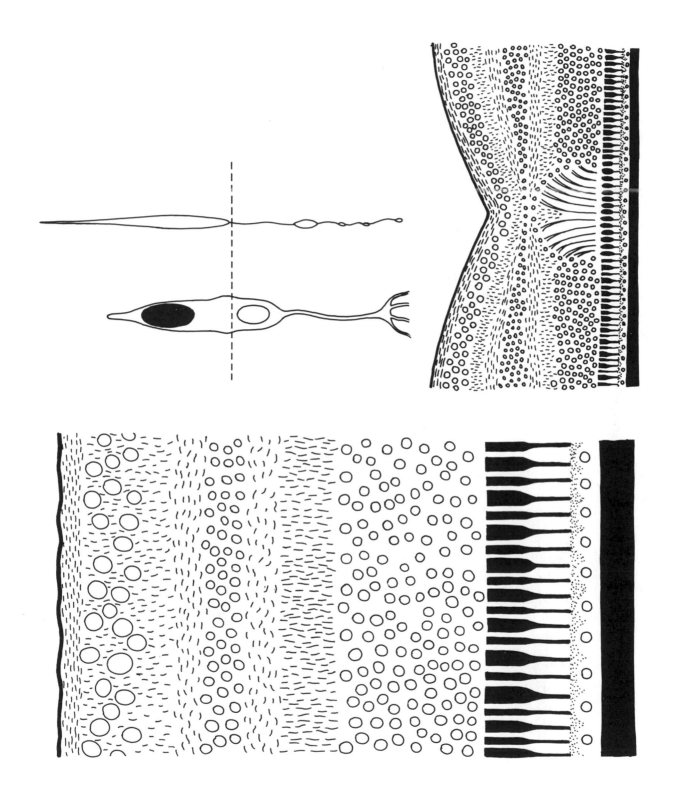

Fig. 11.10 Retina, macula - section, rods, cones

L I G H T

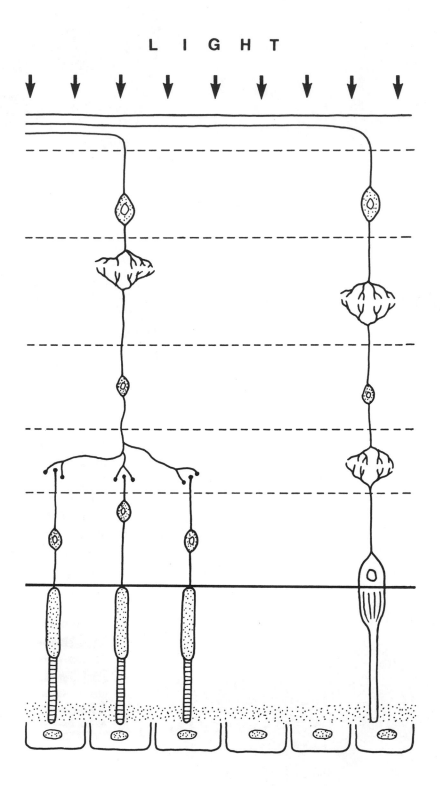

Fig. 11.11 Retinal neurons - scheme

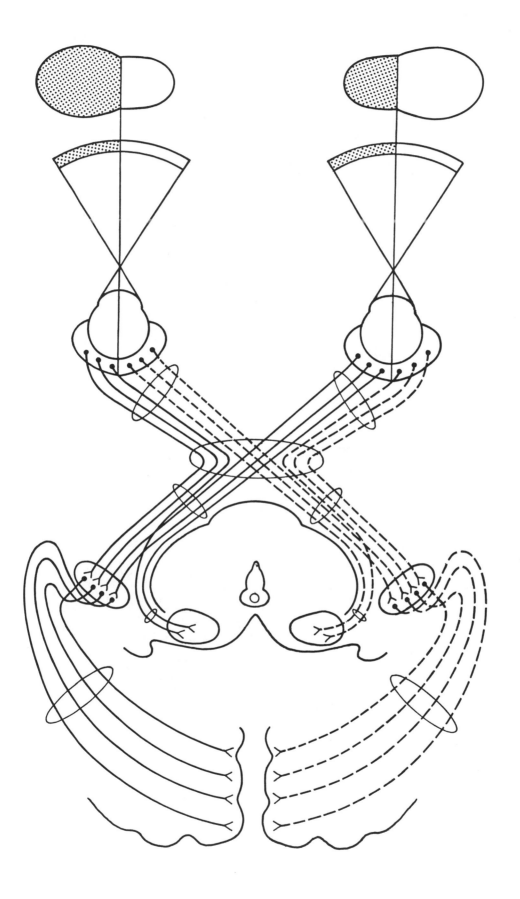

Fig. 11.12 Optic nerves and pathways

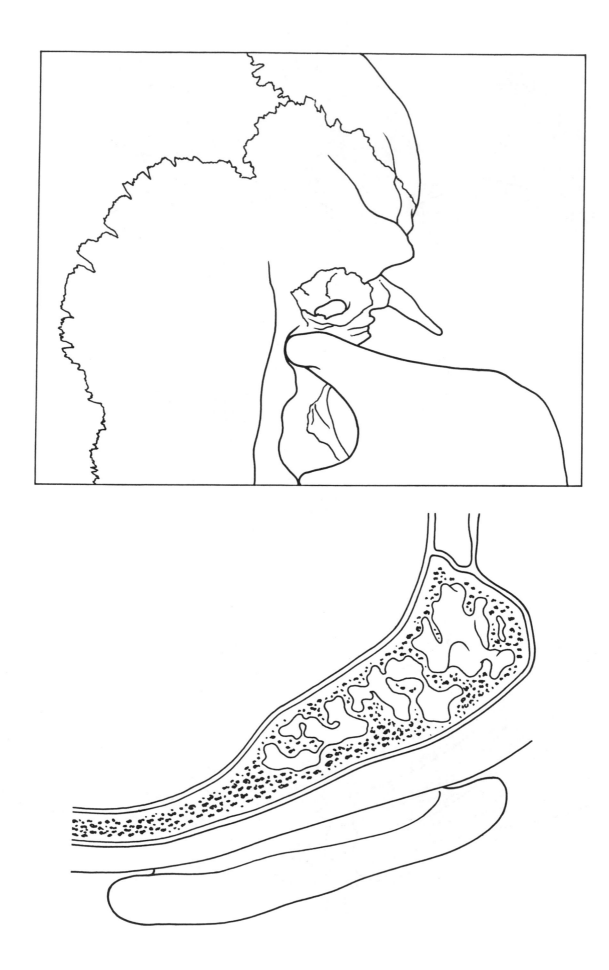

Fig. 11.13 Mastoid process and section

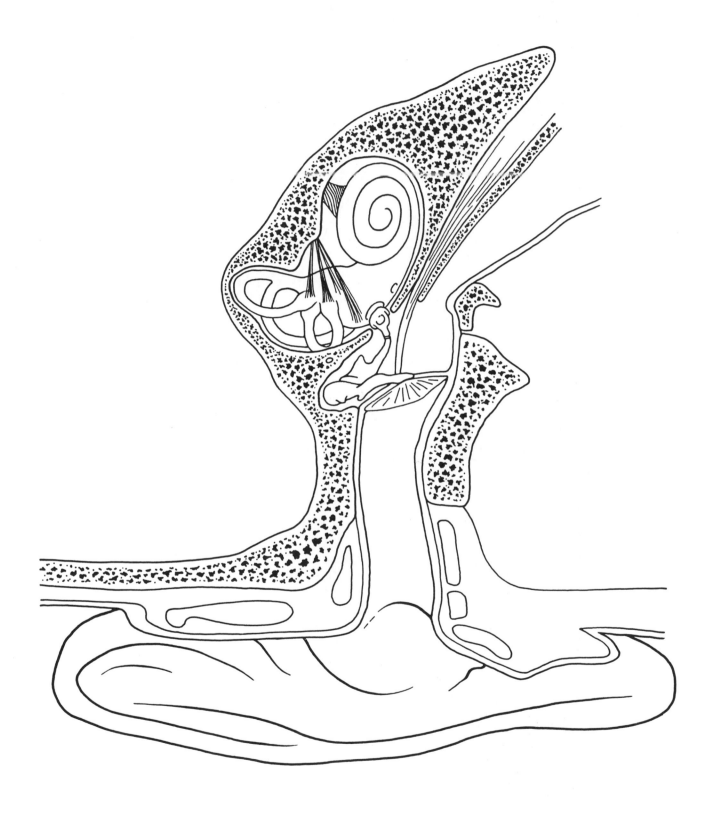

Fig. 11.14 Ear - section

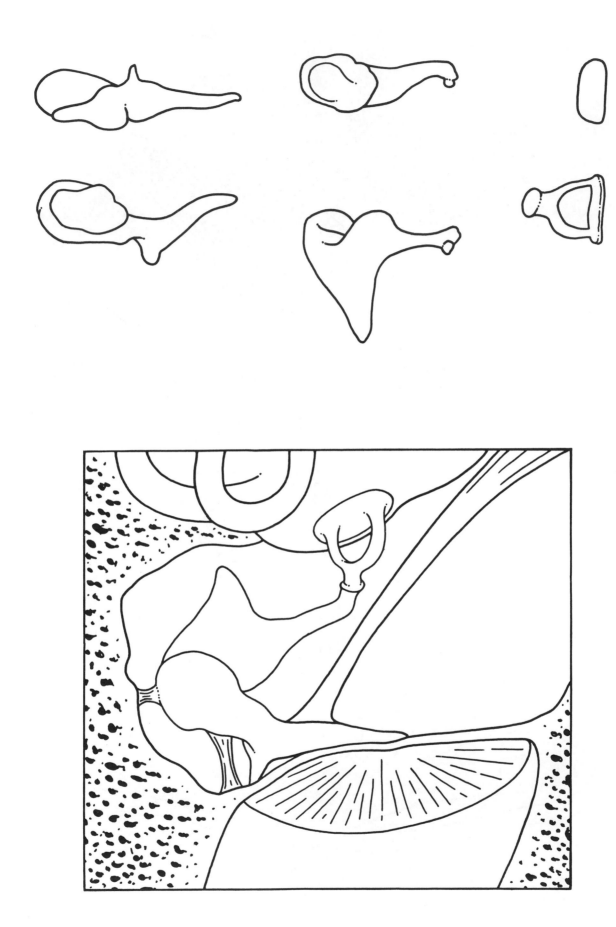

Fig. 11.15 Ear - section, stapes, incus, malleus

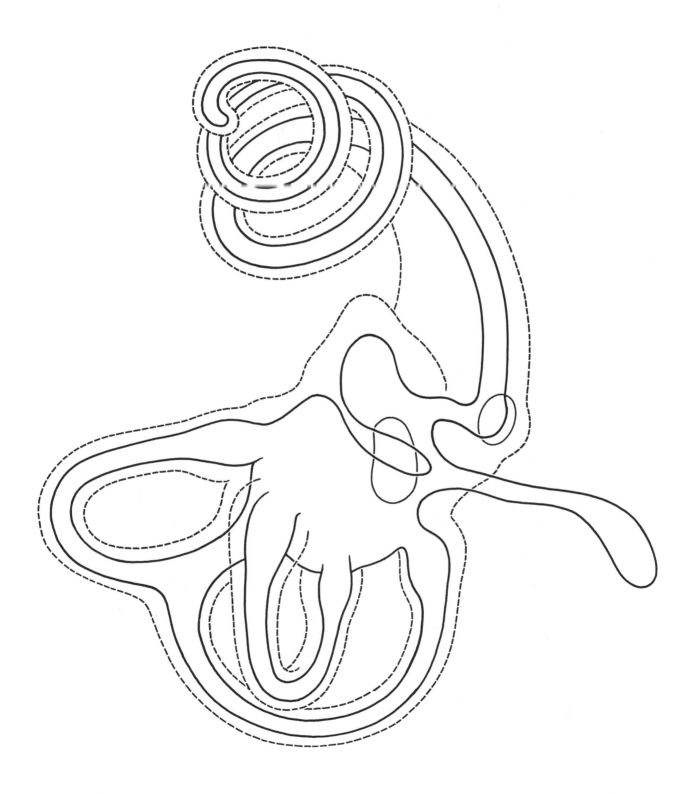

Fig. 11.16 Semi-circular canals, cochlea

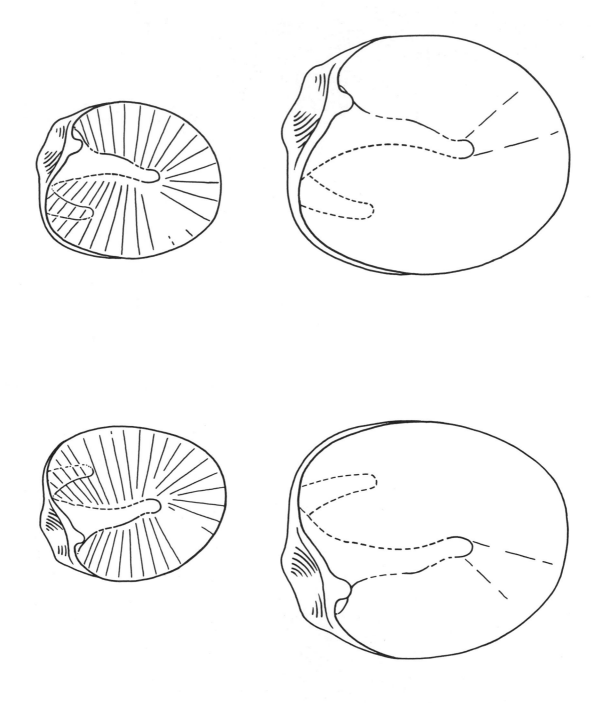

Fig. 11.17 Tympanic membrane

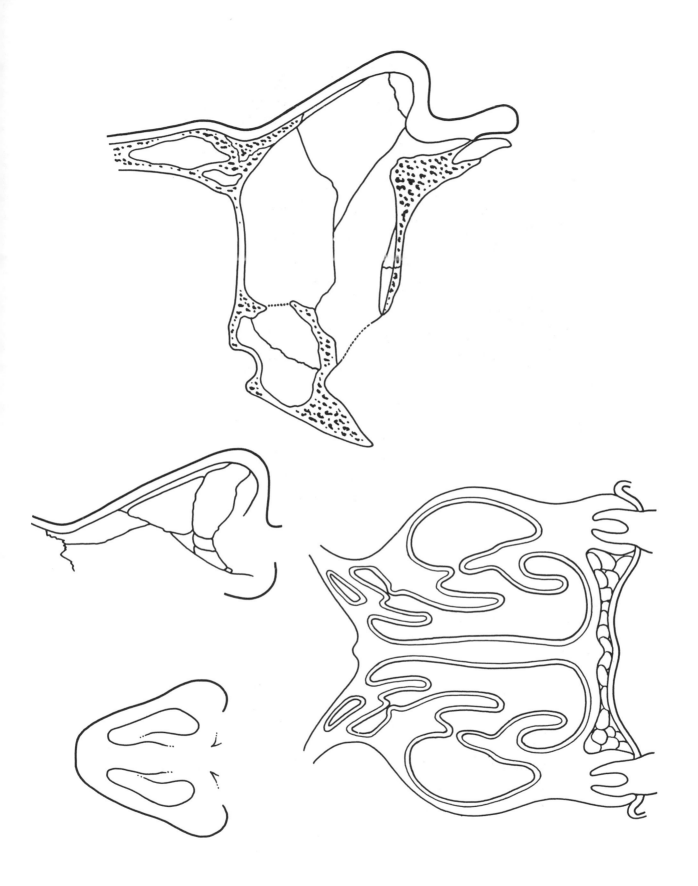

Fig. 11.18 Nose - Bones and cartilages

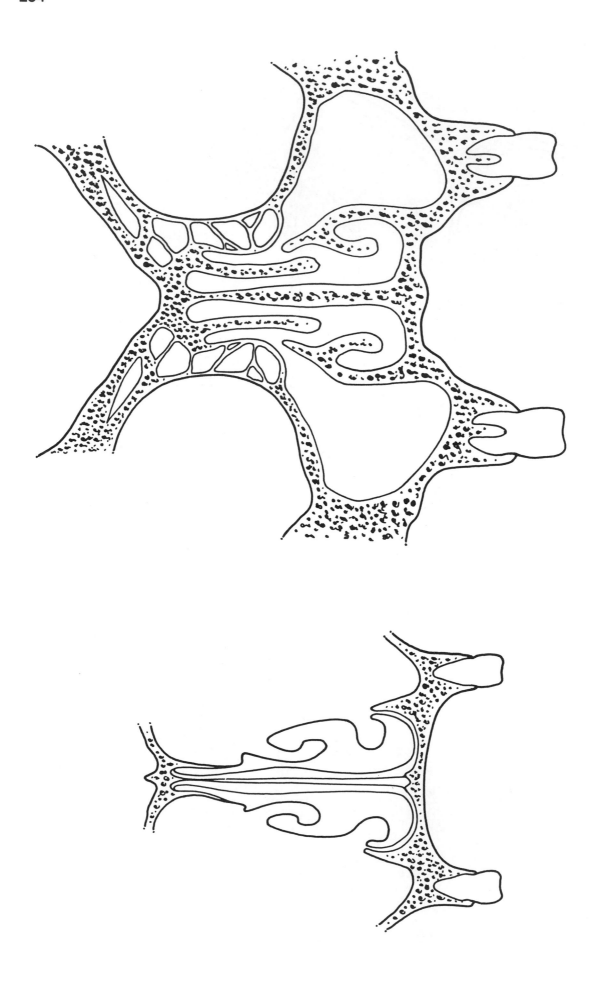

Fig. 11.19 Nose - Nasal cavity and sinuses, coronal section

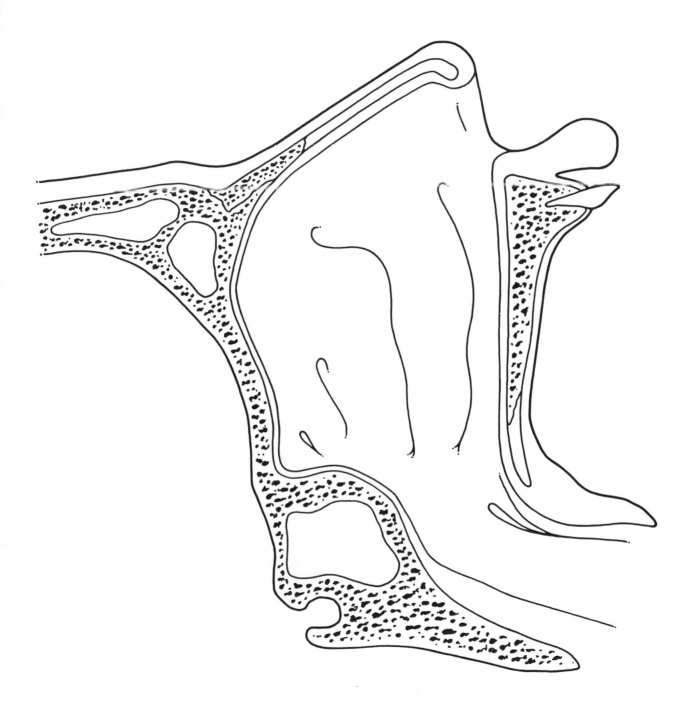

Fig. 11.20 Nose - Nasal cavity and sinuses, sagittal section

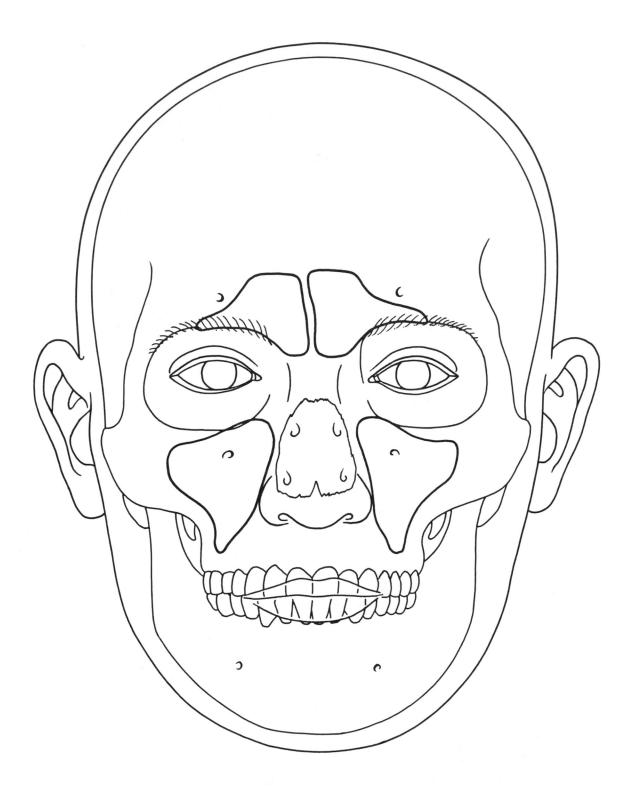

Fig. 11.21 Frontal and maxillary sinuses

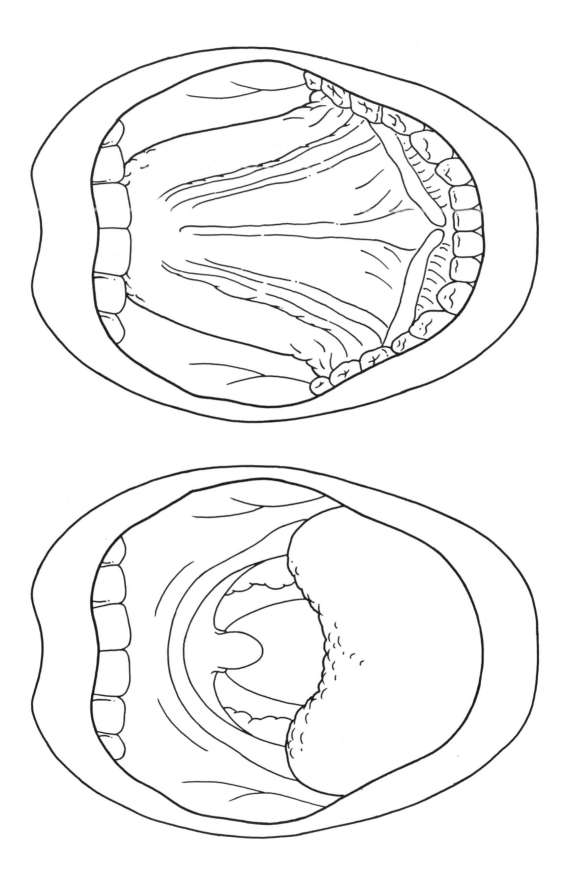

Fig. 11.22 Mouth, open

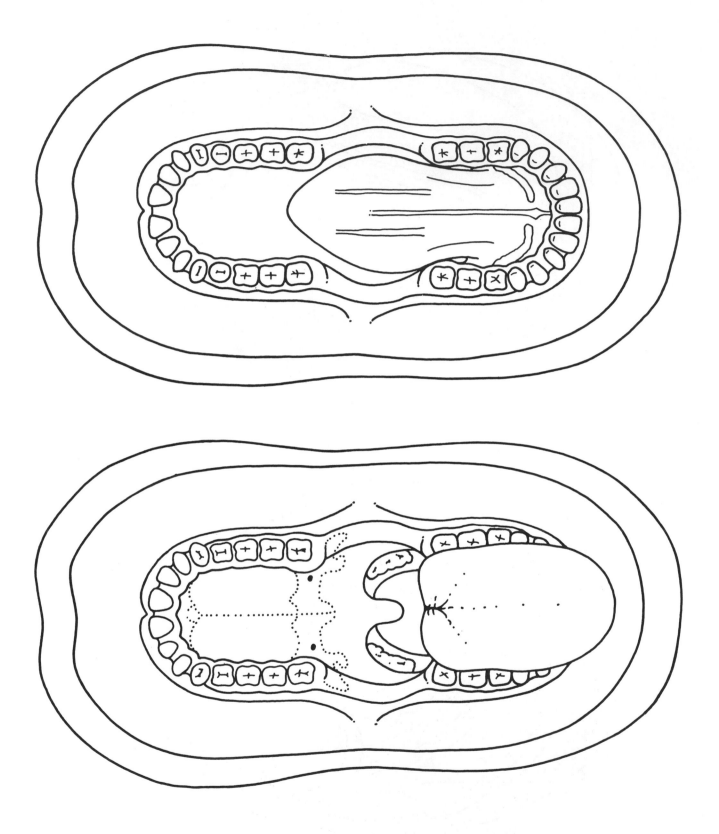

Fig. 11.23 Mouth, open, AP view. Mouth, tongue, teeth - scheme

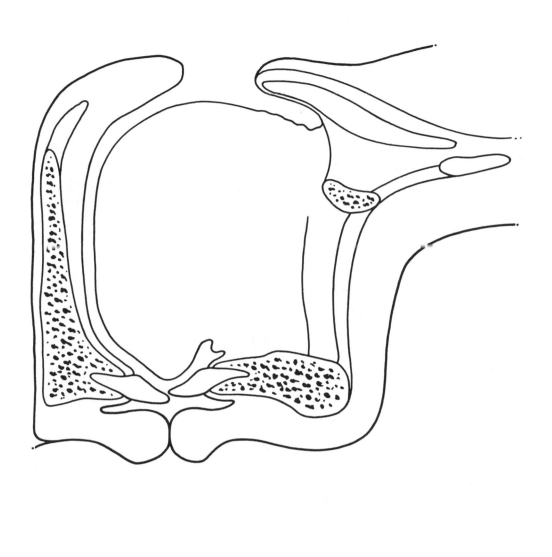

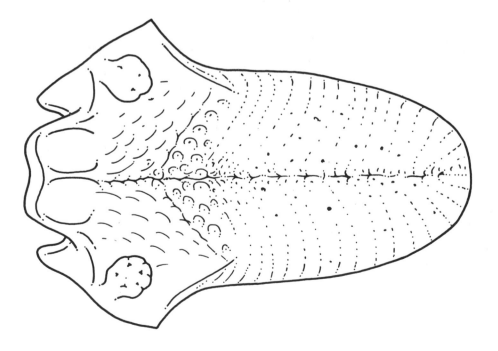

Fig. 11.24 Tongue, superior view, sagittal section

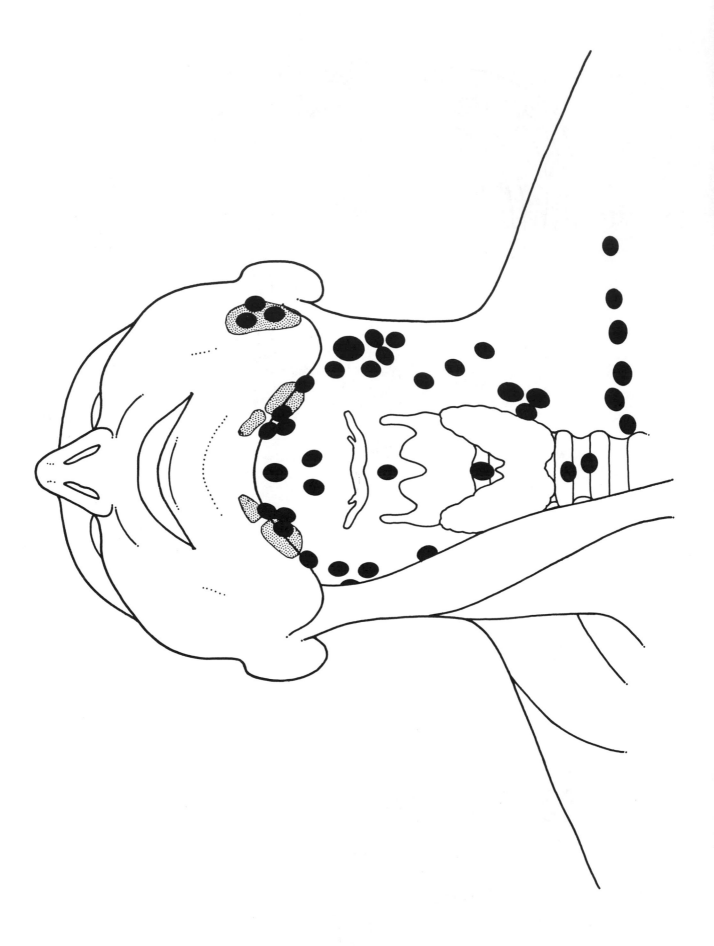

Fig. 11.25 Neck - position of glands, anterior

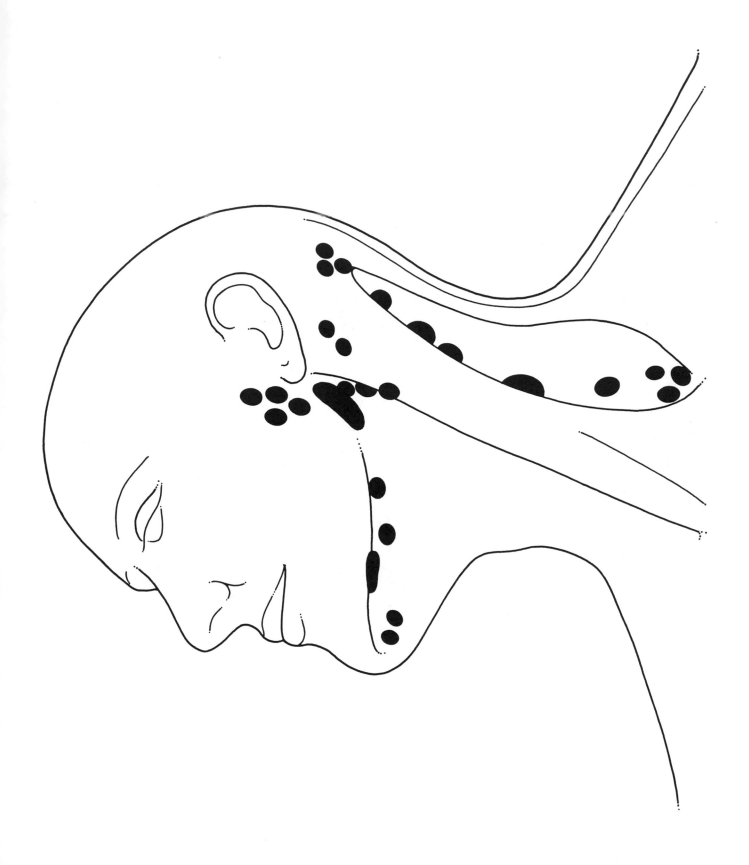

Fig. 11.26 Neck - position of glands, lateral

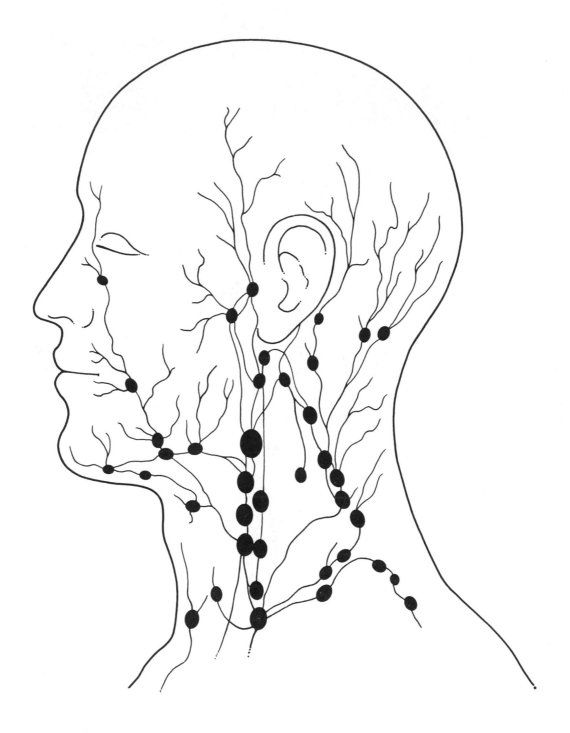

Fig. 11.27 Neck - lymphatic drainage

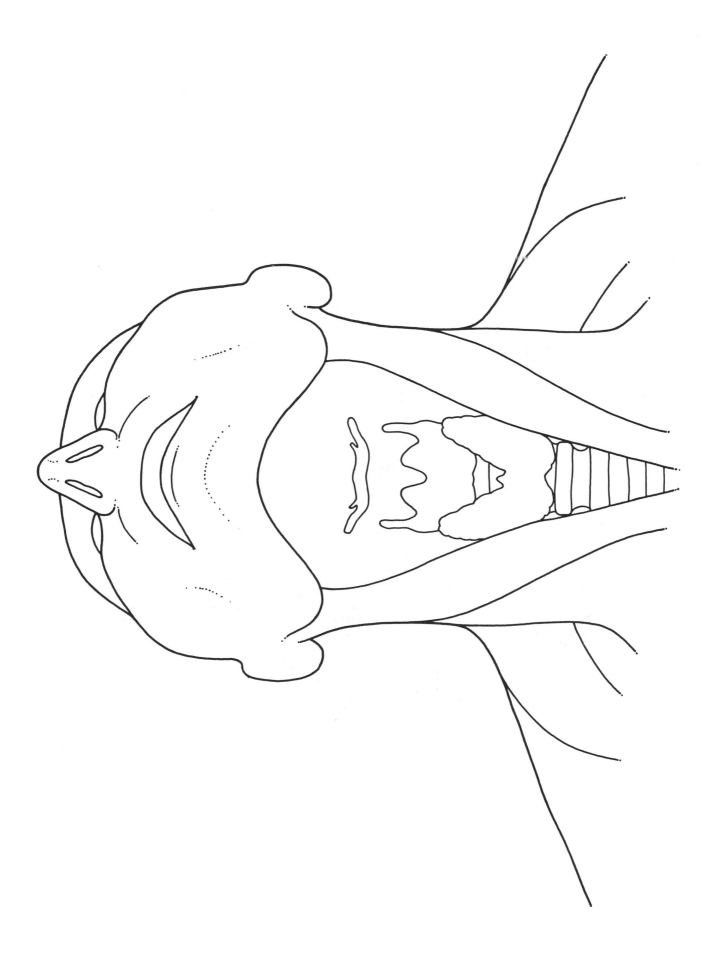

Fig. 11.28 Neck structures, anterior

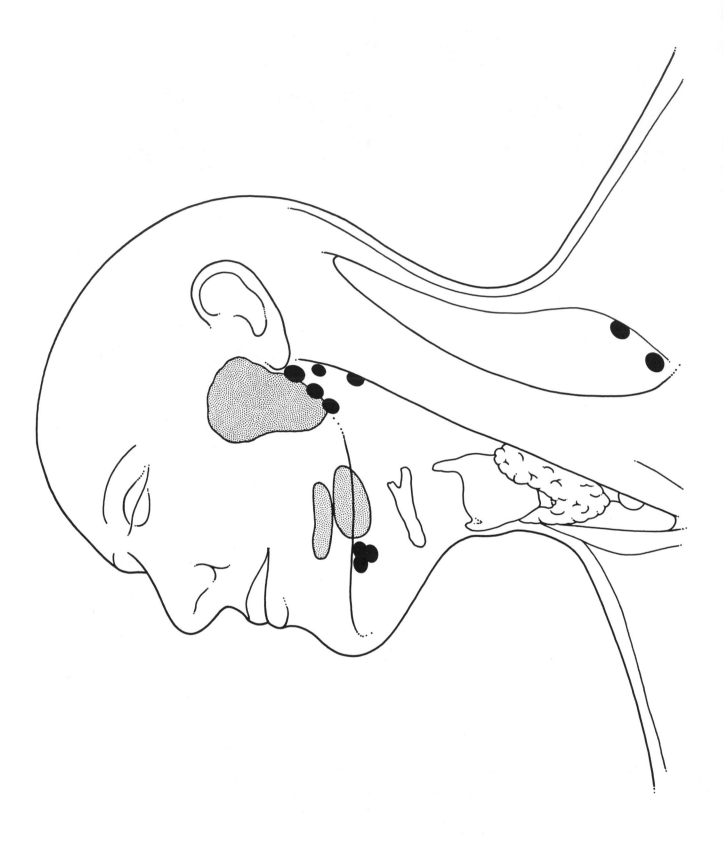

Fig. 11.29 Neck structures, lateral

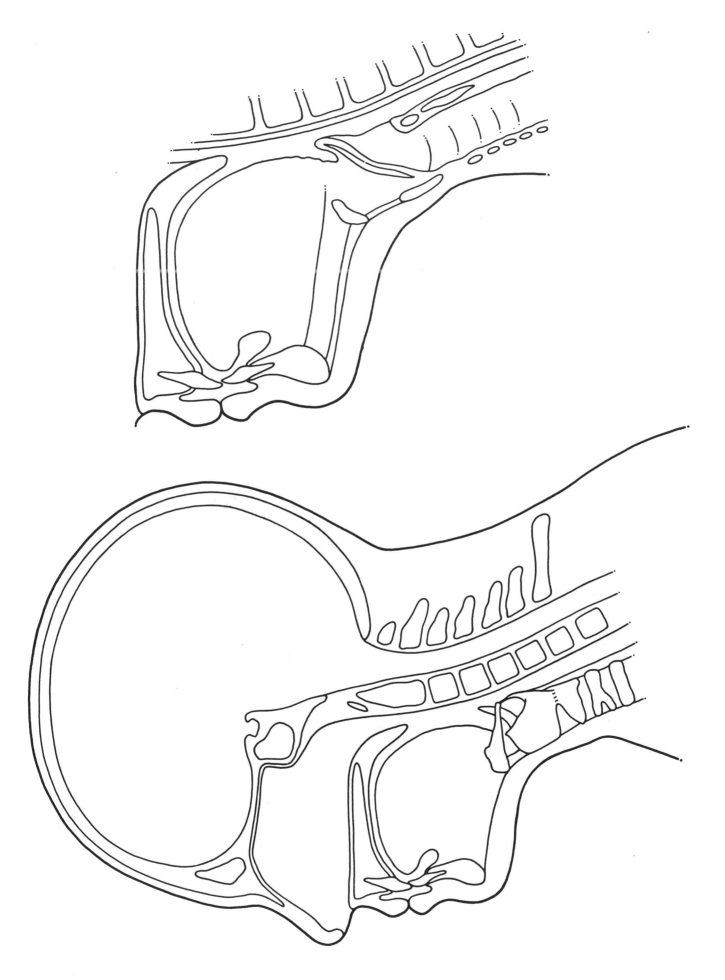

Fig. 11.30 Neck structures, sagittal section

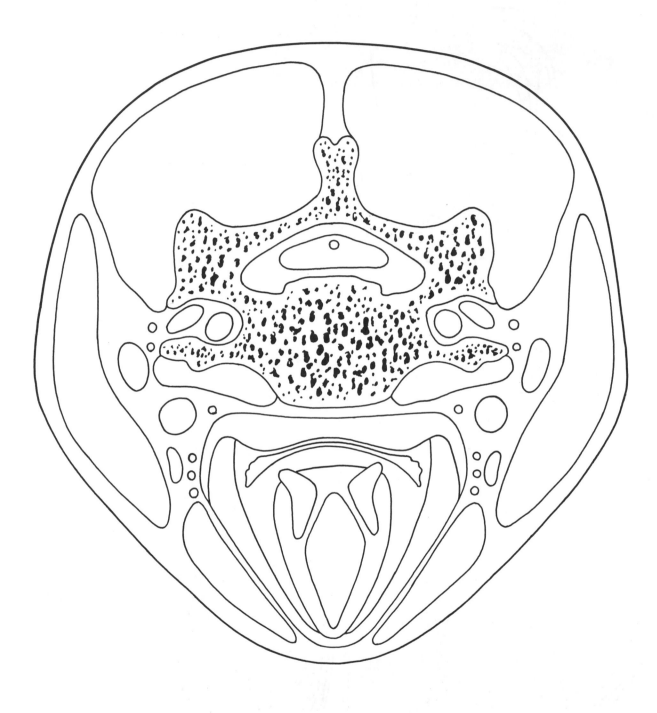

Fig. 11.31 Neck structures - section at level of larynx

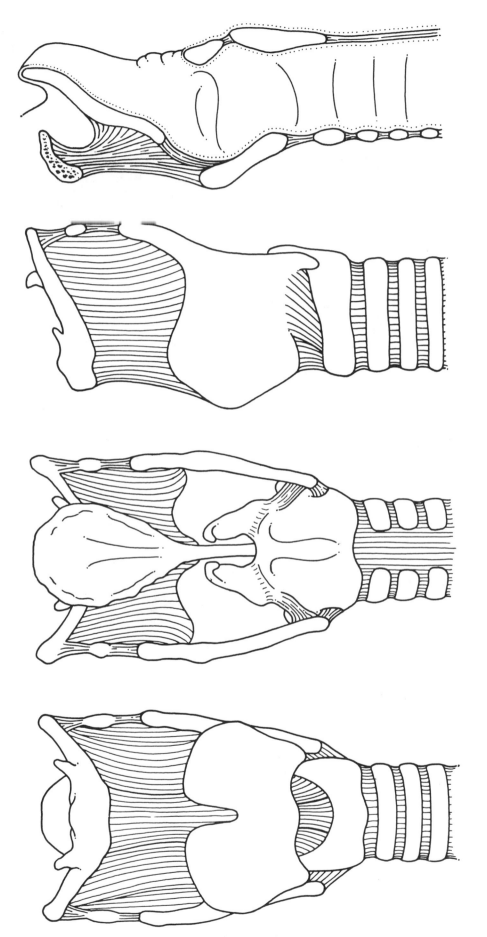

Fig. 11.32 Larynx, AP, PA, lateral, sagittal section

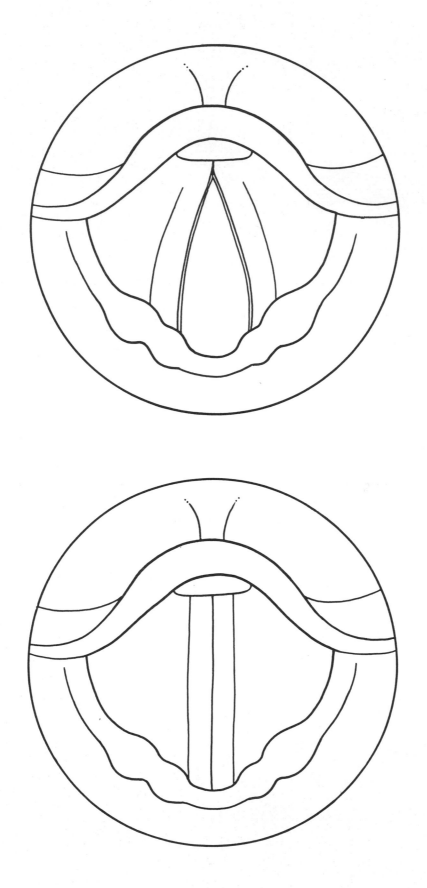

Fig. 11.33 Larynx, mirror view

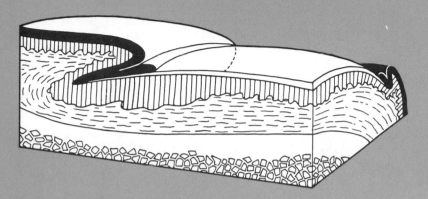

Section 12

Skin

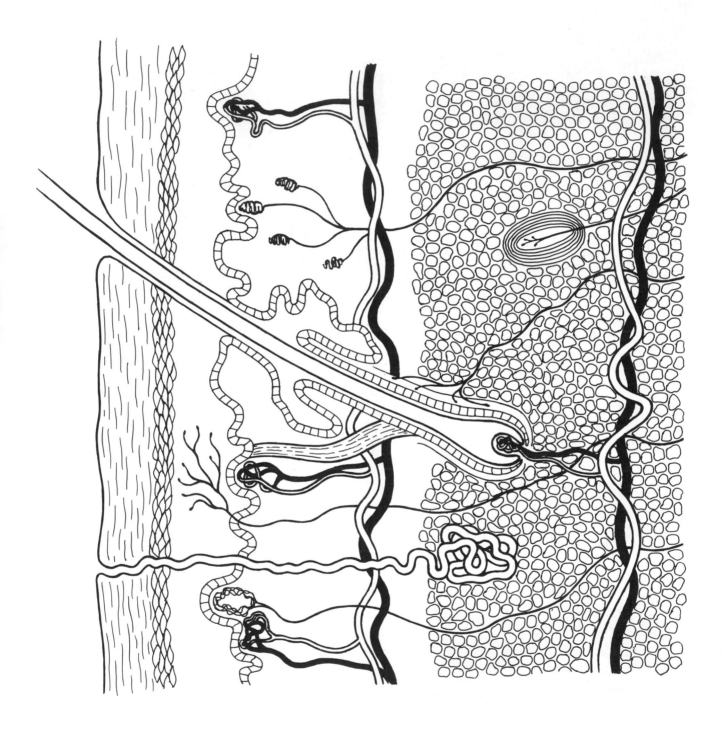

Fig. 12.1 Skin - section

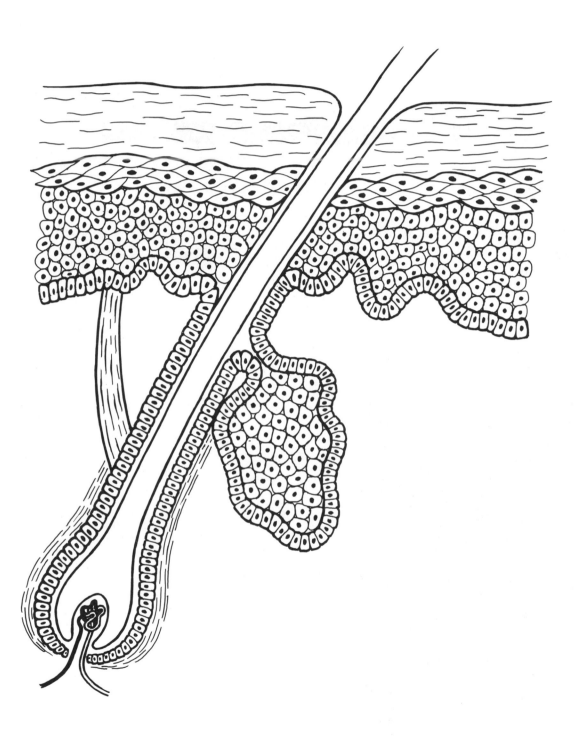

Fig. 12.2 Hair follicle

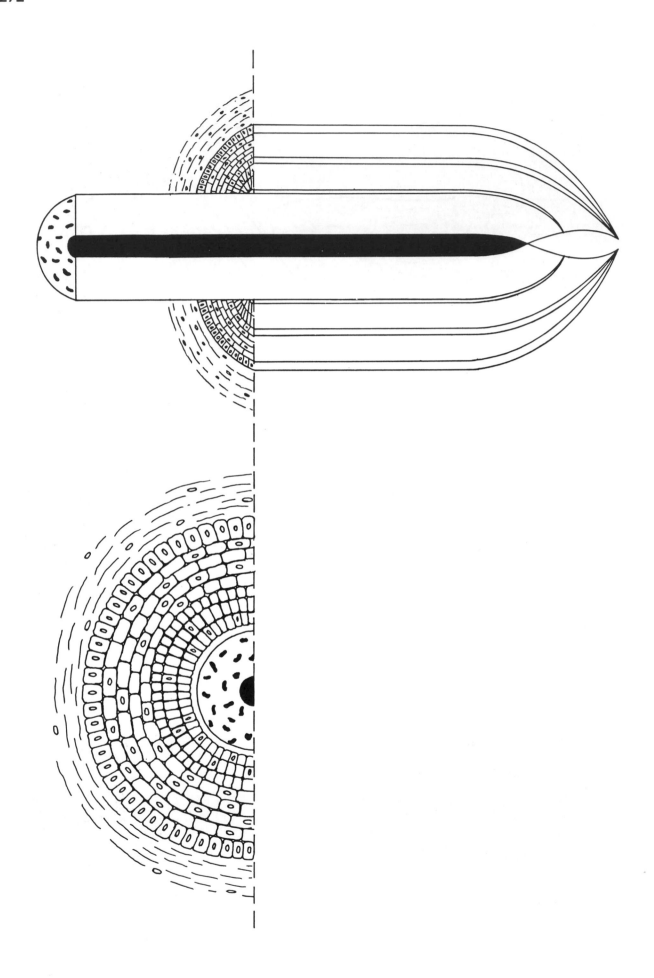

Fig. 12.3 Hair follicle

273

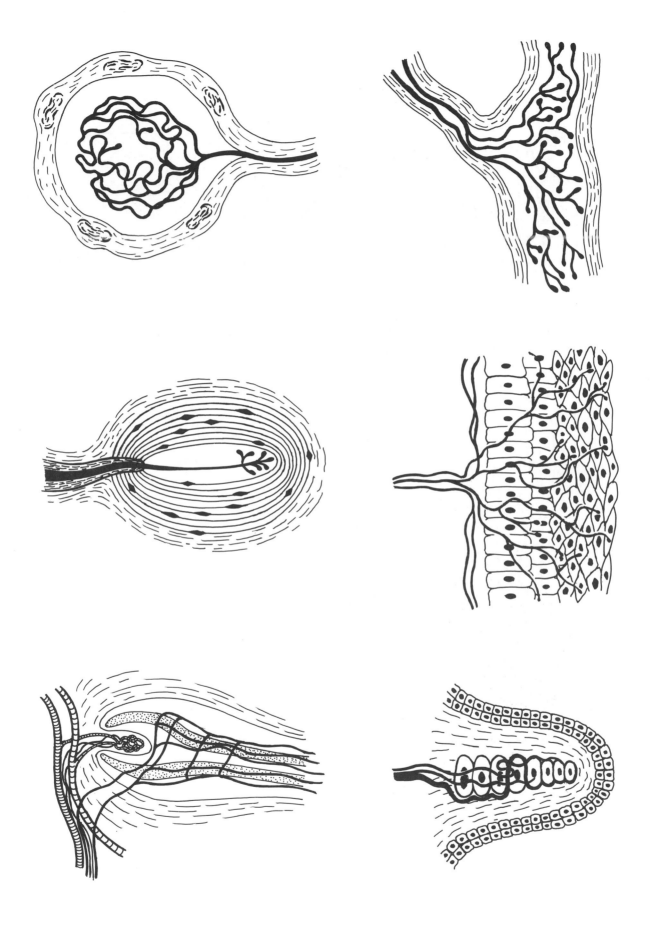

Fig. 12.4 Nerve endings

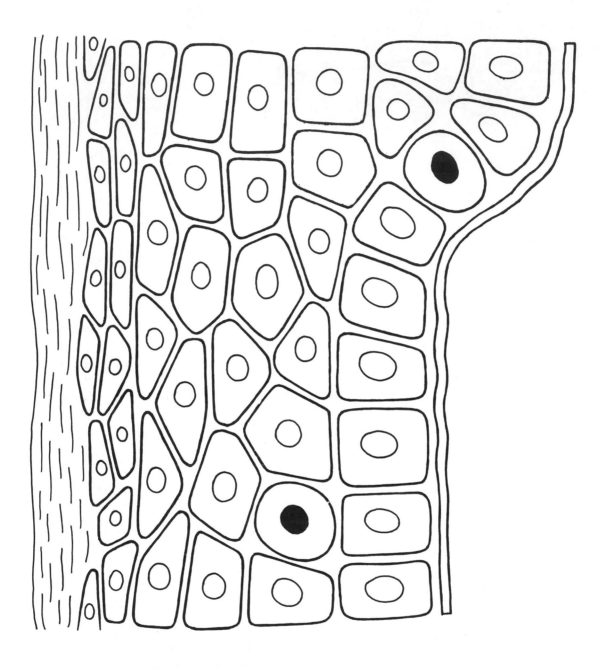

Fig. 12.5 Epidermis - section

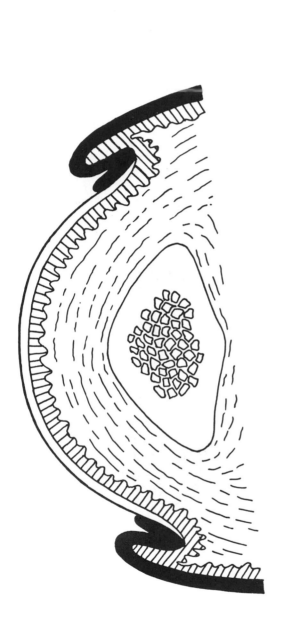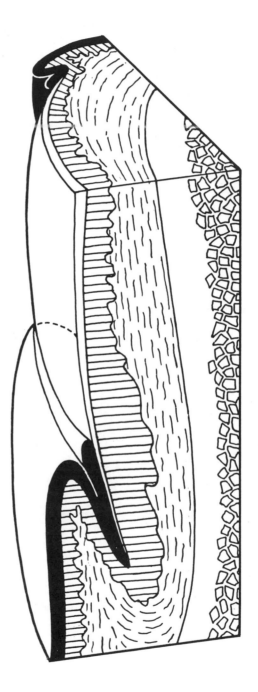

Fig. 12.6 Nail bed

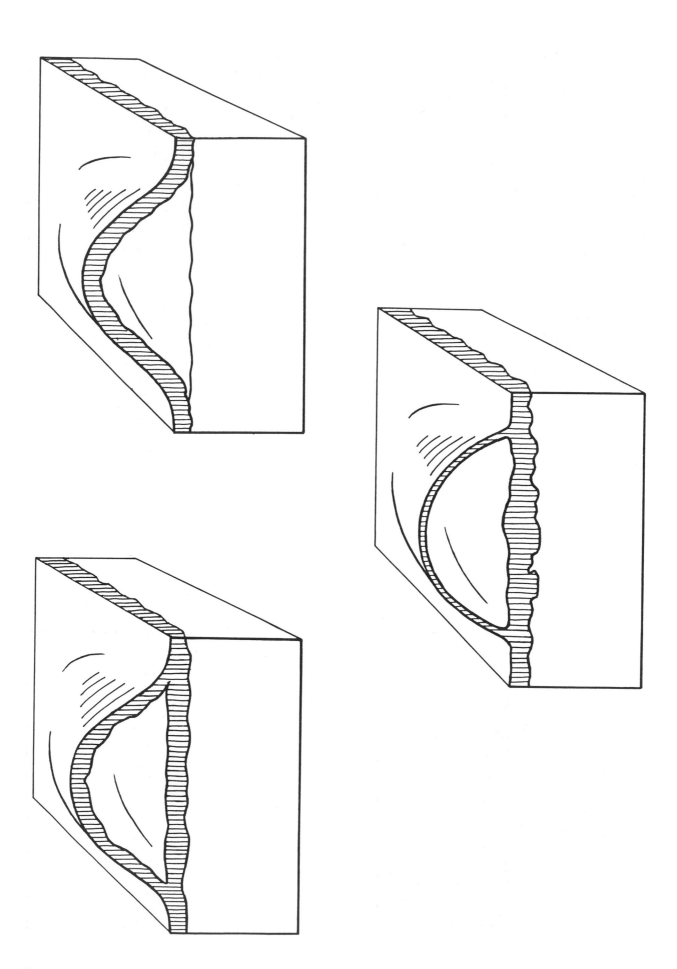

Fig. 12.7 Skin conditions - Blisters

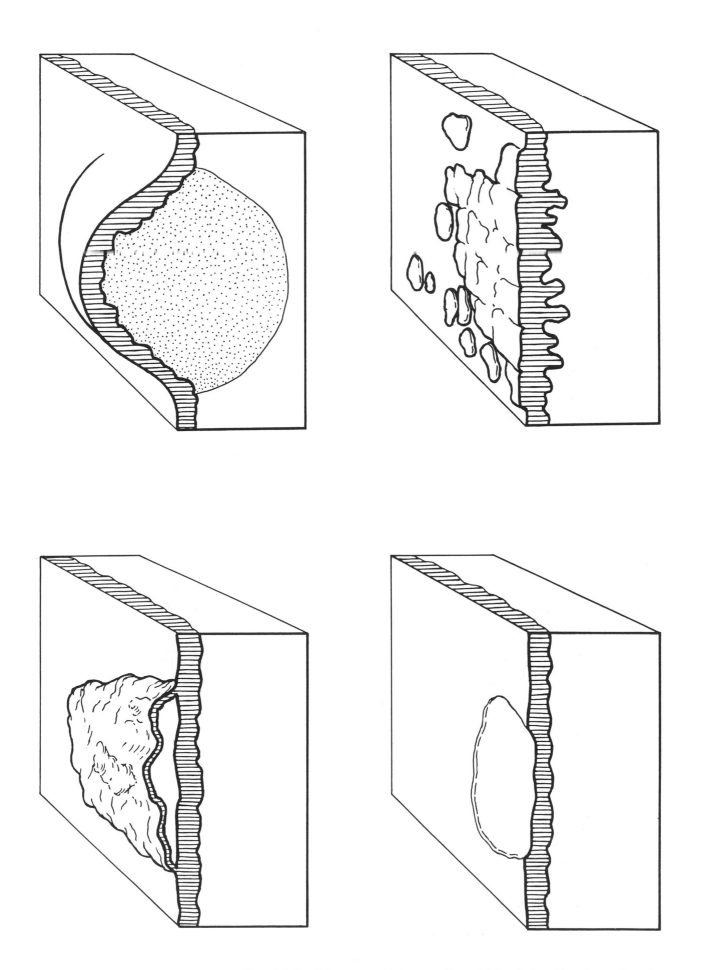

Fig. 12.8 Skin conditions - Crust, Nodule, Erosion, Scale

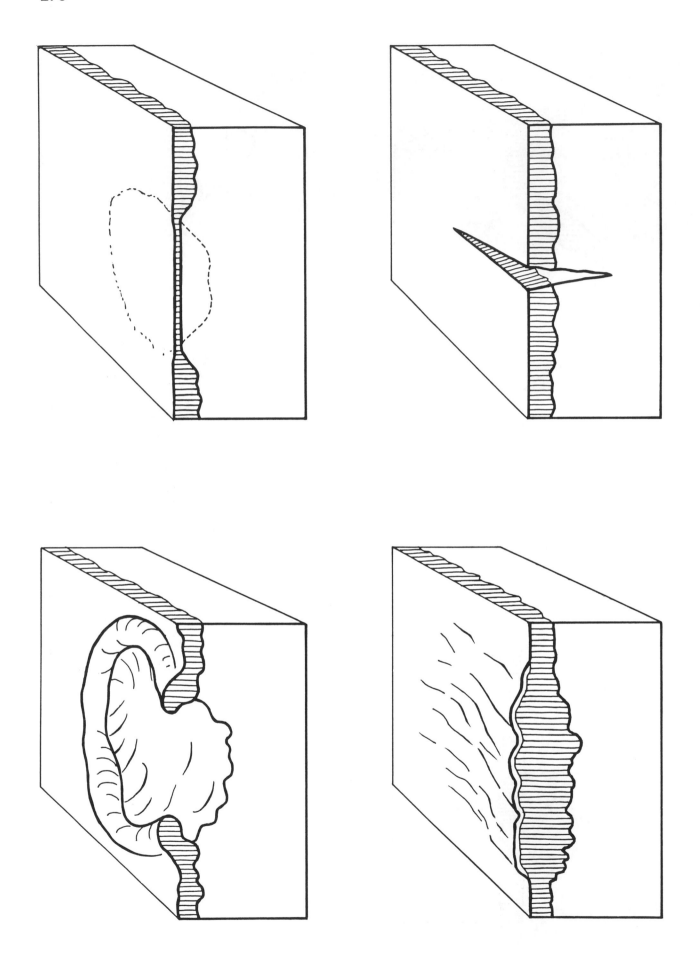

Fig. 12.9 Skin conditions - Ulcers, Atrophy,Lichenification, Fissure

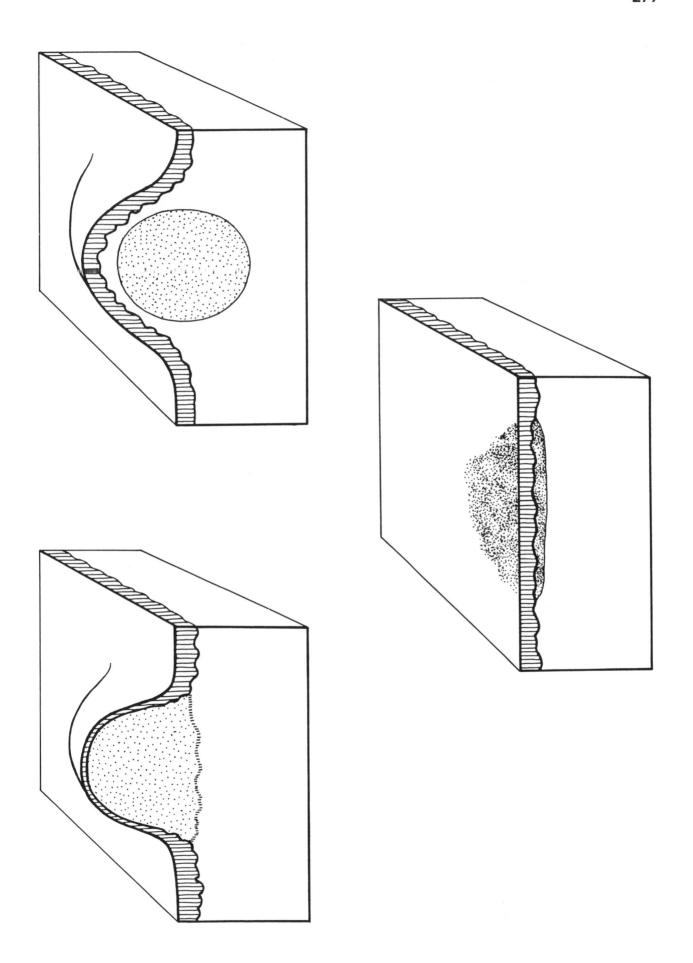

Fig. 12.10 Skin conditions - Pustule, Cyst, Macule

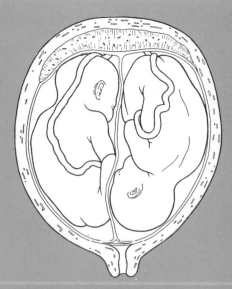

Section 13

Obstetrics

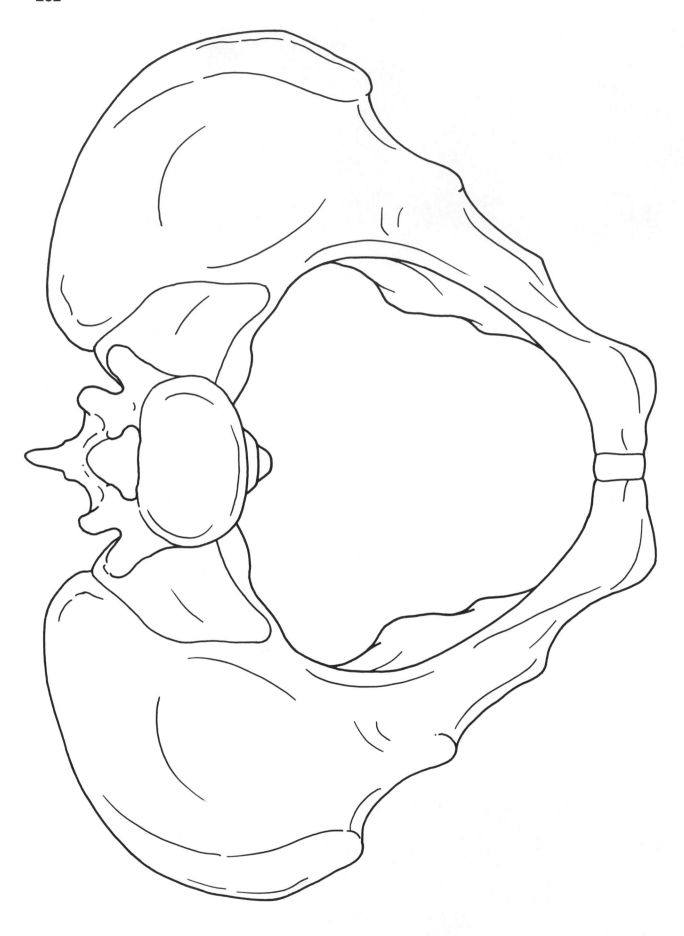

Fig. 13.1 Pelvis, superior

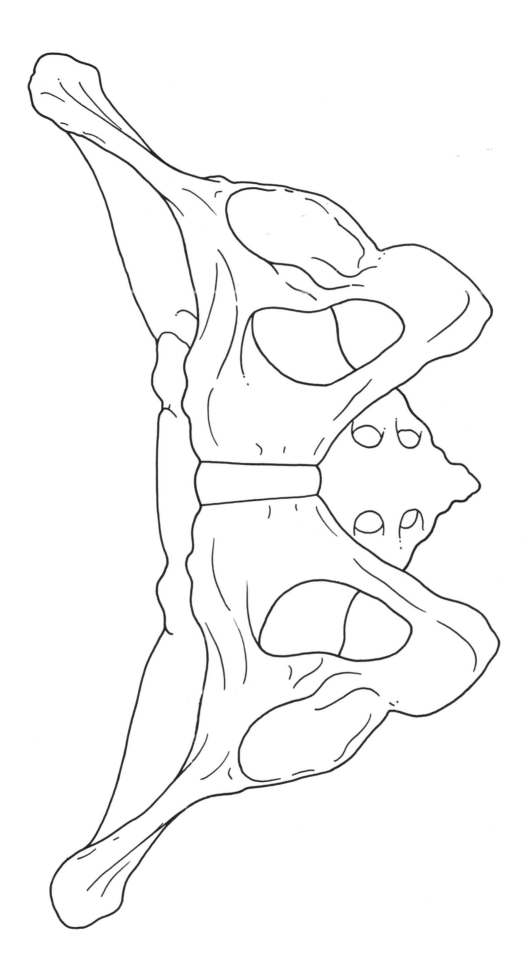

Fig. 13.2 Pelvis, anterior

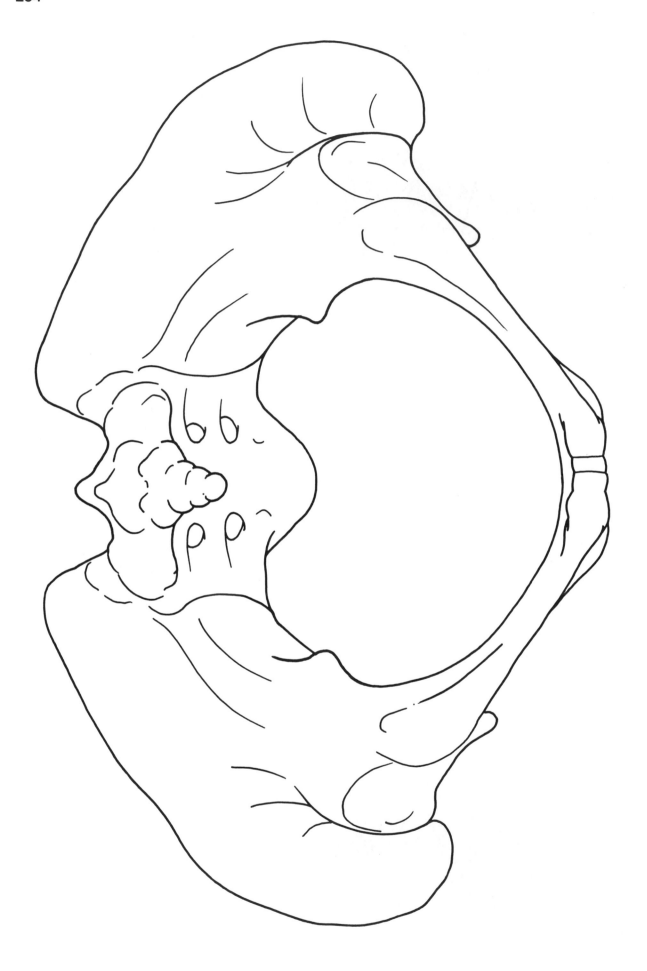

Fig. 13.3 Pelvis, inferior

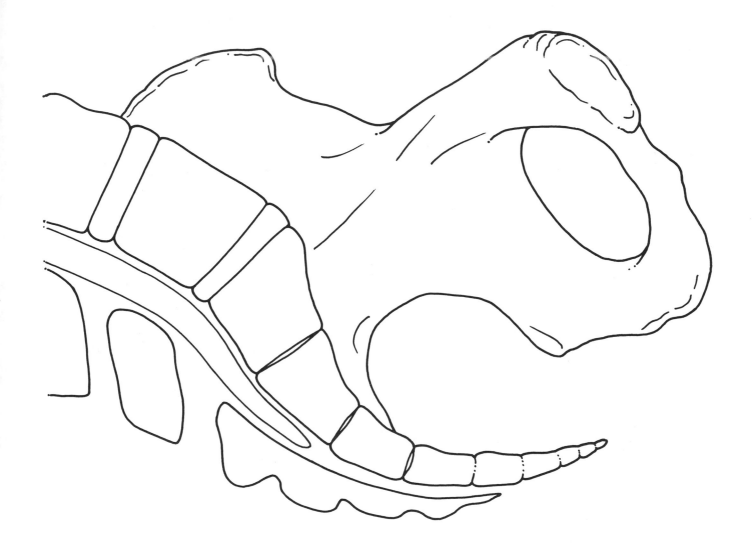

Fig. 13.4 Pelvis, sagittal section

286

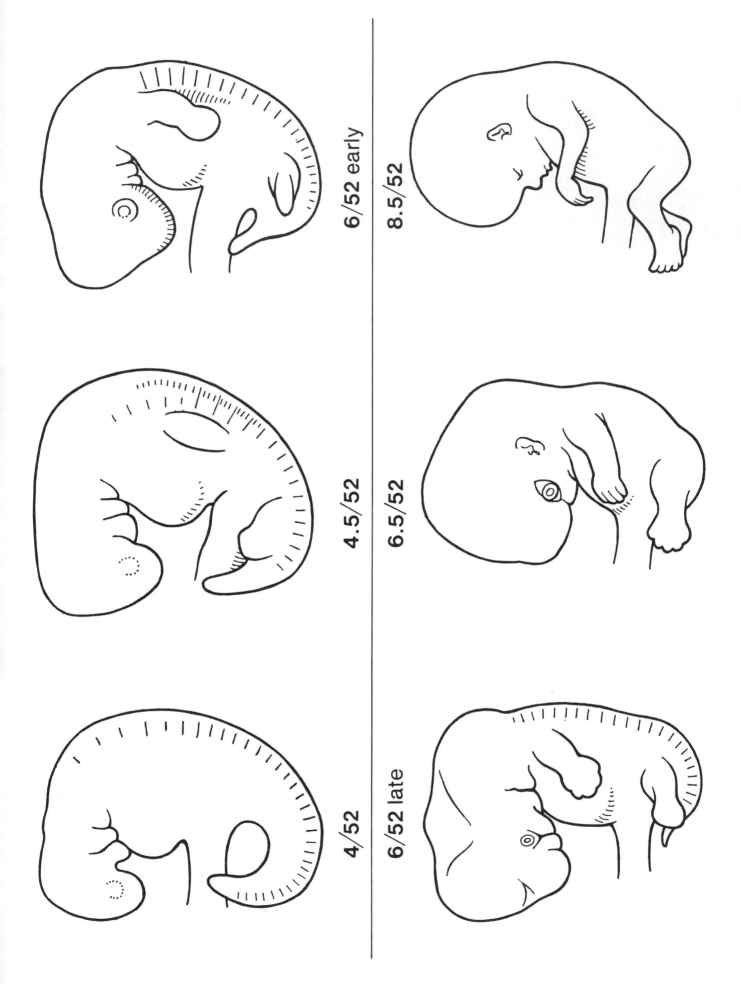

6/52 early

8.5/52

4.5/52

6.5/52

4/52

6/52 late

Fig. 13.5 Fetus, stages of development

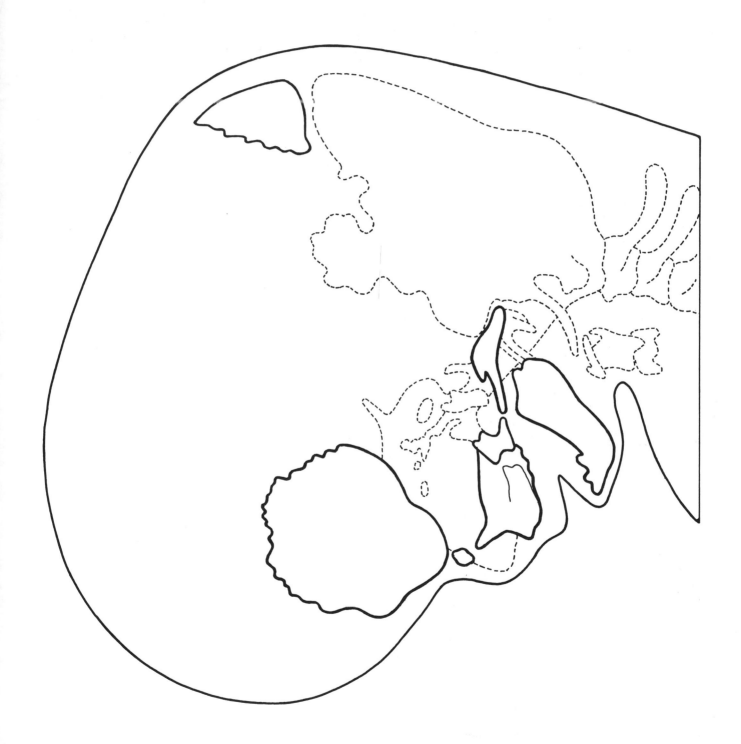

Fig. 13.6 Fetal skull, 3/12

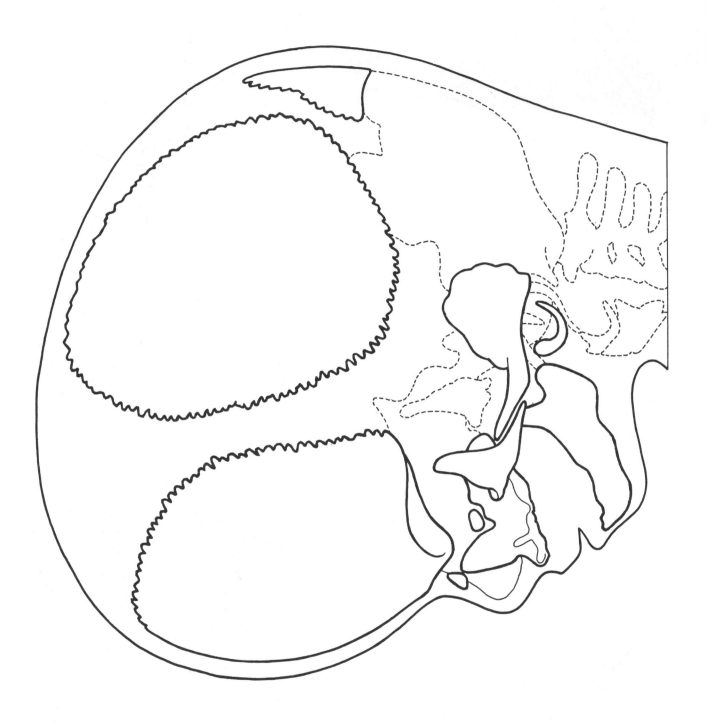

Fig. 13.7 Fetal skull, 4/12

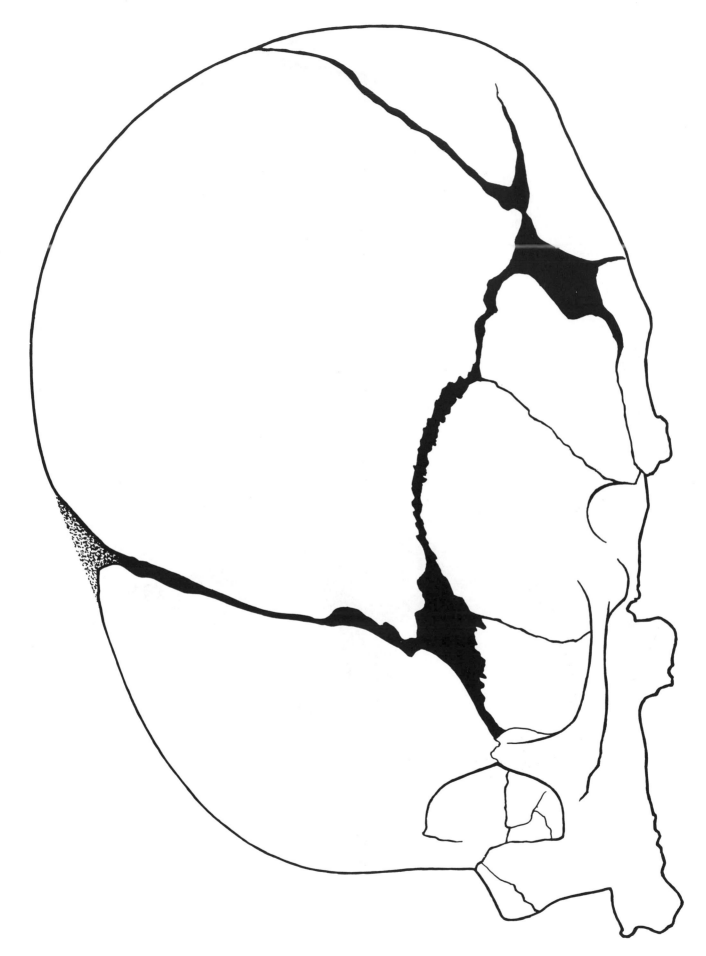

Fig. 13.8 Fetal skull, at term, lateral

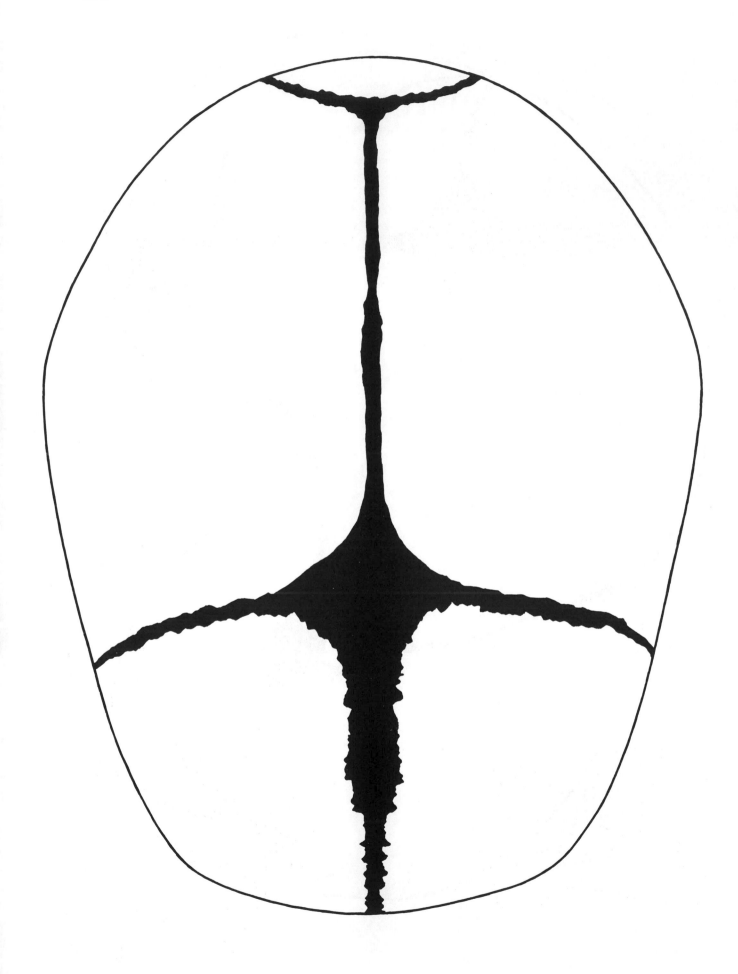

Fig. 13.9 Fetal skull, at term, superior

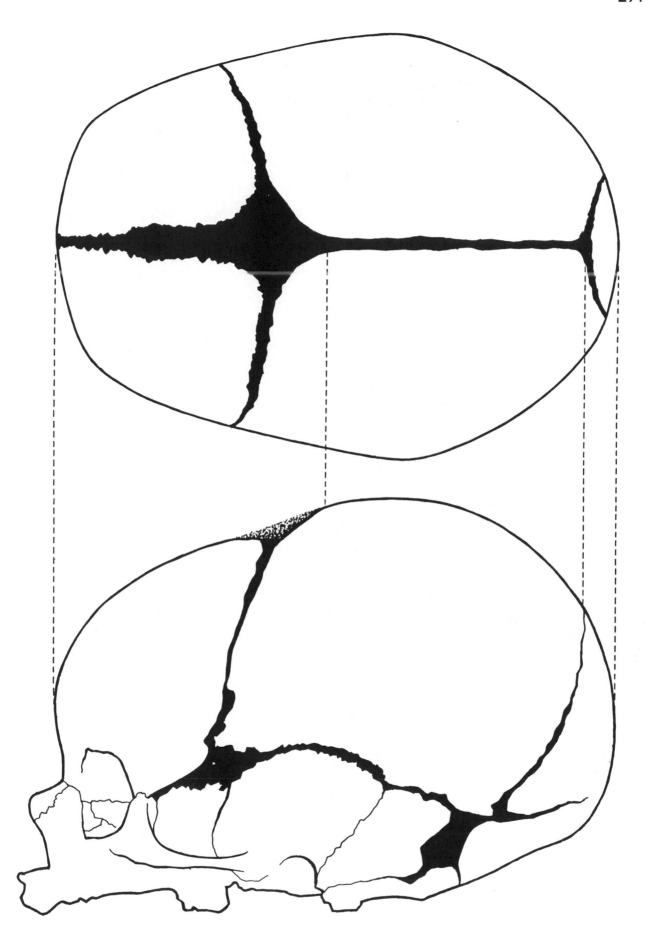

Fig. 13.10 Fetal skull, at term, superior, lateral

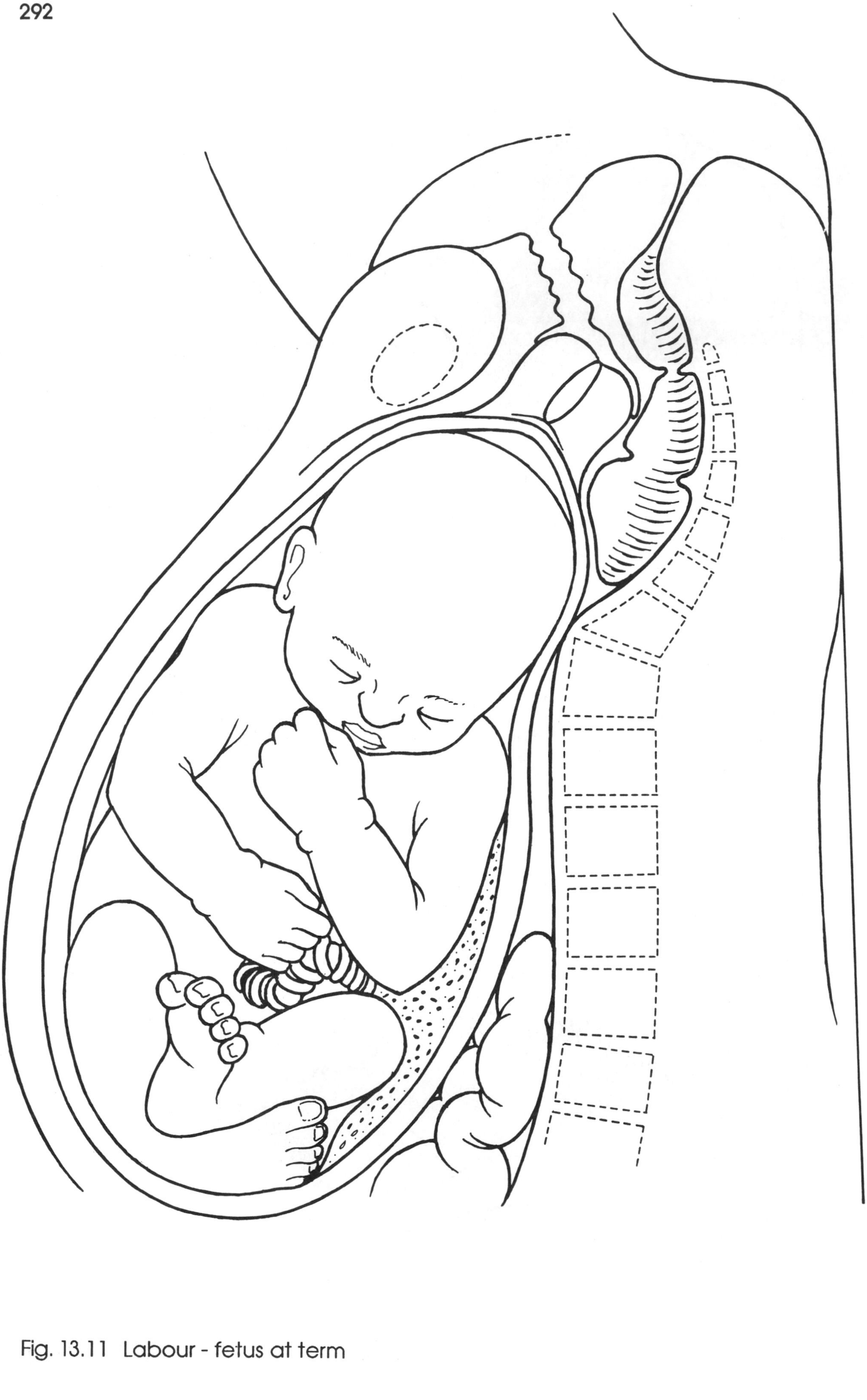

Fig. 13.11 Labour - fetus at term

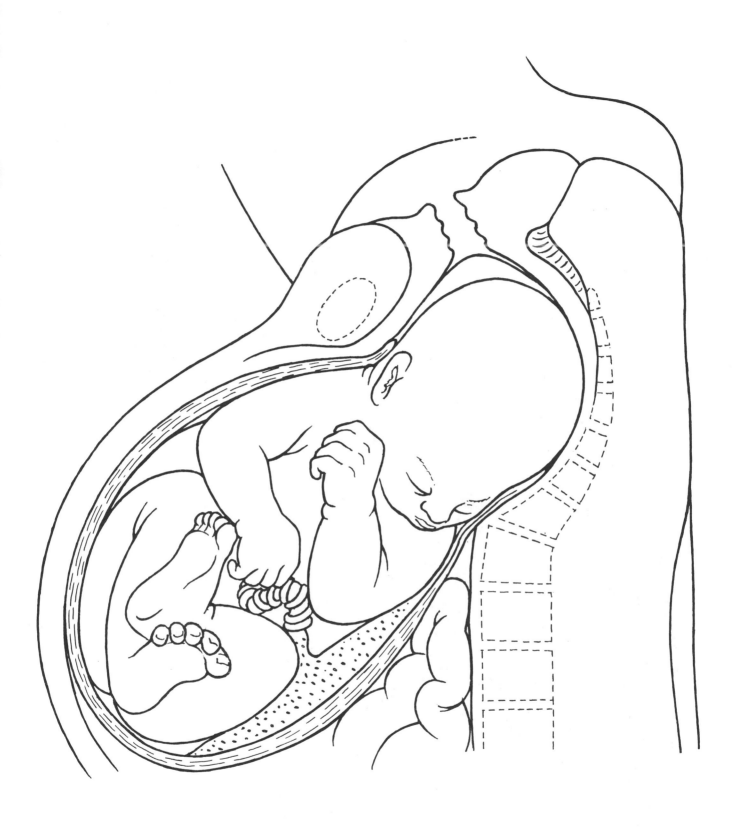

Fig. 13.12 Labour - cervical dilation

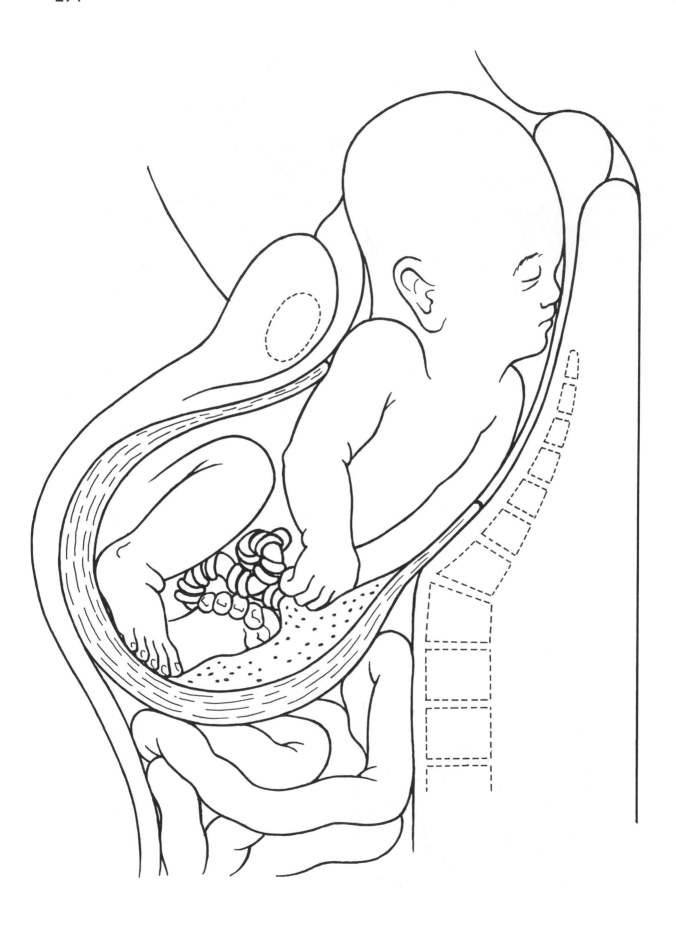

Fig. 13.13 Labour - descent in birth canal

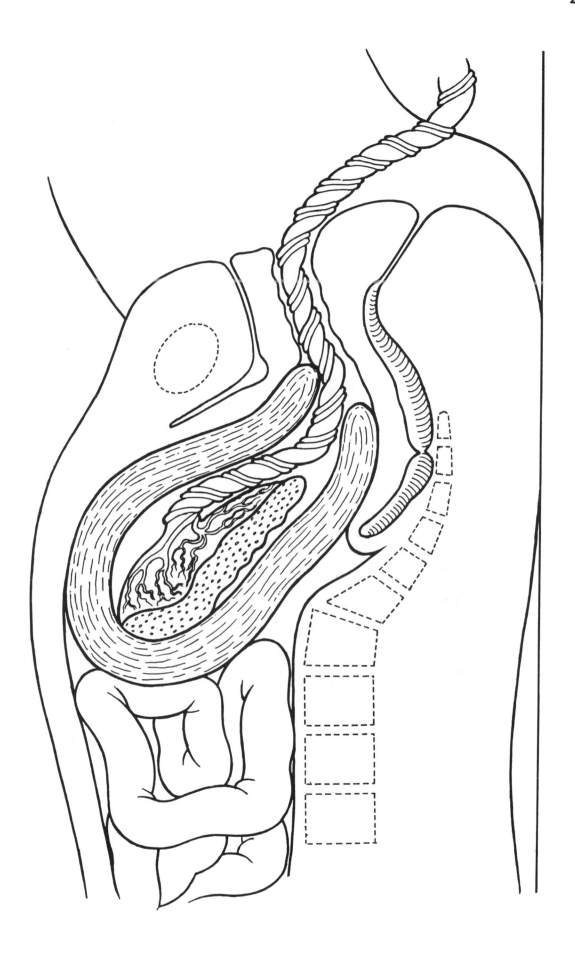

Fig. 13.14 Labour - placental separation

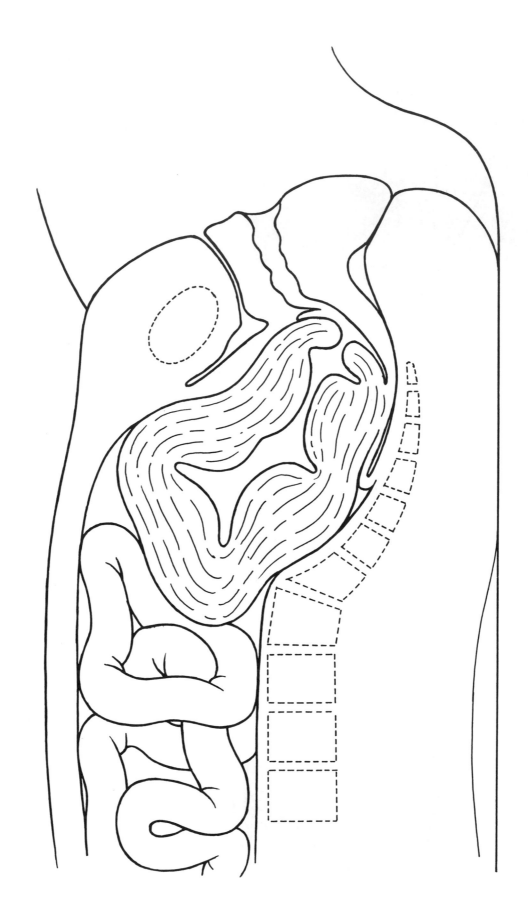

Fig. 13.15 Labour - uterine involution

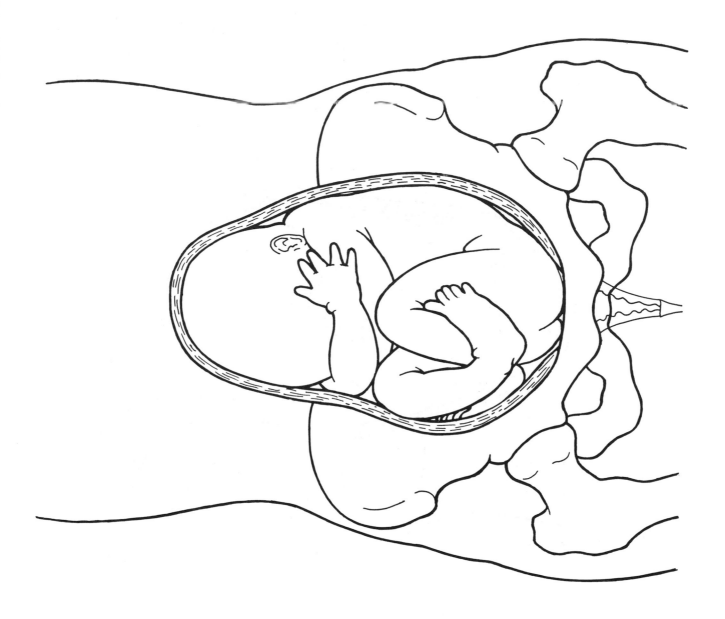

Fig. 13.16 Breech presentation - full

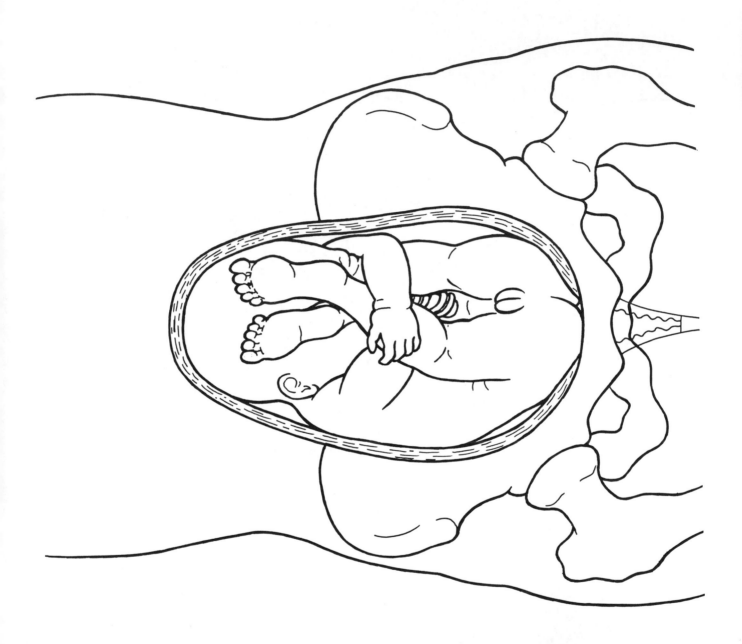

Fig. 13.17 Breech presentation - frank

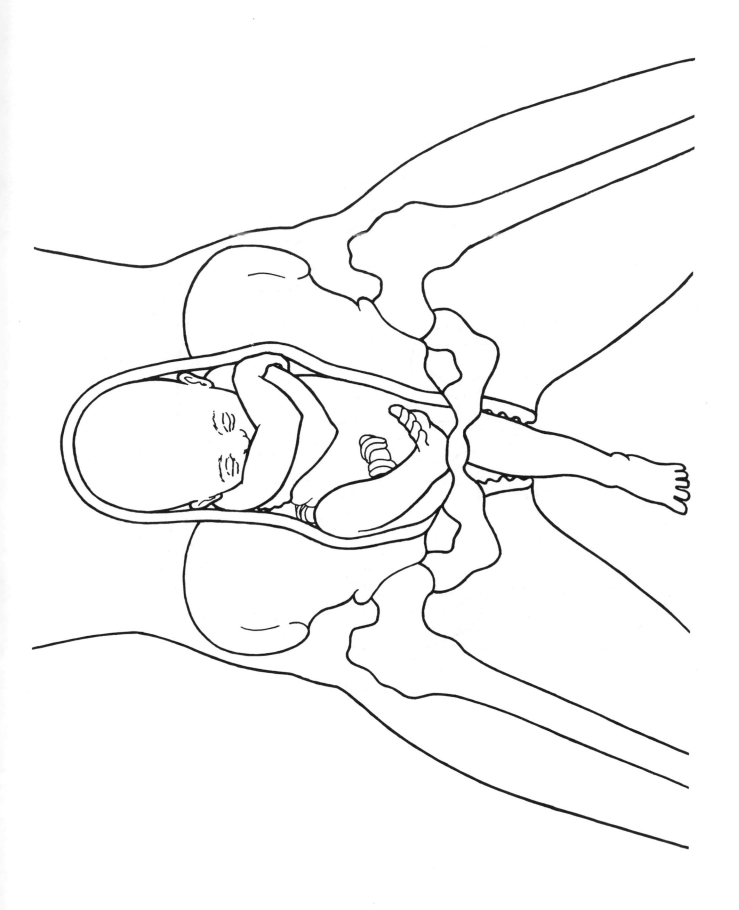

Fig. 13.18 Breech presentation - footling

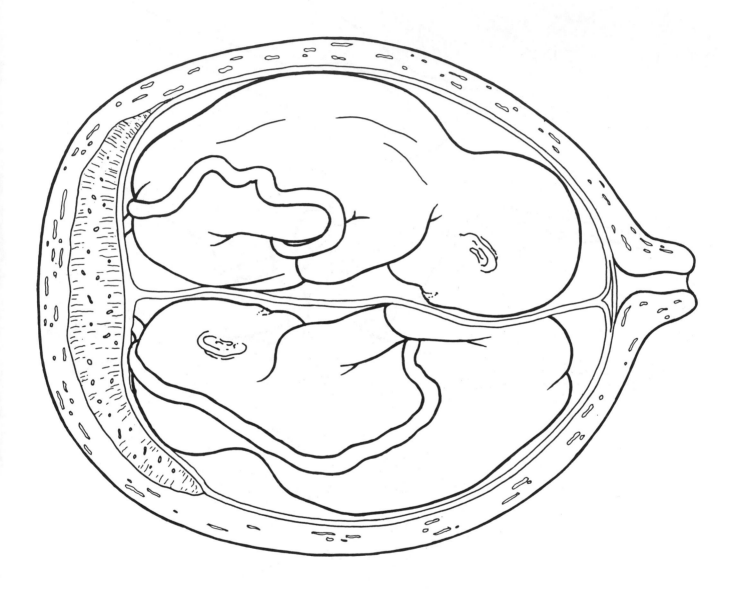

Fig. 13.19 Twins - monovular

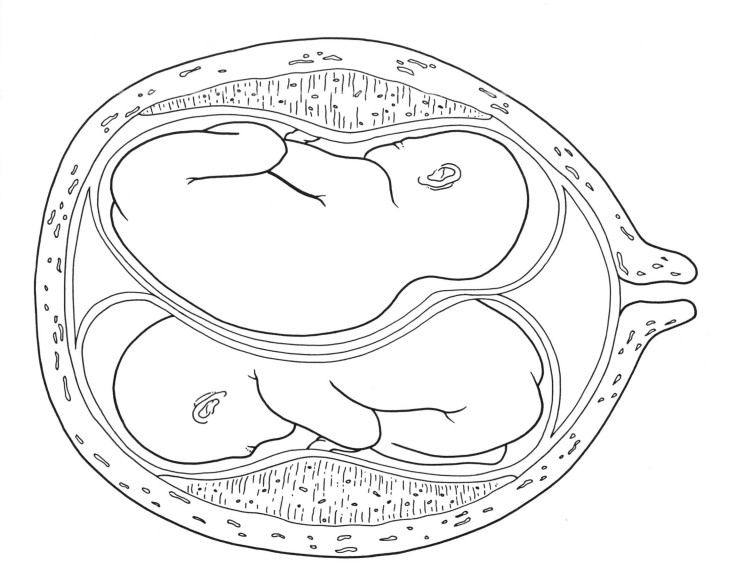

Fig. 13.20 Twins - binovular

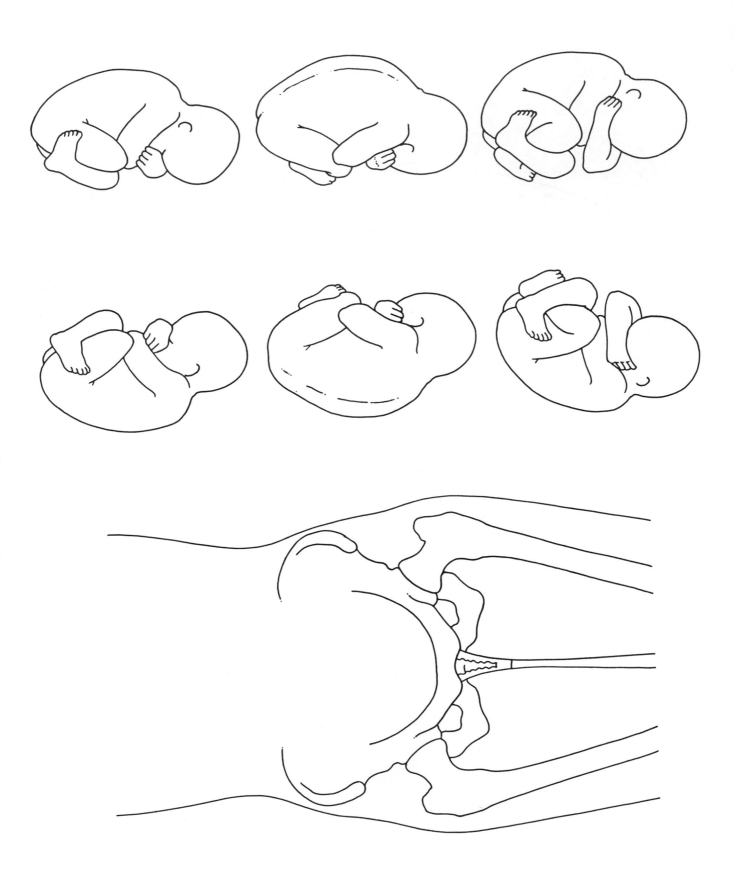

Fig. 13.21 Pelvis with six vertex positions

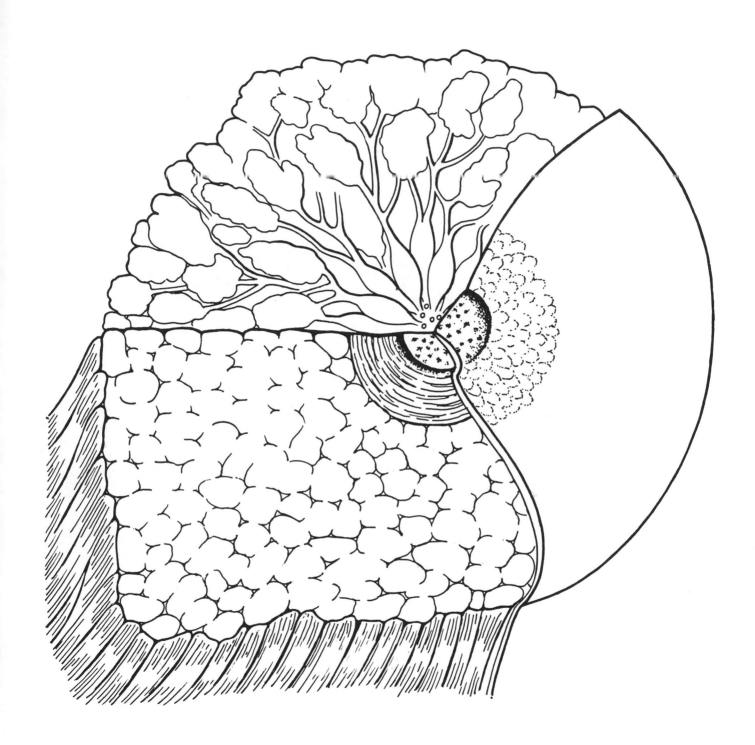

Fig. 13.22 Breast, AP dissection

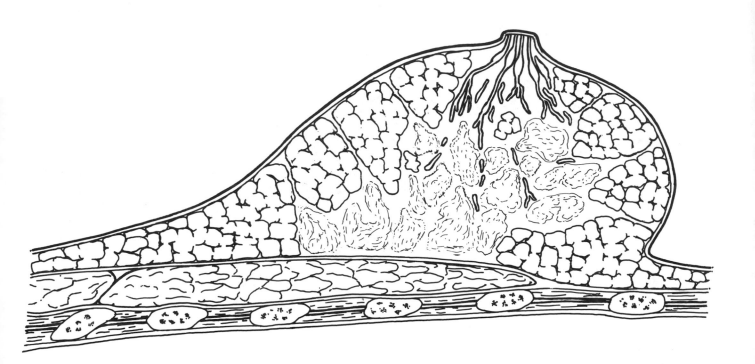

Fig. 13.23 Breast, sagittal section

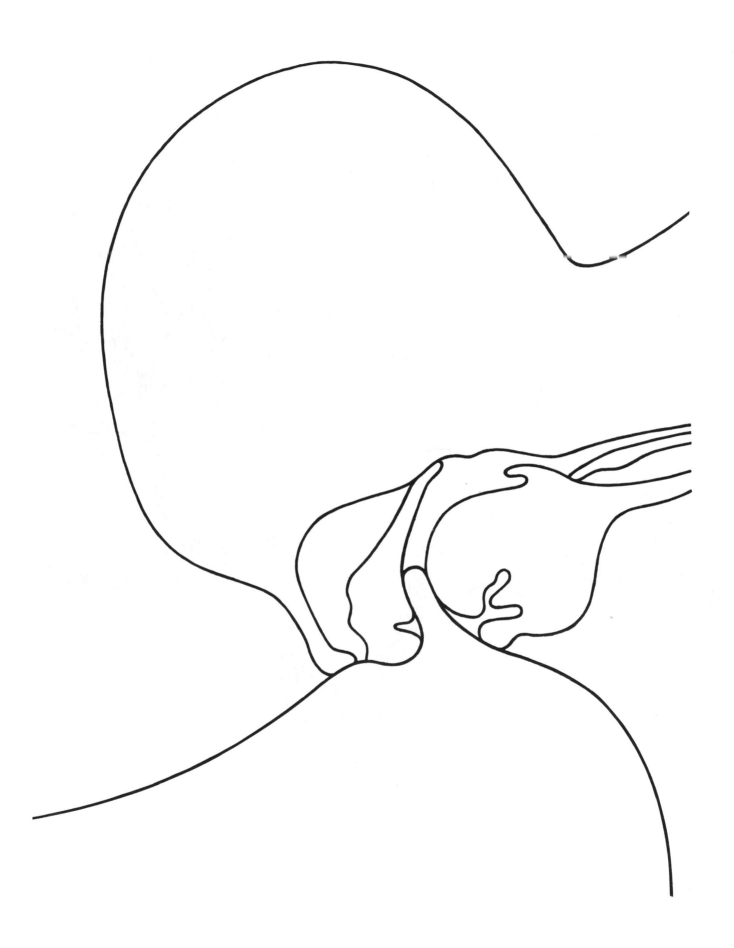

Fig. 13.24 Suckling infant, sagittal section

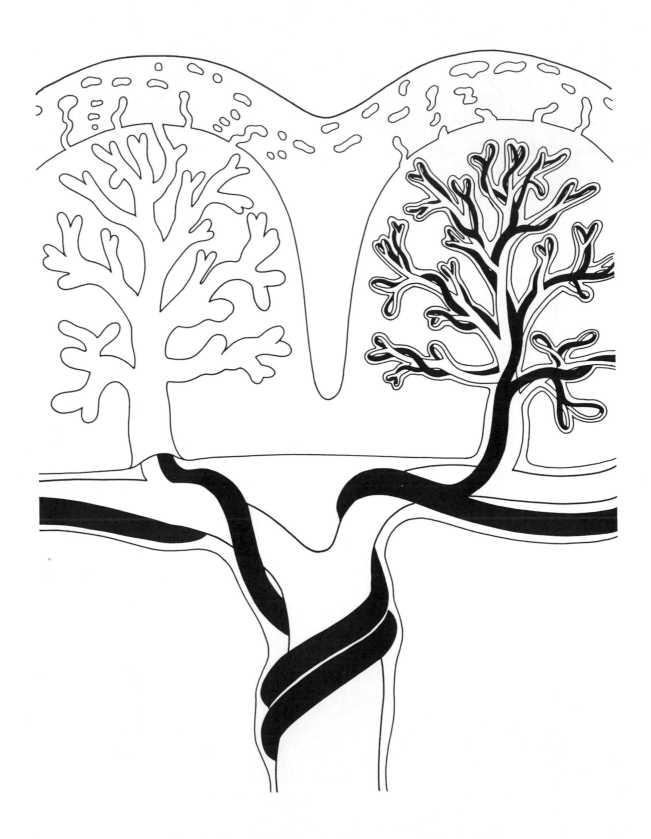

Fig. 13.25 Placenta, cotyledon, - scheme

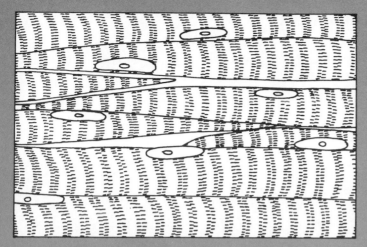

Section 14

Cells and Tissues

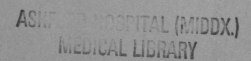

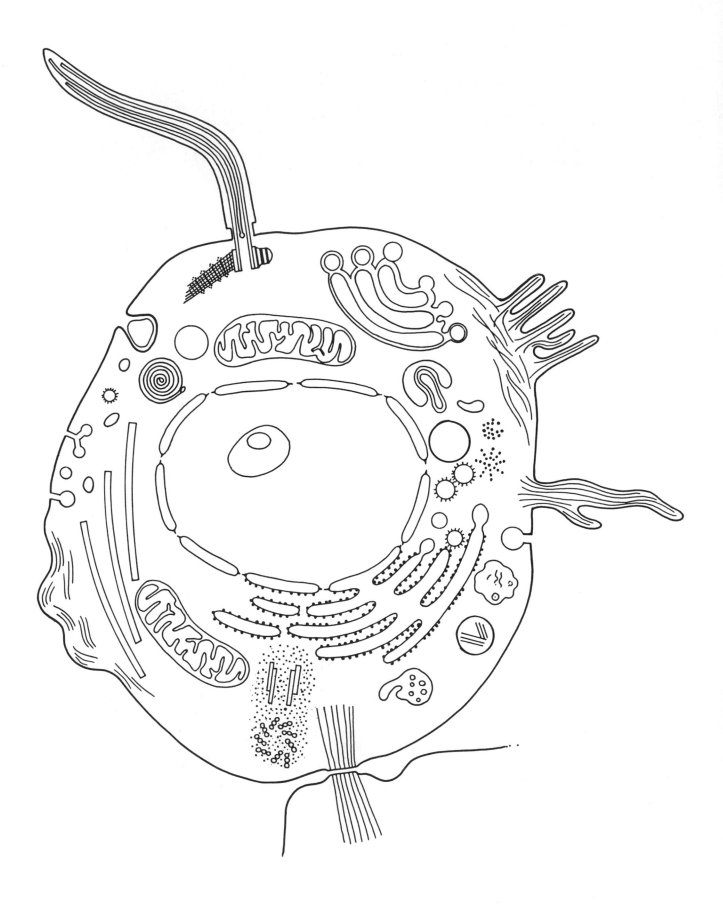

Fig. 14.1 Composite cell

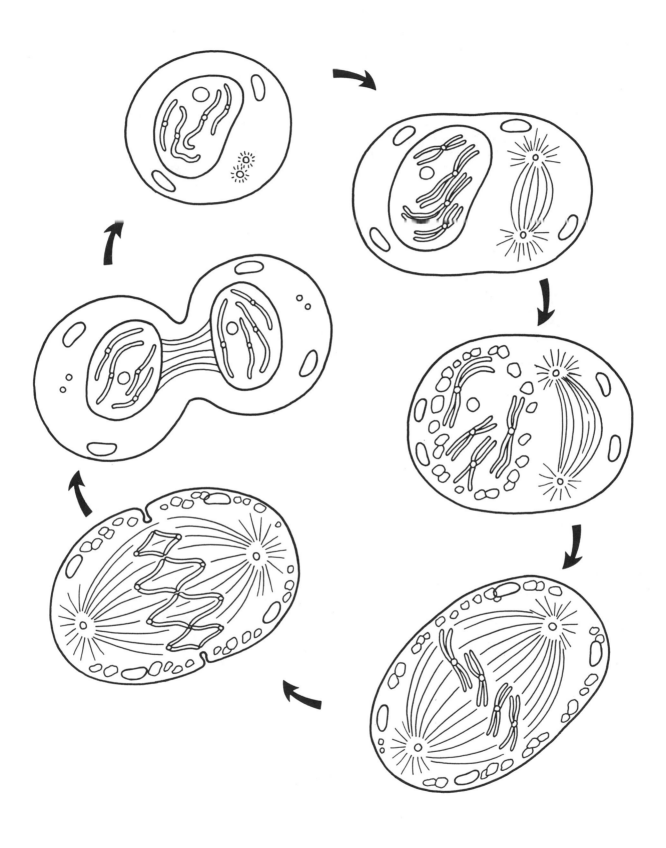

Fig. 14.2 Cell mitosis

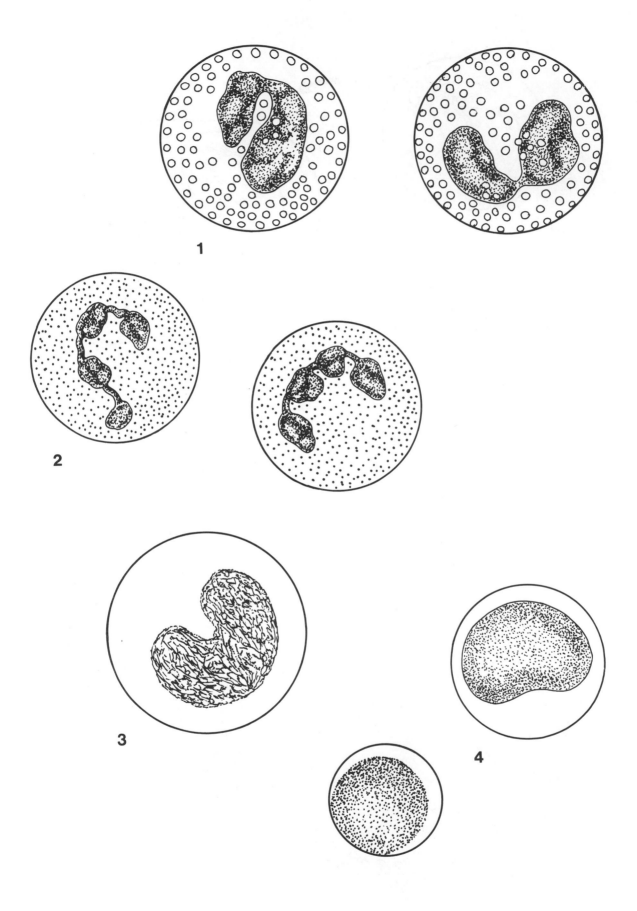

Fig. 14.3   1 - Eosinophils, 2 - Neutrophils, 3 - Monocyte, 4 - Lymphocytes

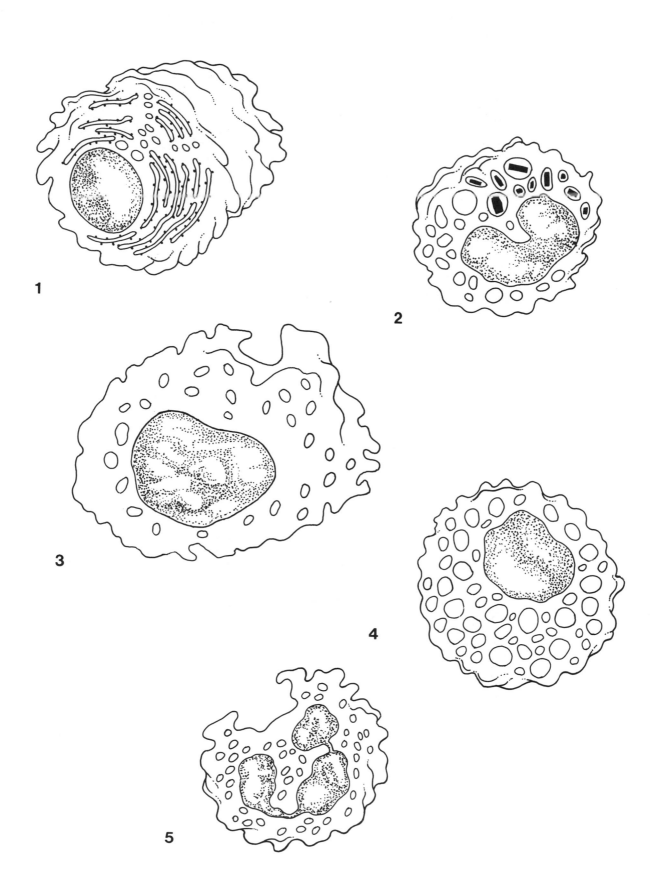

Fig. 14.4 1 - Plasma cell, 2 - Eosinophil, 3 - Macrophage, 4 - Mast cell,
5 - Neutrophil

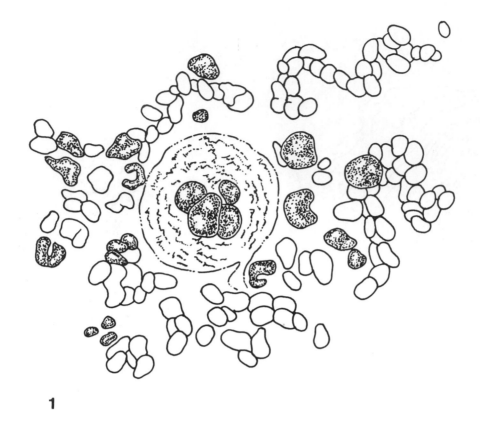

1

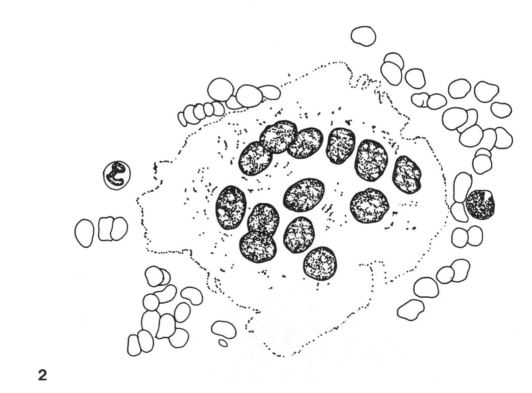

2

Fig. 14.5ˉ 1 - Megakaryocyte, 2 - Osteoclast

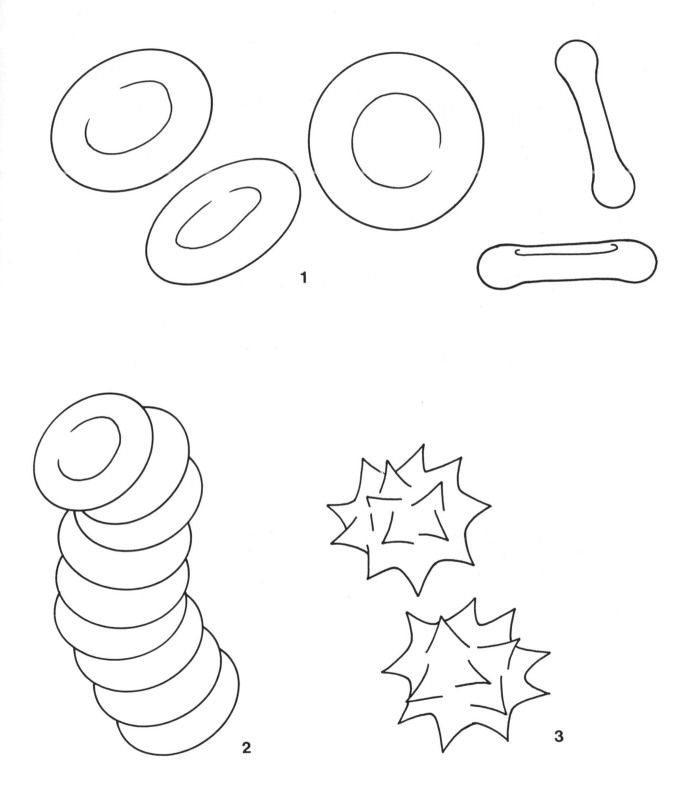

Fig. 14.6 1 - Single red blood cells, 2 - 'packed cells', 3 - Acanthocytes

314

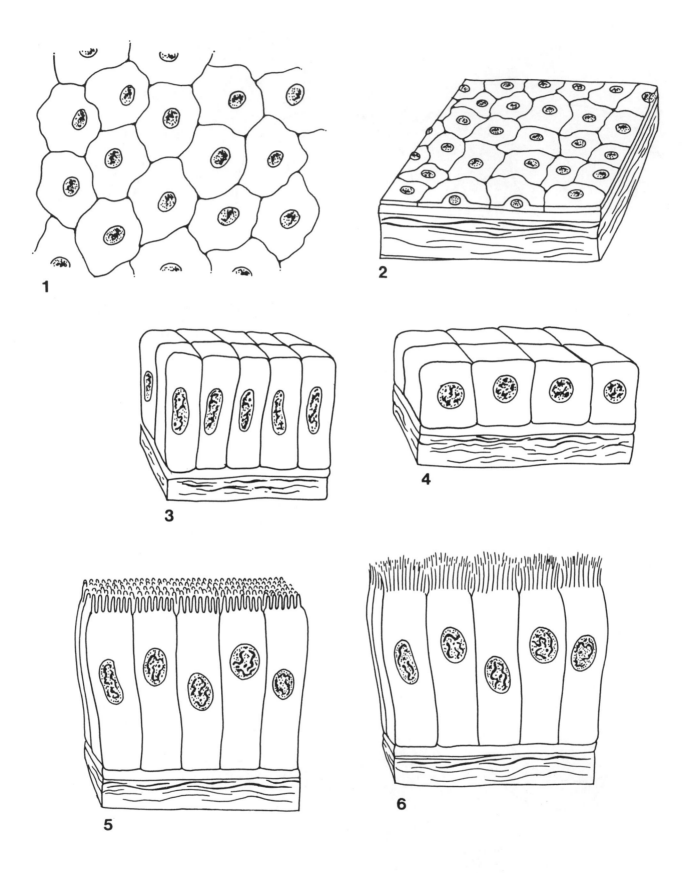

Fig. 14.7 Epithelium, 1 - simple squamous en face, 2 - simple squamous in section, 3 - simple columnar, 4 - simple cuboidal, 5 - simple columnar with microvilli, 6 - simple columnar, ciliated

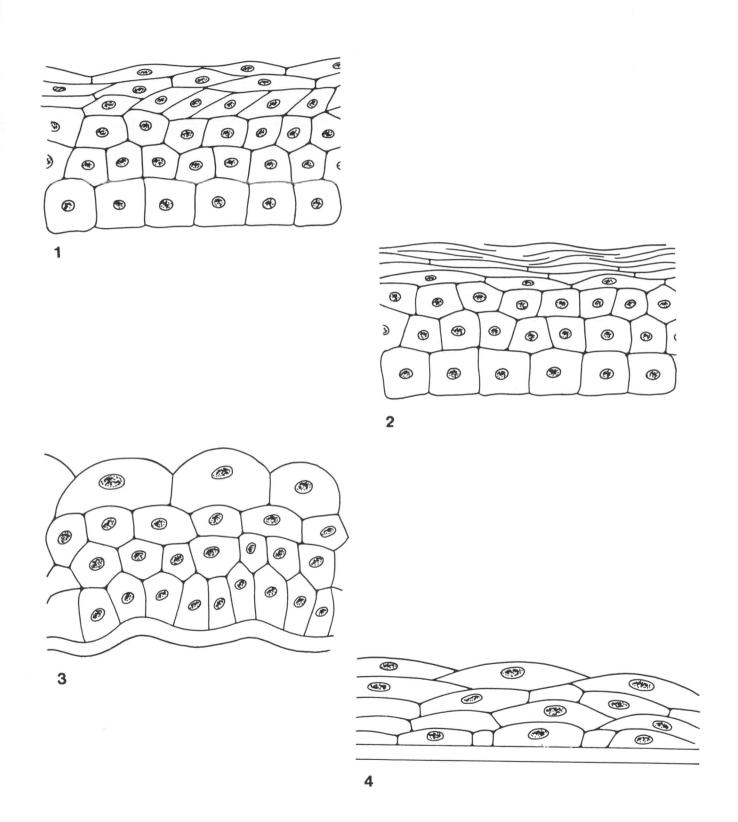

Fig. 14.8 Epithelium, 1 - stratified squamous non-keratinizing,
2 - keratinizing, 3 - transitional relaxed, 4 - transitional stretched

316

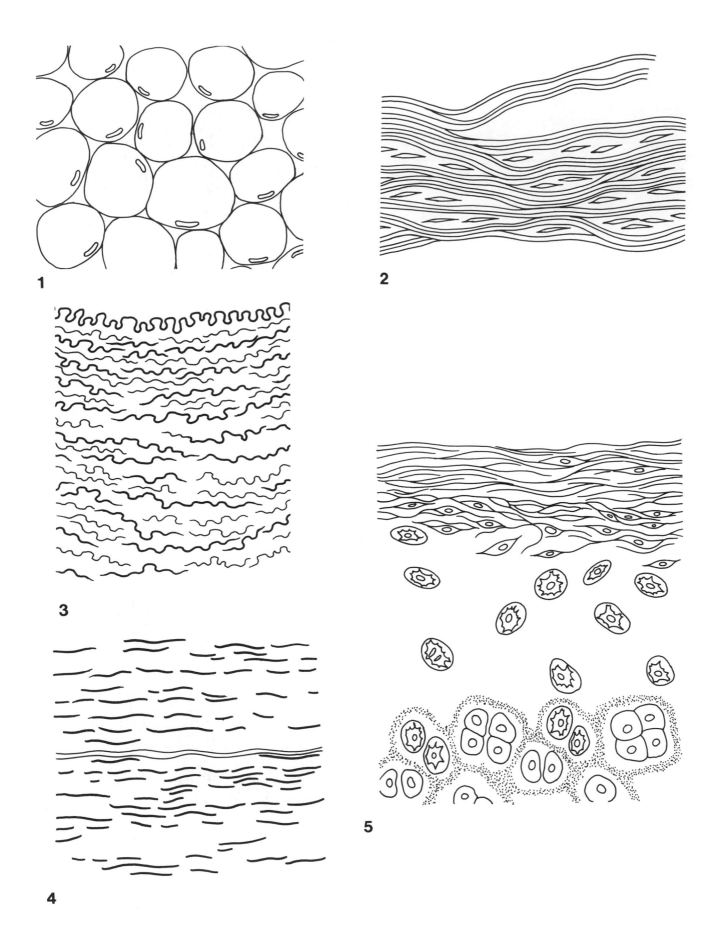

Fig. 14.9   Connective tissue, 1 - adipose, 2 - fibrous, 3 - elastic
(contracted), 4 - tendinous (intercellular), 5 - uncalcified
hyaline cartilage

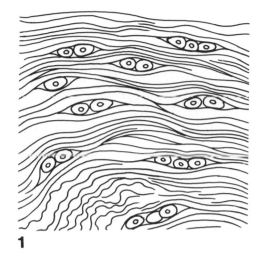

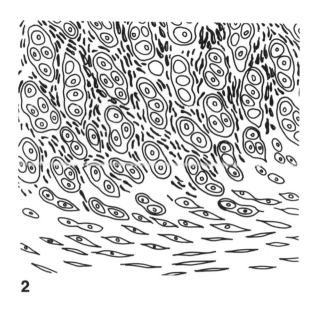

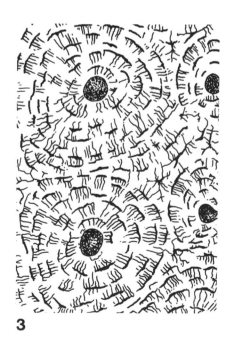

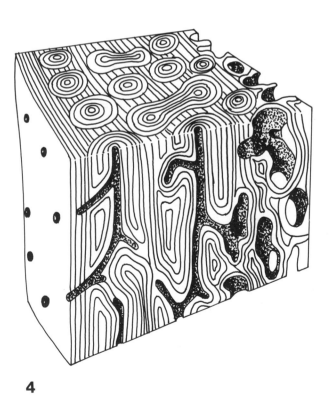

Fig. 14.10 Connective tissue, 1 - fibro-cartilage of an intervertebral disc,
2 - elastic cartilage, 3 - compact bone
4 - compact bone showing Haversian systems

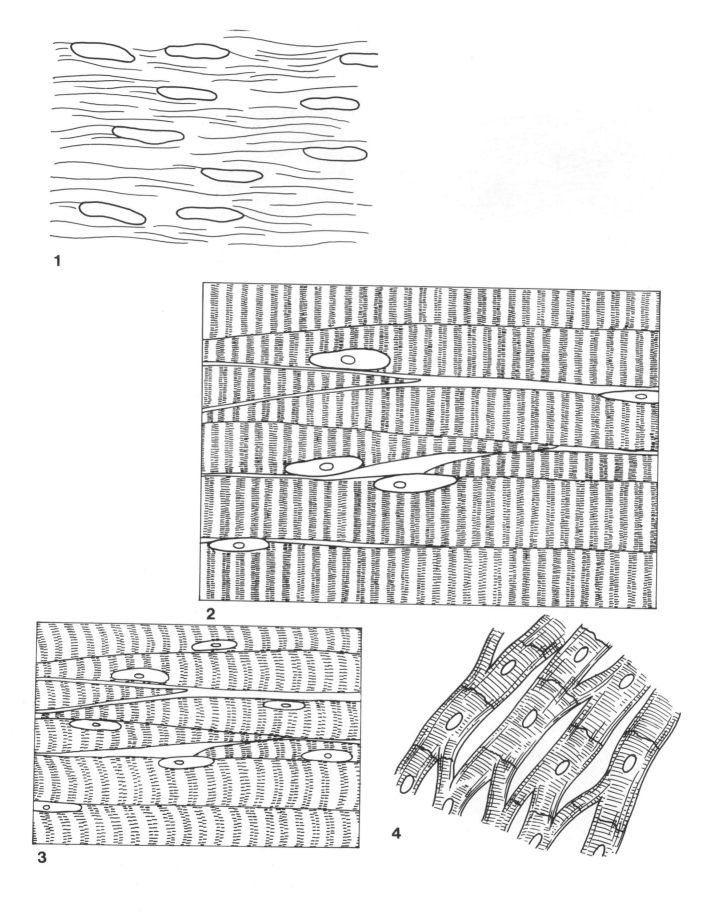

Fig. 14.11 Muscle tissue, 1 - smooth muscle of intestine, 2 - longitudinal section through skeletal (striated) muscle, 3 - cylindrical structure of striated muscle, 4 - cardiac muscle

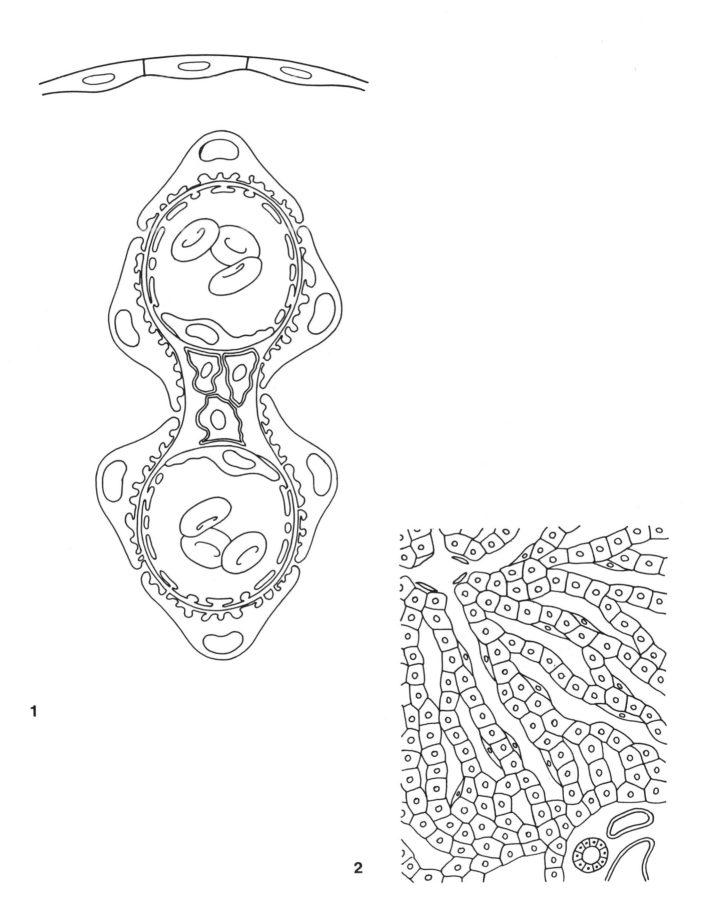

Fig. 14.12 1 - Scheme of capillaries and Bowman's capsule of a glomerulus,
2 - schematic representation of a normal liver lobule

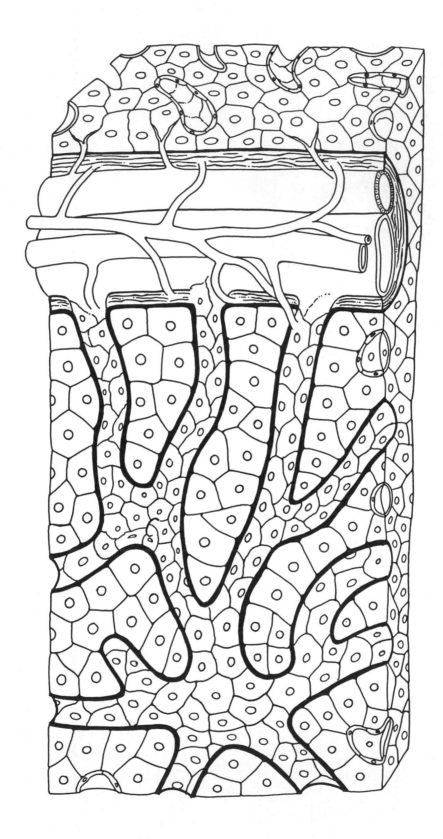

Fig. 14.13 Hepatic section

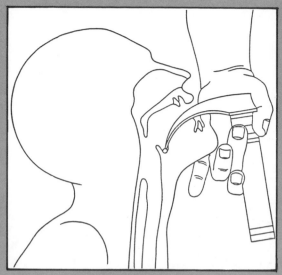

Section 15

Anaesthesia

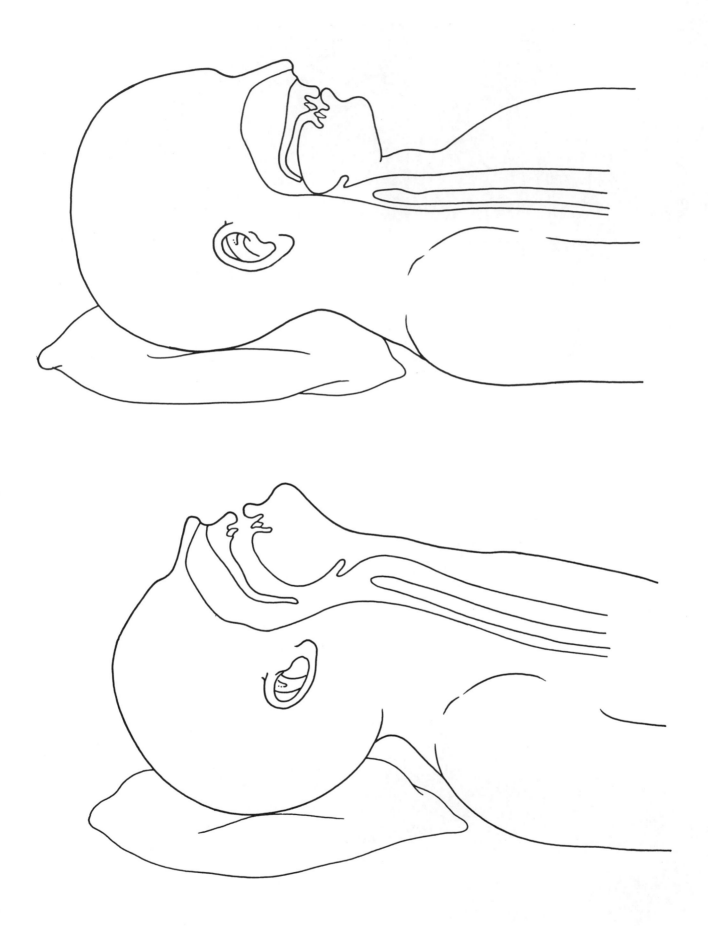

Fig. 15.1 Obstructed and clear airway

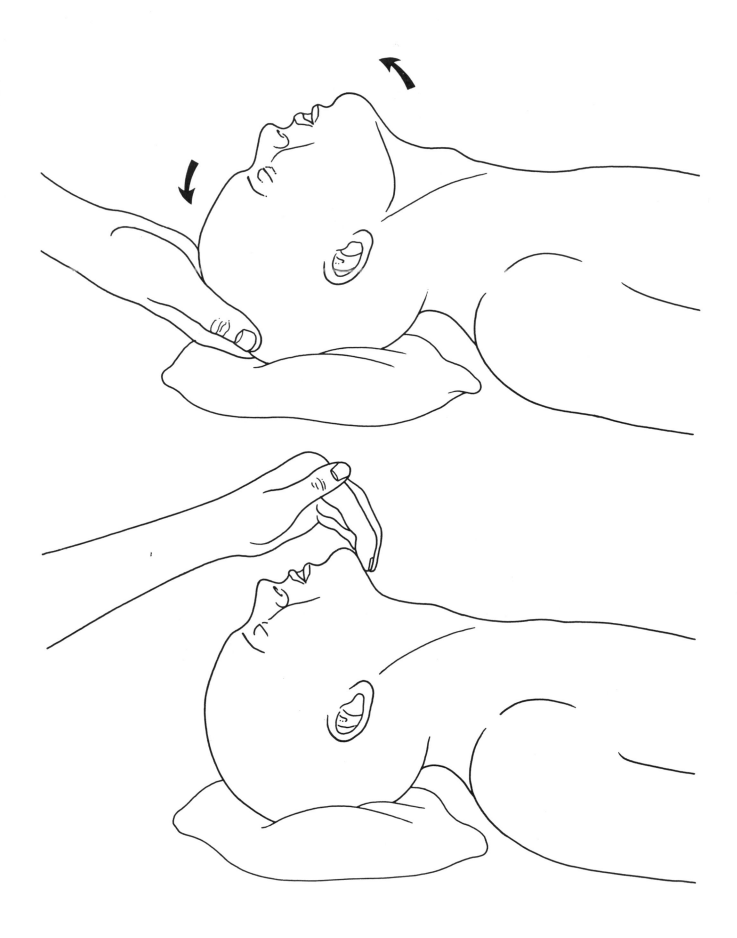

Fig. 15.2 Extension of head, maintenance of clear airway

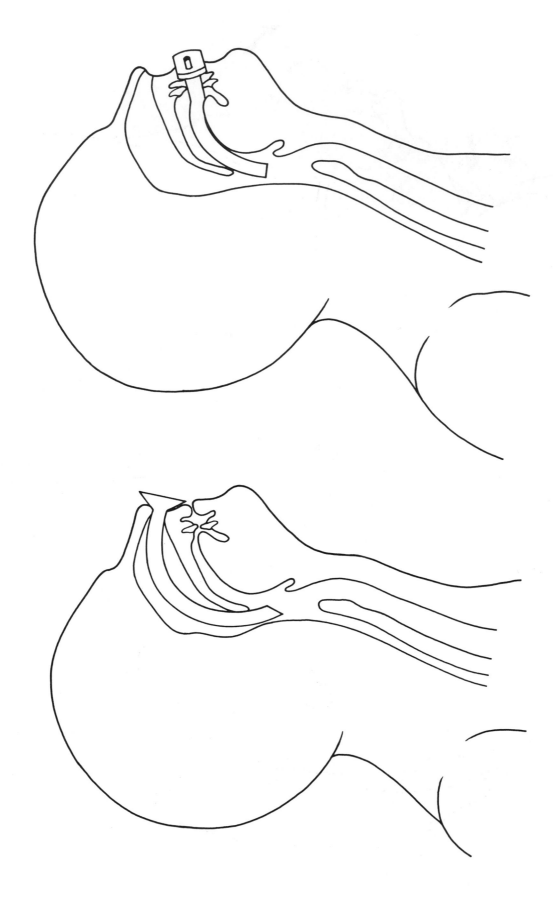

Fig. 15.3 Oropharyngeal and nasopharyngeal airways

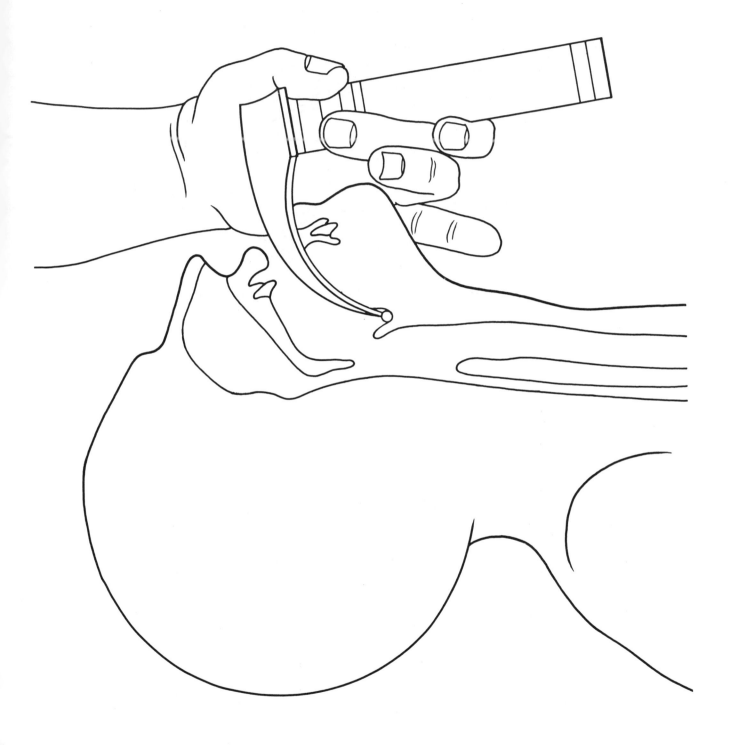

Fig. 15.4 Laryngoscope in situ

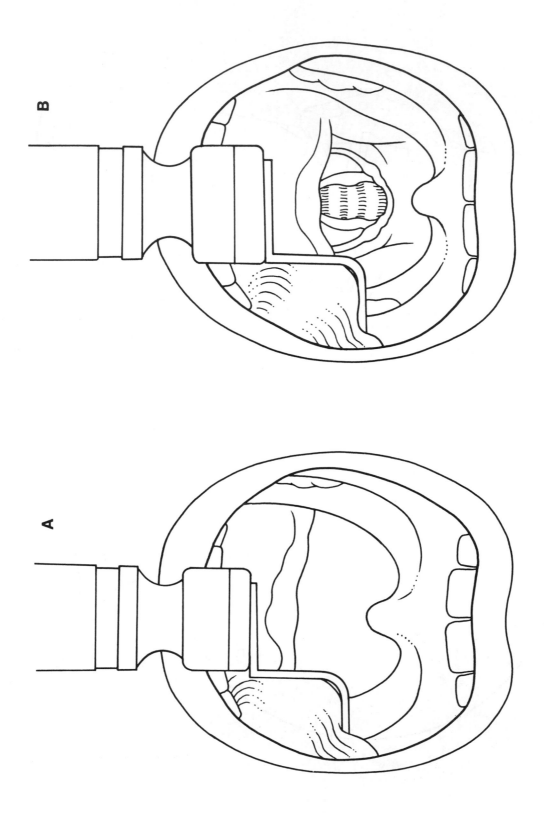

Fig. 15.5 Laryngoscopic view, A - of pharynx and epiglottis, B - of larynx

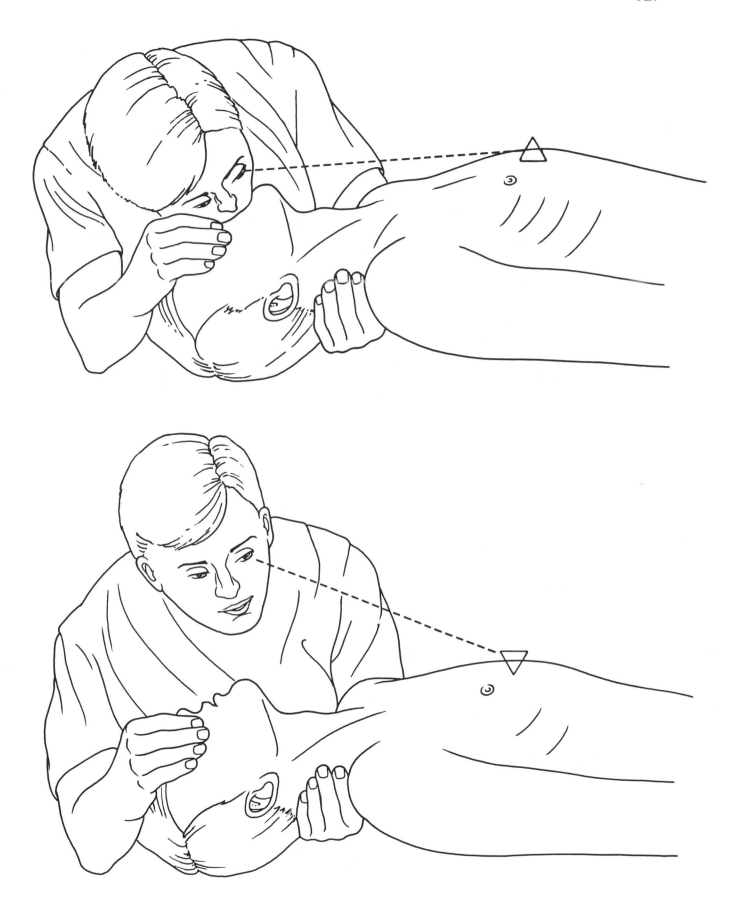

Fig. 15.6 Expired air ventilation

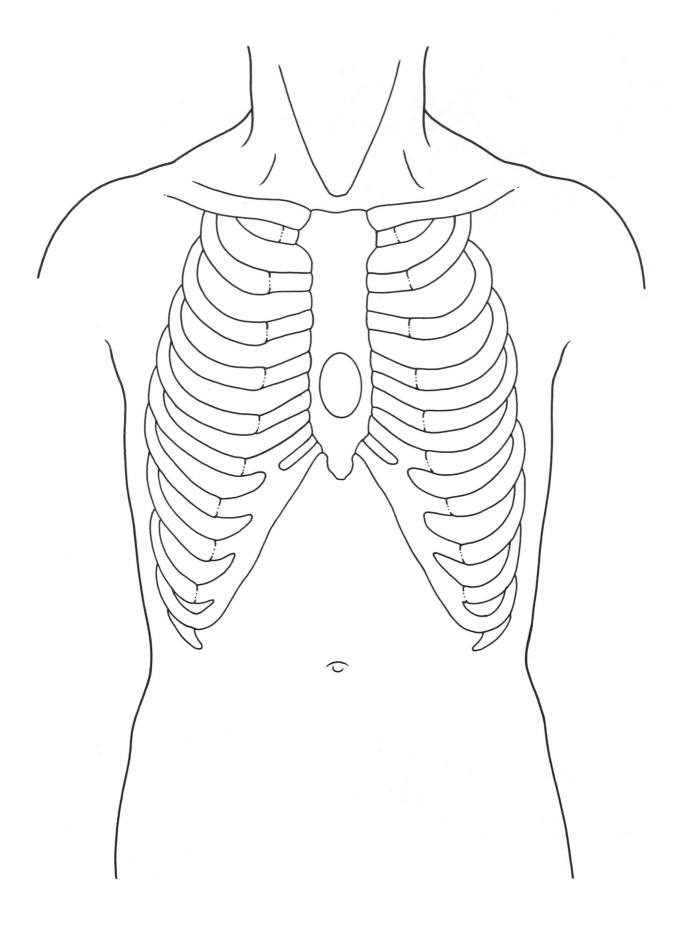

Fig. 15.7 Pressure area for external cardiac massage

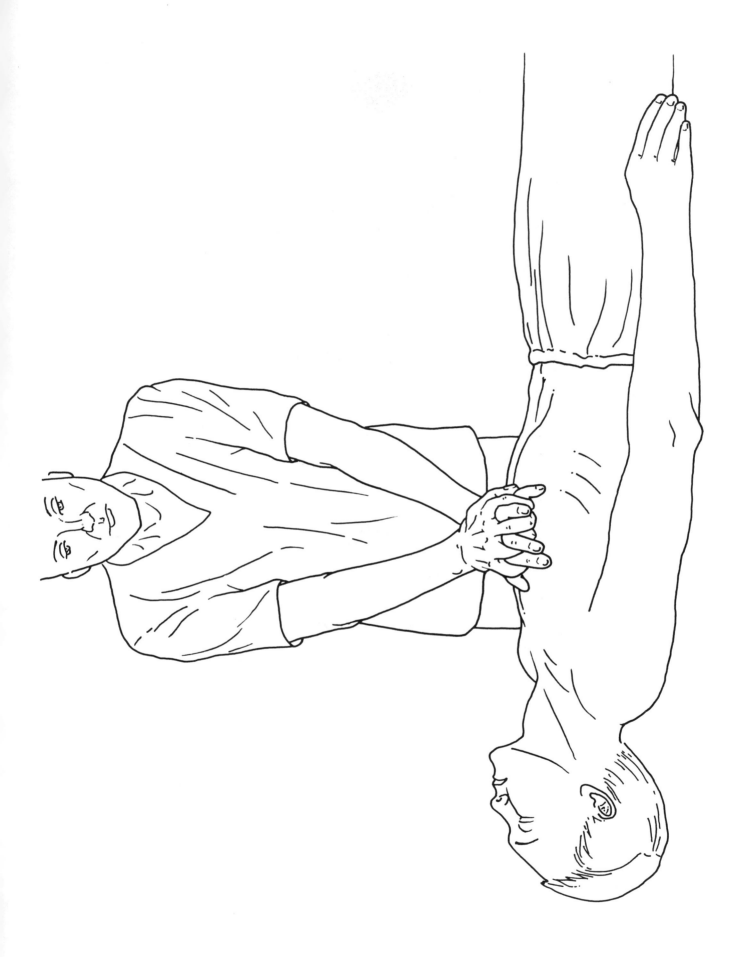

Fig. 15.8 External cardiac massage

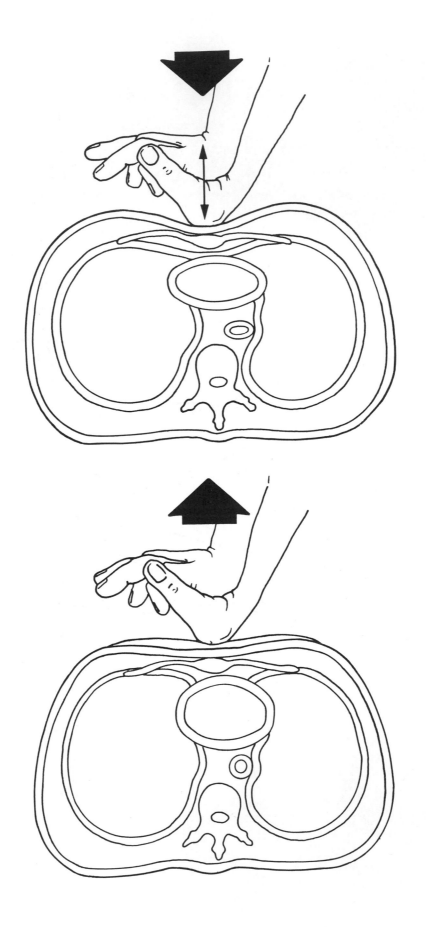

Fig. 15.9 External cardiac massage - section

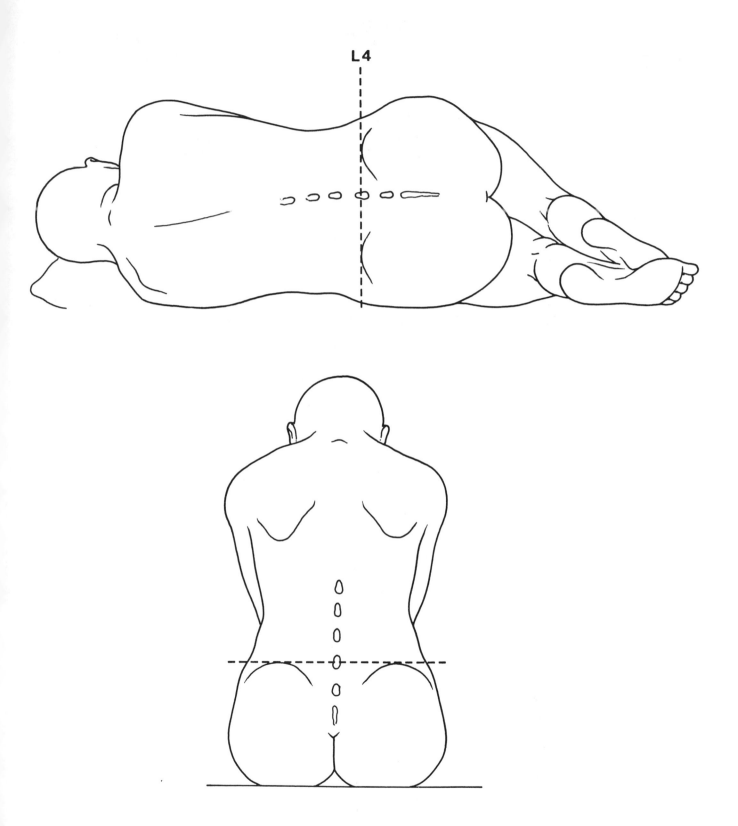

Fig. 15.10 Regions for spinal anaesthesia

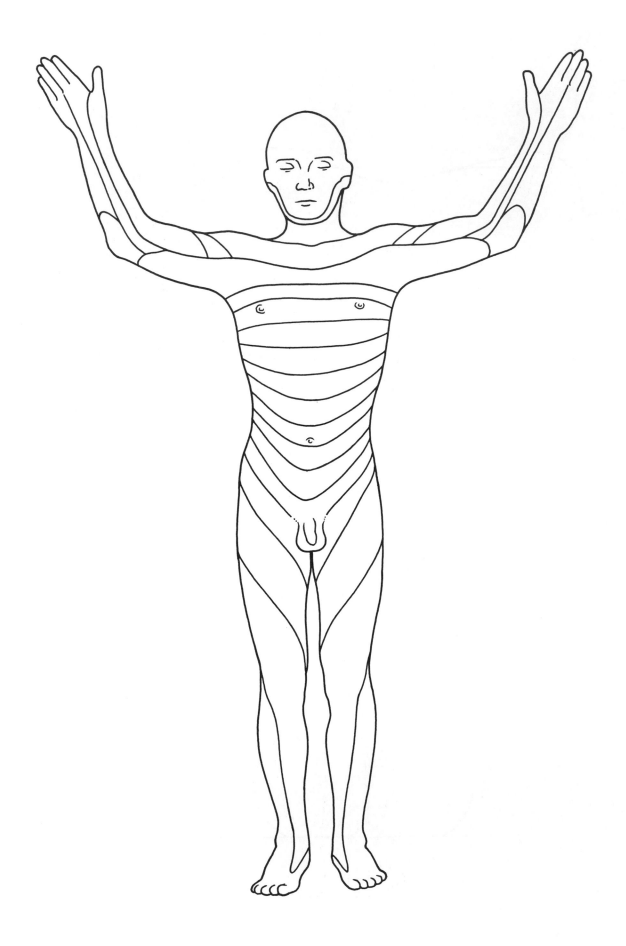

Fig. 15.11 Spinal dermatomes, AP

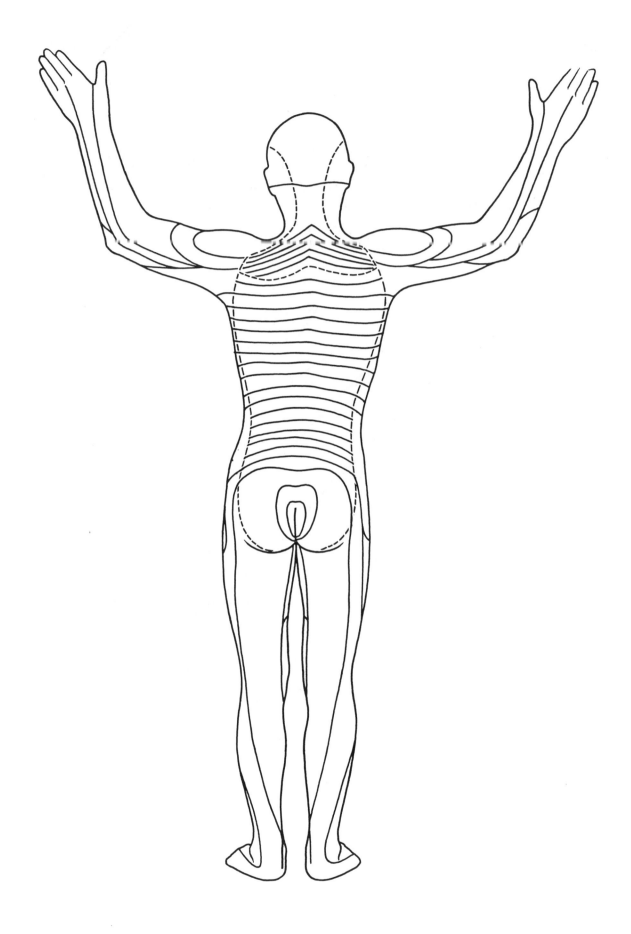

Fig. 15.12 Spinal dermatomes, PA

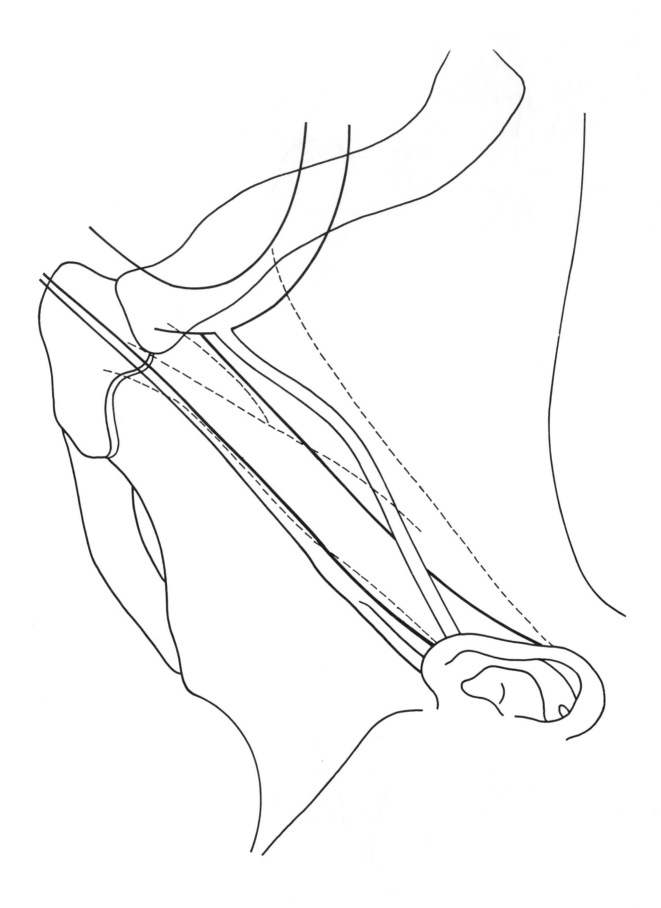

Fig. 15.13 CVP, structures in neck

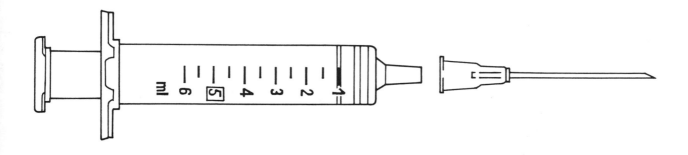

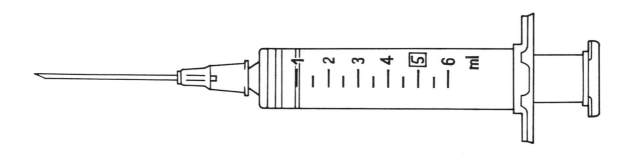

Fig. 15.14 5 ml syringe

Section 16

Bacteria, Yeasts, Protozoans, Helminths, Viruses and Arthropods

16.1   A - Streptococcus D* 0.6 μ
       B - Staphylococcus D 0.9 μ

16.2   A - Clostridium tetani L 7 μ
       B - Vibrio cholerae L 3 μ

16.3   A - Borrelia sp L10 μ
       B - Treponema sp L 10 μ

16.4   A - Salmonella sp L 3 μ
       B - Bacillus anthracis L 6μ

16.5   A - Neisseria gonorrhoeae L 1.5 μ
       B - Streptococcus pneumoniae L 0.8 μ

16.6   A - Campylobacter sp L 3 μ
       B - Clostridium perfringens L 5 μ

16.7   A - Corynebacterium diphtheriae L 6μ
       B - Escherichia coli L 3 μ

16.8   A - Haemophilus influenzae L1 μ
       B - Chlamydia trachomatis D 10 μ - 15 μ

16.9   Mycobacterium tuberculosis L 2.5μ

16.10 Composite bacteria cell: Left - gram negative, Right - gram positive

16.11 Flagella on bacteria

16.12 A - Cryptococcus neoformans
       B - Candida albicans

16.13 A - Pneumocytosis carinii D 5 μ
       B - Trichomonas vaginalis 10μ x 7μ

16.14   Trypanosomes: 4 stages A - Amastigote, B - Promastigote,
       C - Epimastigote, D - Trypomastigote

16.15 Malarial parasites: 1 - P. vivax, 2 - P. malariae,
       3 - P.falciparum, 4 - P. ovale.
       A - Early trophozoites, B - Mature schizonts,
       C - Macrogametocytes

16.16 A - Entamoeba histolytica: cyst, B - Leishmania: amastigote, promastigote, intracellular amastigotes, C - Toxoplasma gondii: trophozoites, cyst, D - Giardia lamblia: trophozoite,

16.17 Fasciola hepatica: A - ovum 140 μ x 75 μ, B - adult 2.5cm x 1cm, C - Redia, D - Cercaria

16.18 Strongyloides stercoralis: A - ♀ L 2.2mm, B - Rhabditiform larva, C - ♂ L 0.7mm
       Schistoma sp: D - ♀ L 1 - 2cm, E - ♂ L 1 - 2cm
       Ova: A - S. haematobium, B - S. mansoni, C - S. japonicum

       *D = Diameter   L = Length

16.19 Filarial Worms, A - Mansonella ozzardi 175 - 240 x 4.5 µ
B - Dipetalonema (Acanthocheilonema) perstans 200 x 4.5 µ
C - Dipetalonema streptocera 180 - 240 x 3 µ
D - ♂ Wuchereria bancrofti 40 x 0.1 µ
E - ♀ Wuchereria bancrofti 100 x 0.25mm
F - Onchocerca volvulus 400 x 0.3mm
G - ♀ Loa loa 40 x 0.3mm
16.20 A - Roundworms ♂ and ♀ , Ascaris L 15 - 35cms, ovum 70 x
50 µ
B - Thread/Pin/Seat worms ♂ and ♀ Enterobius L 1cm,
ovum 55 x 25 µ
C - Whipworm ♂ and ♀ Trichuris L 40mm, ovum 50 x 22 µ
D - Hookworm ♂ and ♀ Ancylostoma and Necator
L 1cm, ovum 58 x 36 µ
16.21 Tapeworms: A - Taenia saginata L up to 30ft, scolex and
gravid proglottid, B - Taenia solium L up to 30ft, scolex and
gravid proglottid, C - Hymenolepis nana L 2.5 - 5 cms
16.22 Trichinella spiralis: A - larva, B - ♀ , C - ♂ , D - larva in skeletal
tissue, Dracunculus medinensis: E - larva, F - ♀ , G - ♂
16.23 Echinococcal cysts: A - Hydatid, B - Multilocular
16.24 Virus size chart
16.25 HIV
16.26 HBV
16.27 A - Calicivirus, B - Reovirus
16.28 A - Bunyavirus, B - Paramyxovirus
16.29 A - Orthomyxovirus, B - Arenavirus
16.30 Adenovirus
16.31 A - Toga/Papova/Parvo/Picorna virus, B - Bacteriophage
C - Pox virus
16.32 Herpes virus
16.33 A - Retrovirus, B - Rhabdovirus
16.34 Corona virus: capiscid and section
16.35 Human louse, Pediculus humanus humanus, egg and adults
16.36 Pubic or crab louse, Phthirus pubis
16.37 Bedbugs, Cimicidae, dorsal and ventral views
16.38 Scabies, Sarcoptes scabii
16.39 Soft ticks, Argas persicus and Ornithodorus moubata
16.40 Soft ticks, Ornithodorus moubata, larva, nymph and adult
16.41 Hard ticks, Ixodes
16.42 Cockroach, Blatella orientalis
16.43 Cockroach, Periplaneta americana
16.44 Housefly, Musca domestica
16.45 Bluebottle, Calliphora, pupa and adult
16.46 Tsetse fly, Glossina
16.47 Biting midge, Culicoides
16.48 A - Black fly, Simulium, and B - Sandfly,Phlebotomus
16.49 Jigger flea, Tunga penetrans, gravid ♀ ♀ and ♂
16.50 Plague flea, Xenopsylla cheopis
16.51 Triatomine bugs, Reduviidae
16.52 Mosquito, A - Anopheles and B - Culicine: larva and adult
16.53 Mosquito, Anopheles

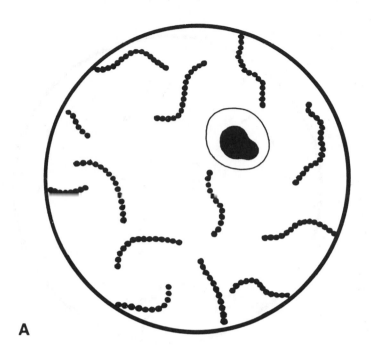

A

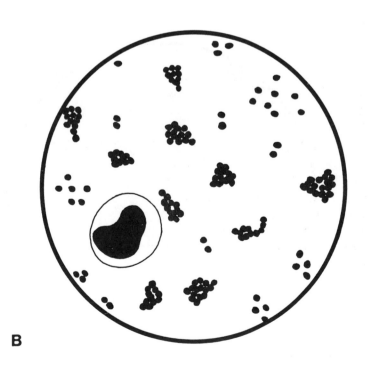

B

Fig. 16.1　A - Streptococcus D 0.6 μ
　　　　　　B - Staphylococcus D 0.9 μ

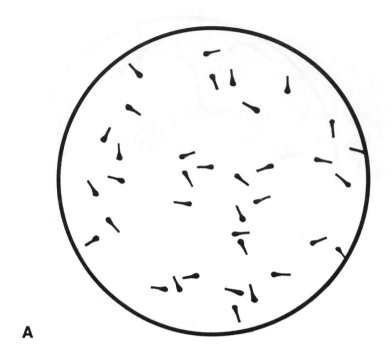

A

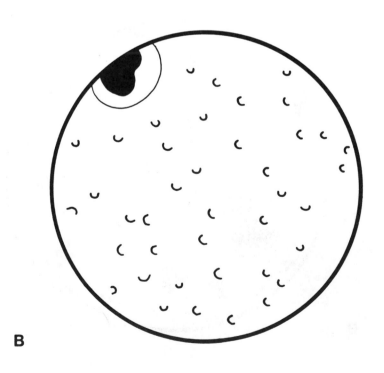

B

Fig.16.2   A - Clostridium tetani L 7 μ
            B - Vibrio cholerae L 3 μ

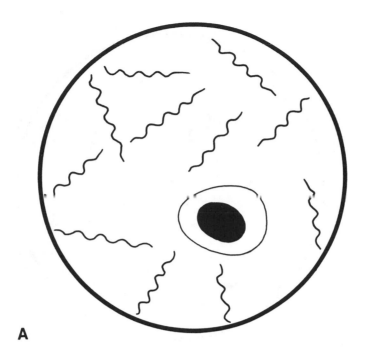

A

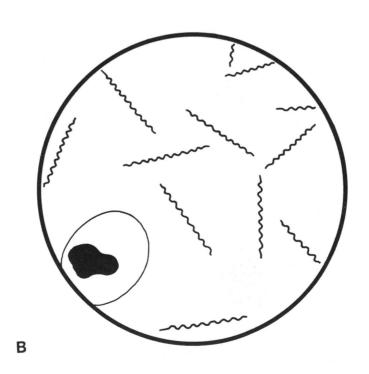

B

Fig.16.3   A - Borrelia sp L10 μ
          B - Treponema sp L 10 μ

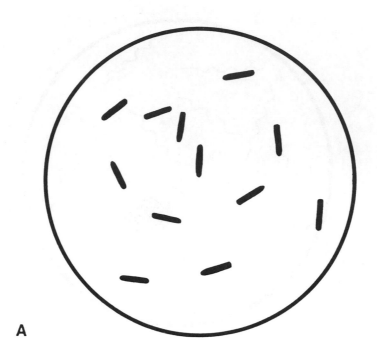

A

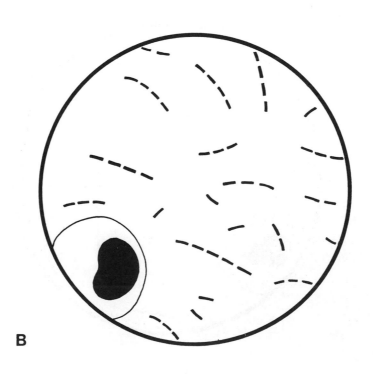

B

Fig.16.4   A - Salmonella sp L 3 μ
          B - Bacillus anthracis L 6μ

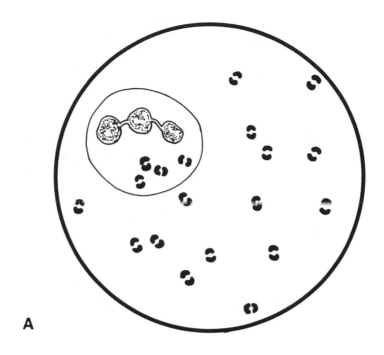

A

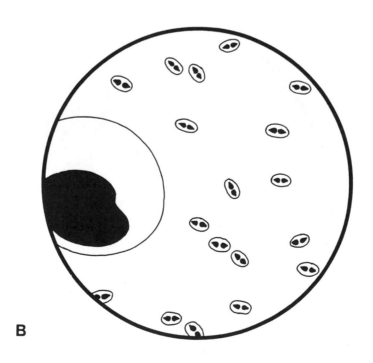

B

Fig. 16.5 A - Neisseria gonorrhoeae L 1.5 μ
          B - Streptococcus pneumoniae L 0.8 μ

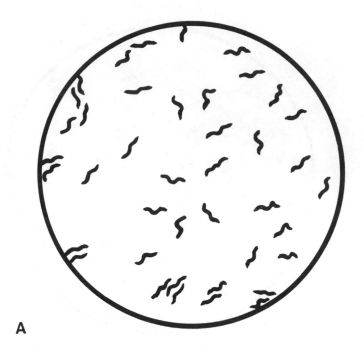

A

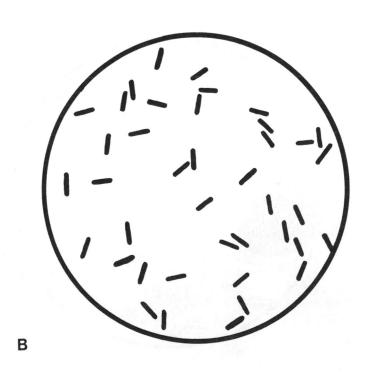

B

Fig. 16.6   A - Campylobacter sp L 3 μ
            B - Clostridium perfringens L 5 μ

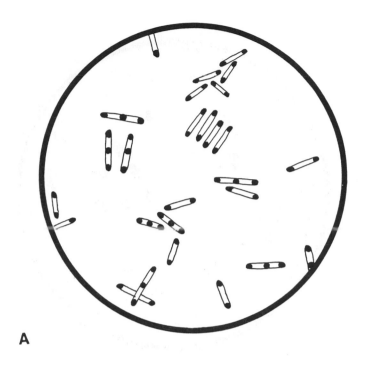

A

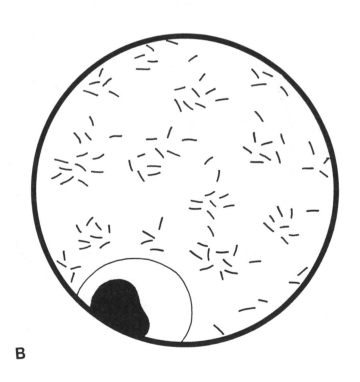

B

Fig.16.7   A - Corynebacterium diphtheriae L 6μ
B - Escherichia coli L 3 μ

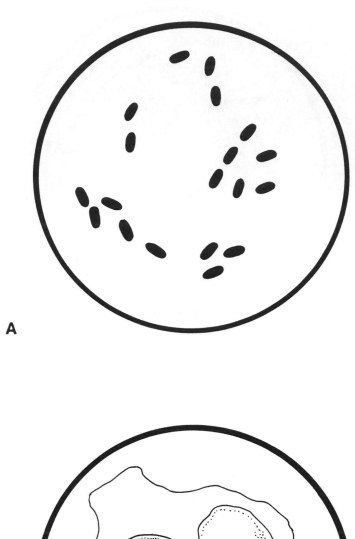

A

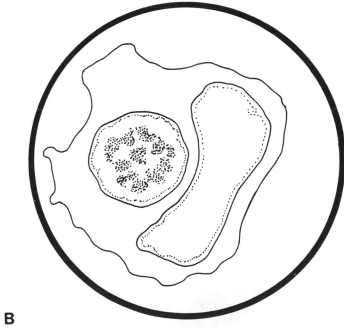

B

Fig.16.8   A - Haemophilus influenzae L1 μ
            B - Chlamydia trachomatis D 10 μ - 15 μ

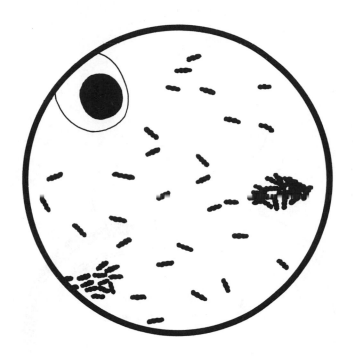

16.9   Mycobacterium tuberculosis L 2.5μ

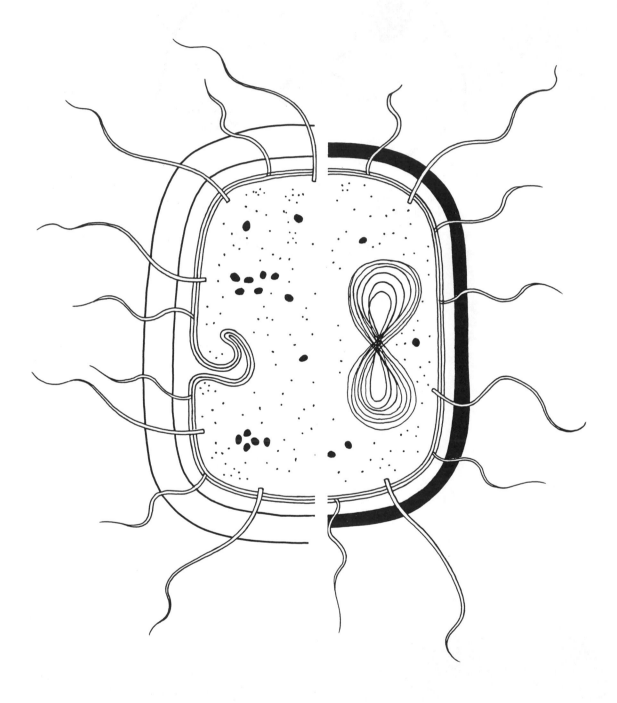

Fig.16.10 Composite bacteria cell: Left - gram negative, Right - gram positive

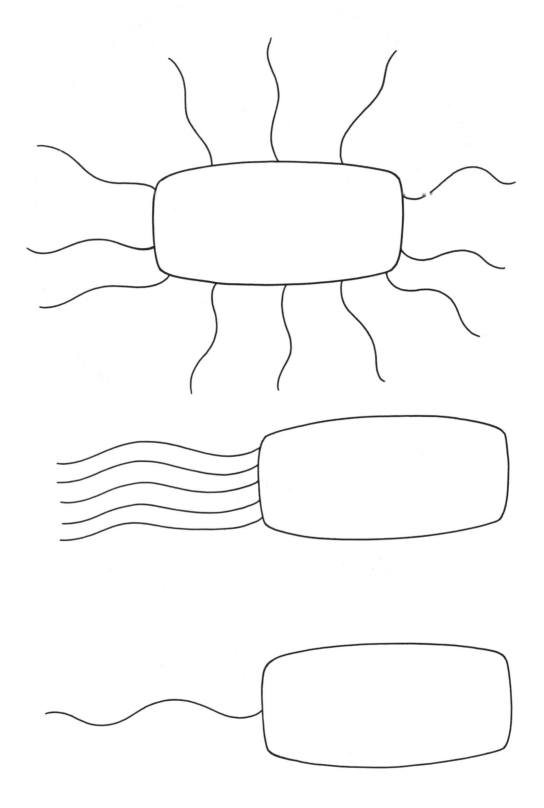

Fig.16.11 Flagella on bacteria

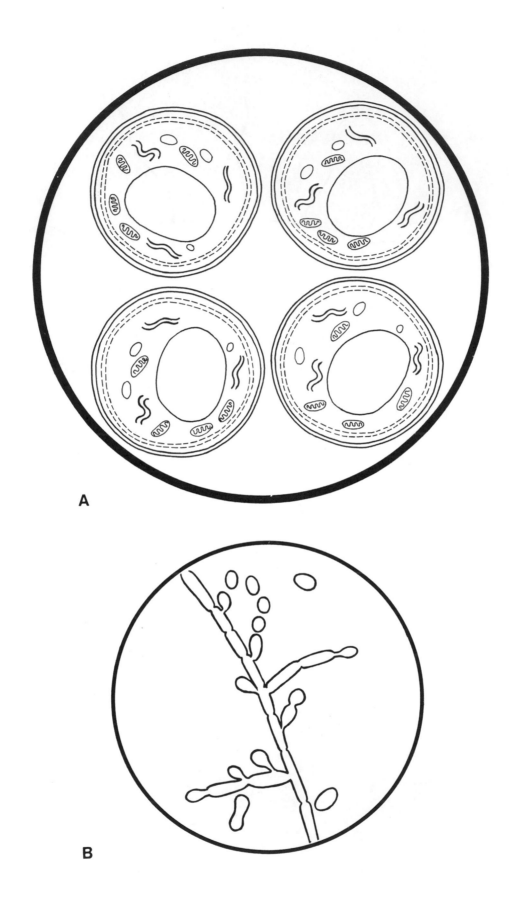

A

B

Fig.16.12 A - Cryptococcus neoformans
           B - Candida albicans

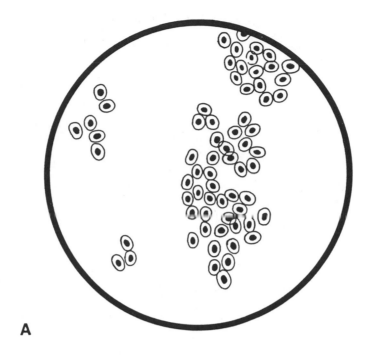

A

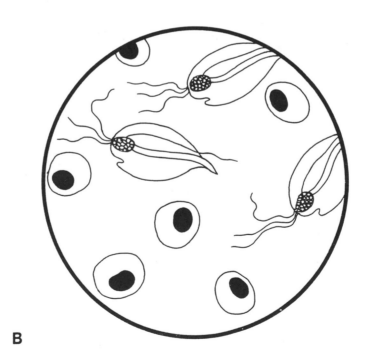

B

Fig.16.13   A - Pneumocytosis carinii D 5 μ
             B - Trichomonas vaginalis 10μ x 7μ

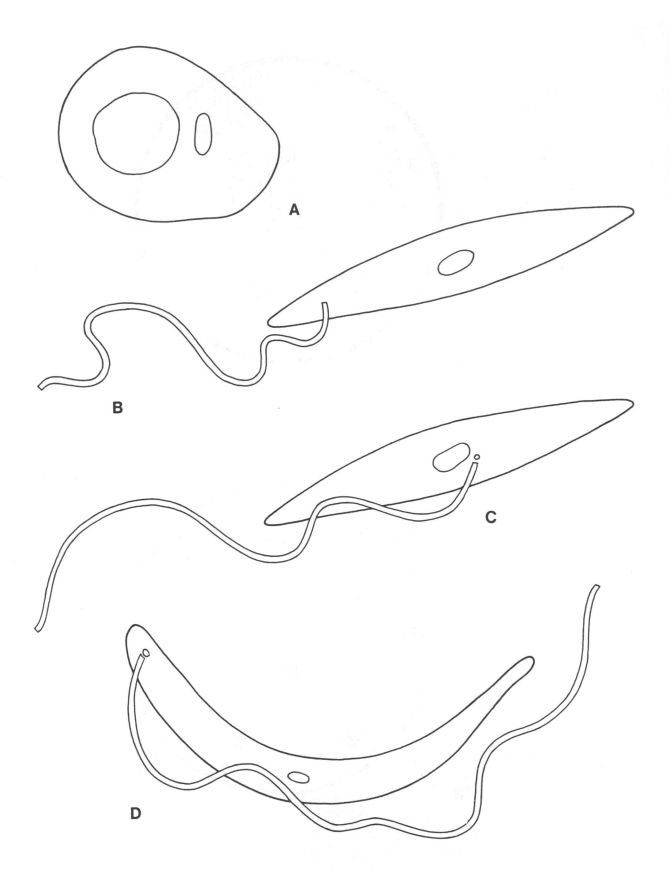

Fig.16.14   Trypanosomes: 4 stages, A - Amastigote, B - Promastigote,
C - Epimastigote, D - Trypomastigote

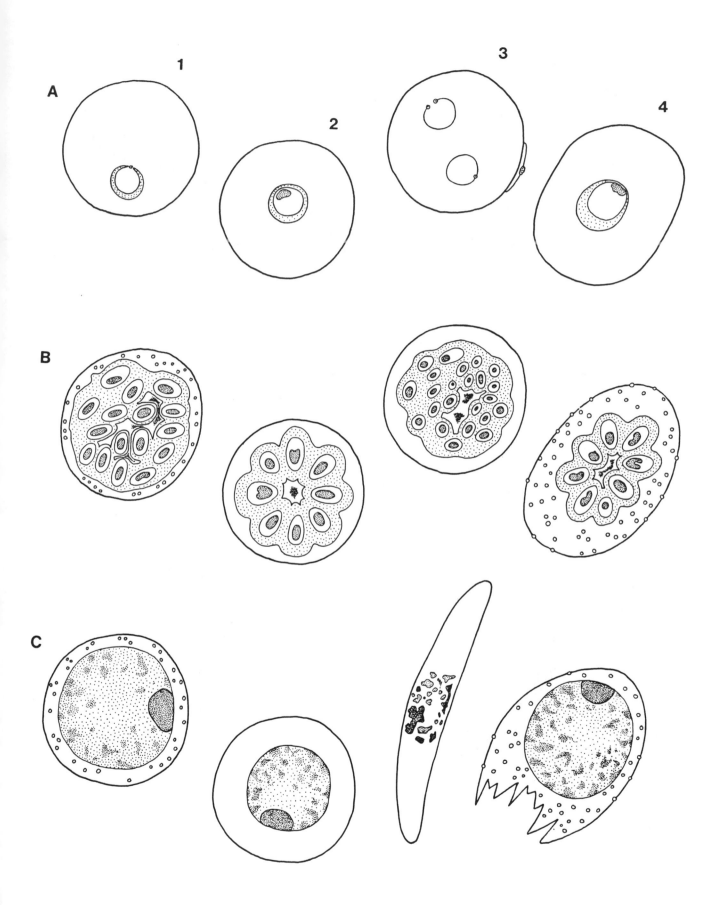

Fig.16.15 Malarial parasites: 1 - P. vivax, 2 - P. malariae,
3 - P.falciparum, 4 - P. ovale.
A - Early trophozoites, B - Mature schizonts,
C - Macrogametocytes

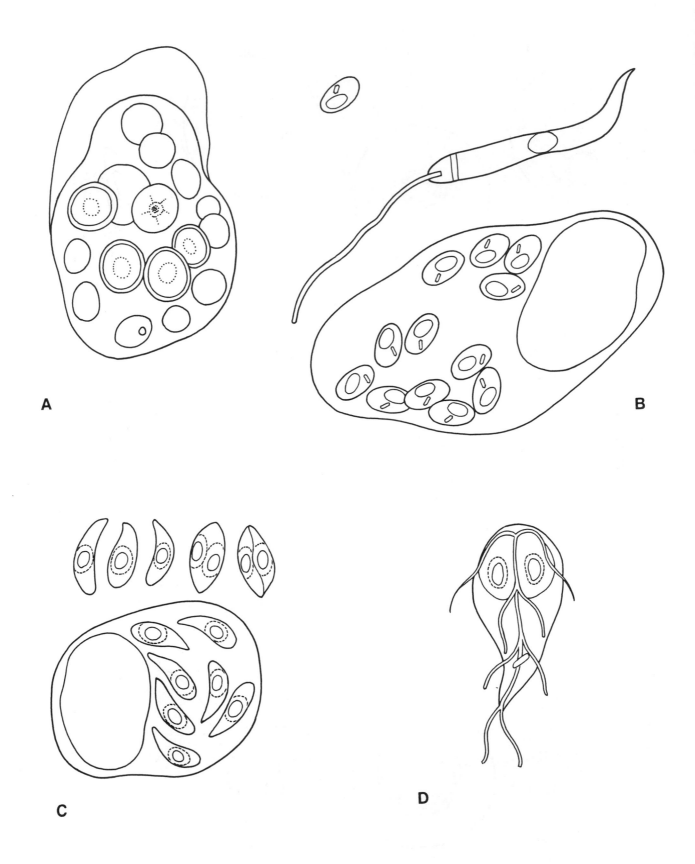

Fig.16.16 A - Entamoeba histolytica: cyst, B - Leishmania: amastigote,
         promastigote, intracellular amastigotes, C - Toxoplasma
         gondii: trophozoites, cyst, D - Giardia lamblia: trophozoite,

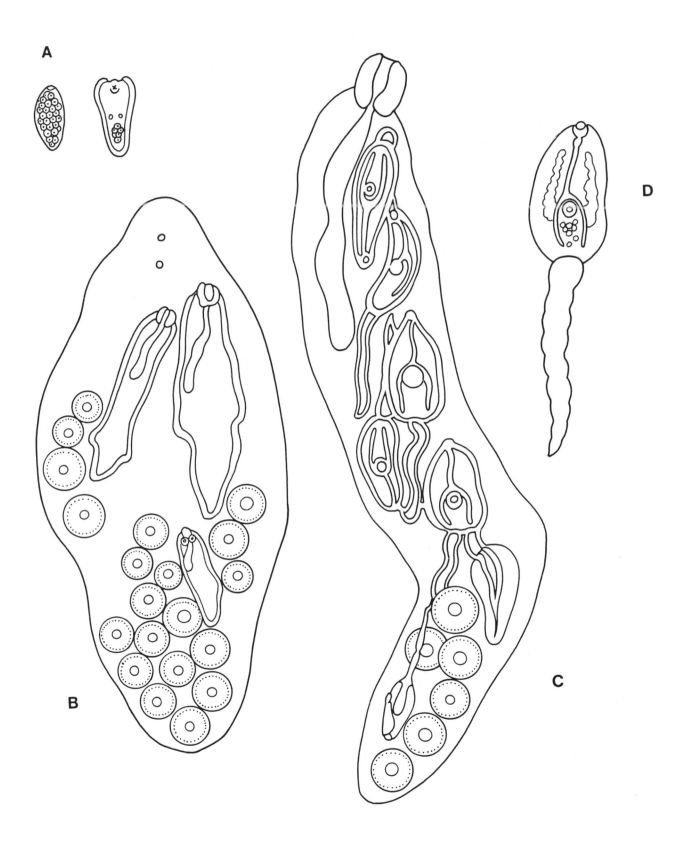

Fig.16.17 Fasciola hepatica: A - ovum 140 μ x 75 μ, B - adult 2.5cm x 1cm,
C - Redia, D - Cercaria

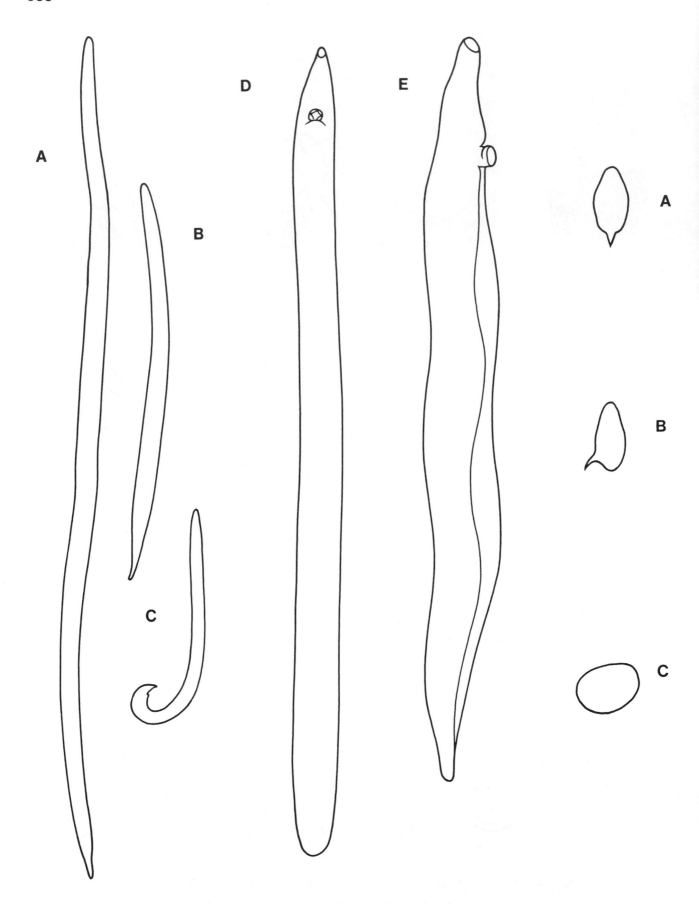

Fig.16.18 Strongyloides stercoralis: A - ♀ L 2.2mm, B - Rhabditiform larva,
    C - ♂ L 0.7mm
    Schistoma sp: D - ♀ L 1 - 2cm, E - ♂ L 1 - 2cm
    Ova: A - S. haematobium, B - S. mansoni, C - S. japonicum

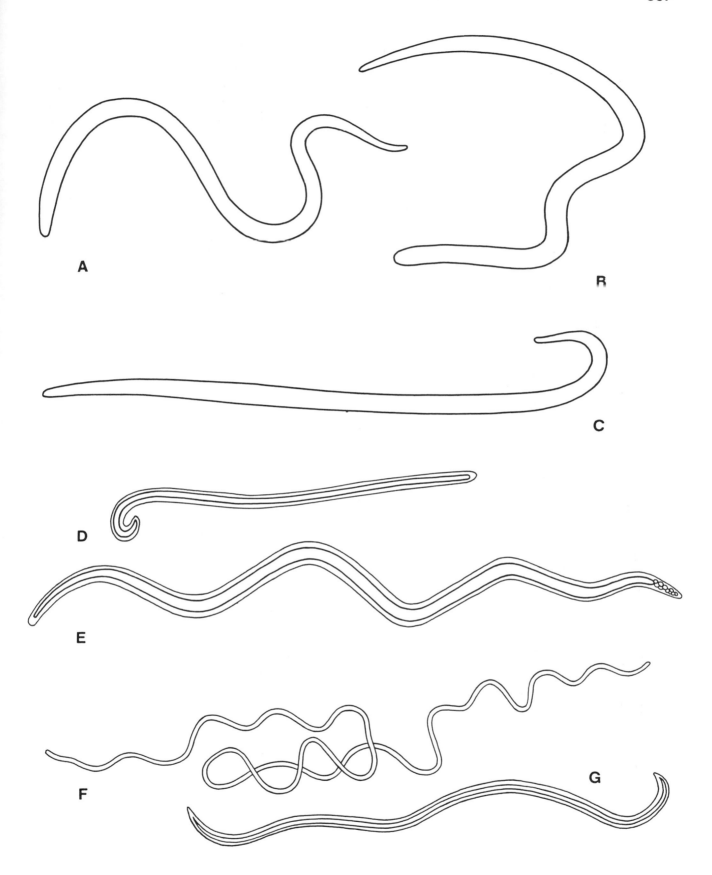

Fig.16.19 Filarial Worms, A - Mansonella ozzardi 175 - 240 x 4.5 μ
B - Dipetalonema (Acanthocheilonema) perstans 200 x 4.5 μ
C - Dipetalonema streptocera 180 - 240 x 3 μ
D - ♂ Wuchereria bancrofti 40 x 0.1 μ
E - ♀ Wuchereria bancrofti 100 x 0.25mm
F - Onchocerca volvulus 400 x 0.3mm
G - ♀ Loa loa 40 x 0.3mm

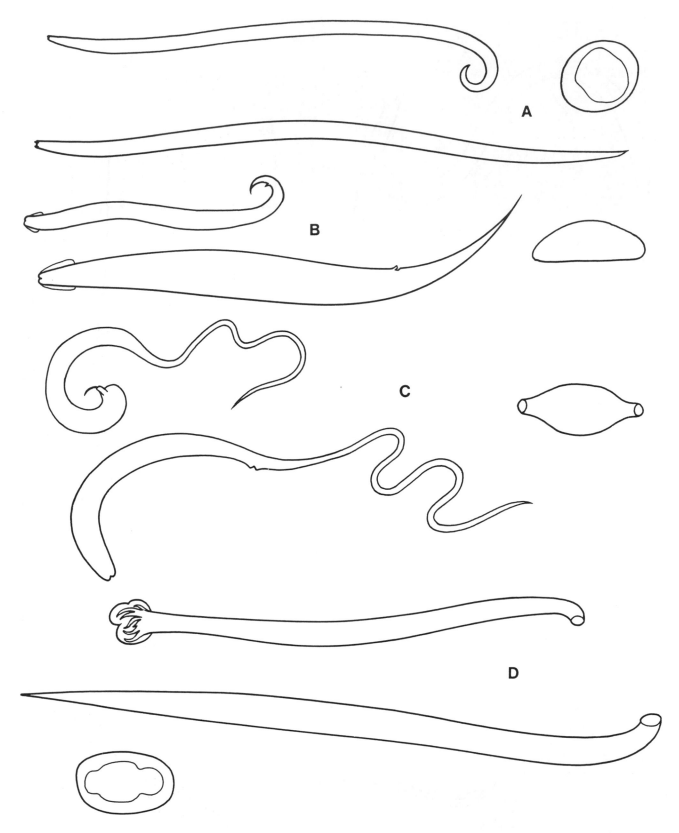

Fig.16.20 A - Roundworms ♂ and ♀ , eg. Ascaris L 15 - 35cms, ovum 70 x 50 μ

B - Thread/Pin/Seat worms ♂ and ♀ eg. Enterobius L 1cm, ovum 55 x 25 μ

C - Whipworm ♂ and ♀ eg. Trichuris L 40mm, ovum 50 x 22 μ

D - Hookworm ♂ and ♀ eg. Ancylostoma and Necator L 1cm, ovum 58 x 36 μ

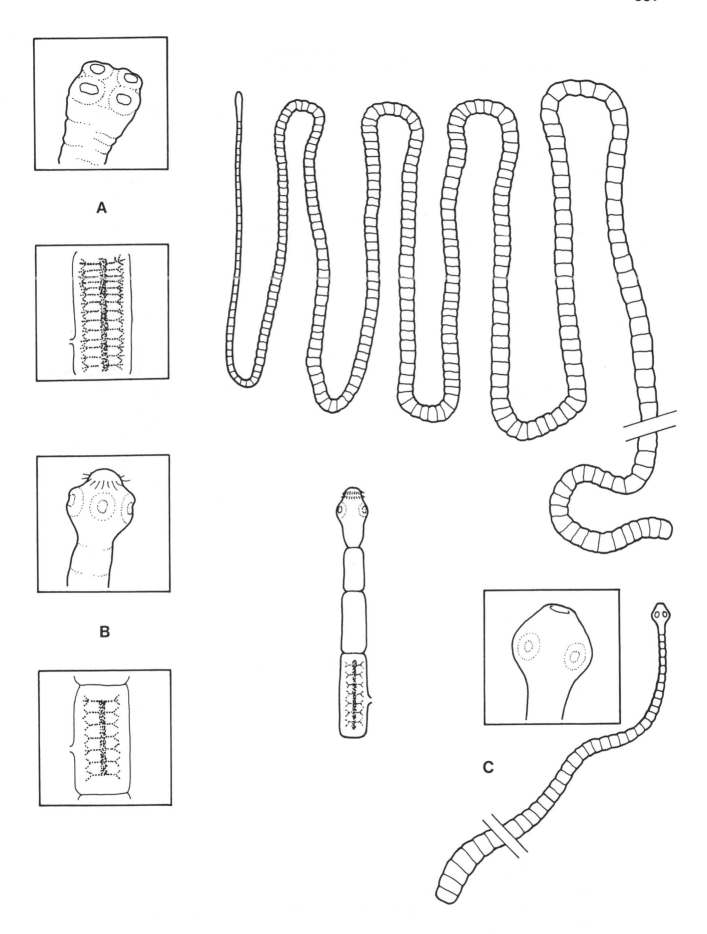

Fig.16.21 Tapeworms: A - Taenia saginata L up to 30ft, scolex and gravid proglottid, B - Taenia solium L up to 30ft, scolex and gravid proglottid, C - Hymenolepis nana L 2.5 - 5 cms

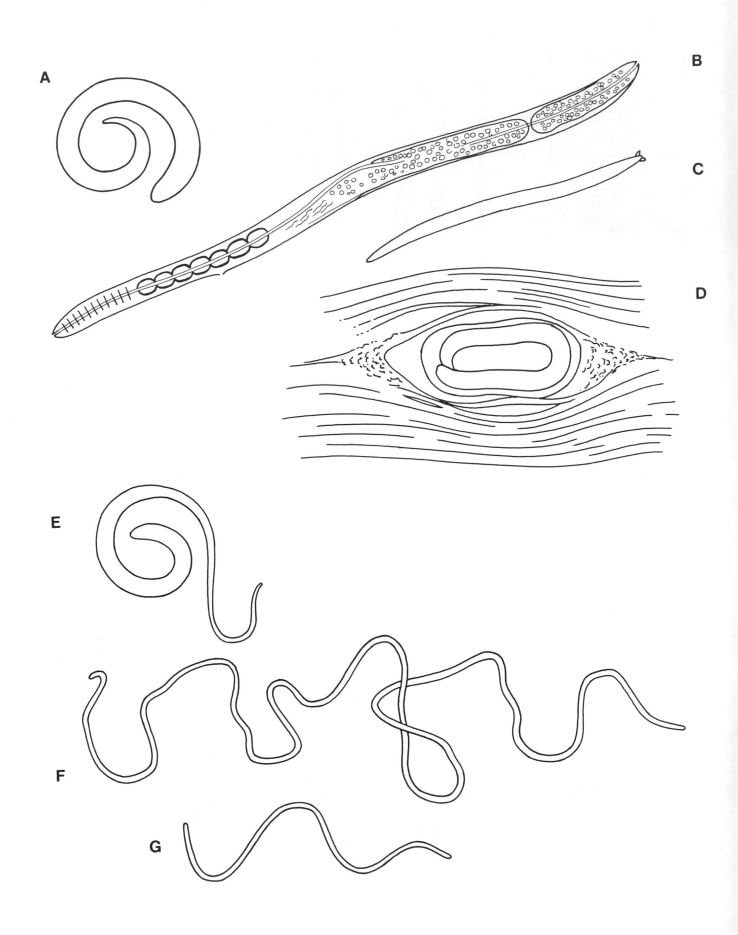

Fig. 16.22 Trichinella spiralis: A - larva, B - ♀ , C - ♂ , D - larva in skeletal tissue, Dracunculus medinensis: E - larva, F - ♀ , G - ♂

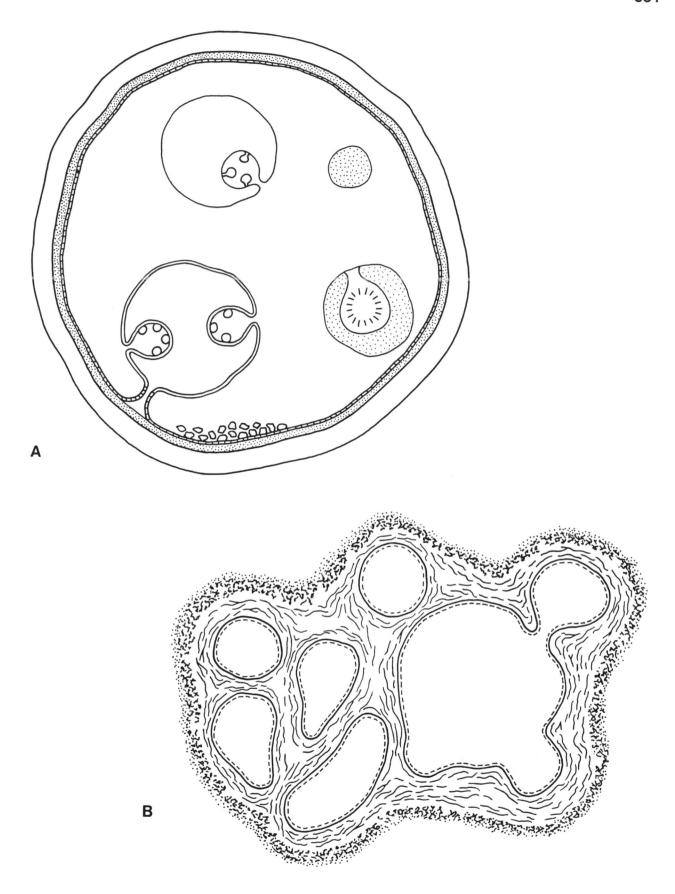

Fig.16.23 Echinococcal cysts: A - Hydatid, B - Multilocular

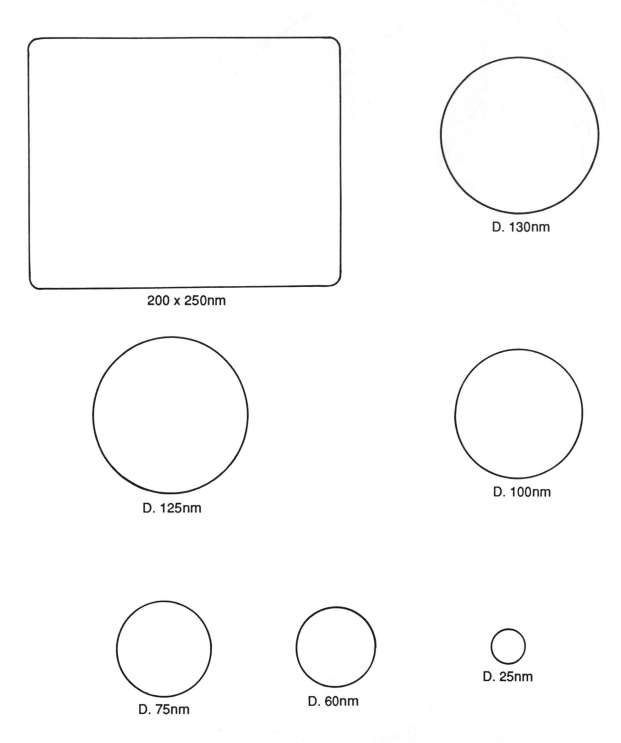

200 x 250nm

D. 130nm

D. 125nm

D. 100nm

D. 75nm

D. 60nm

D. 25nm

Fig.16.24 Virus size chart

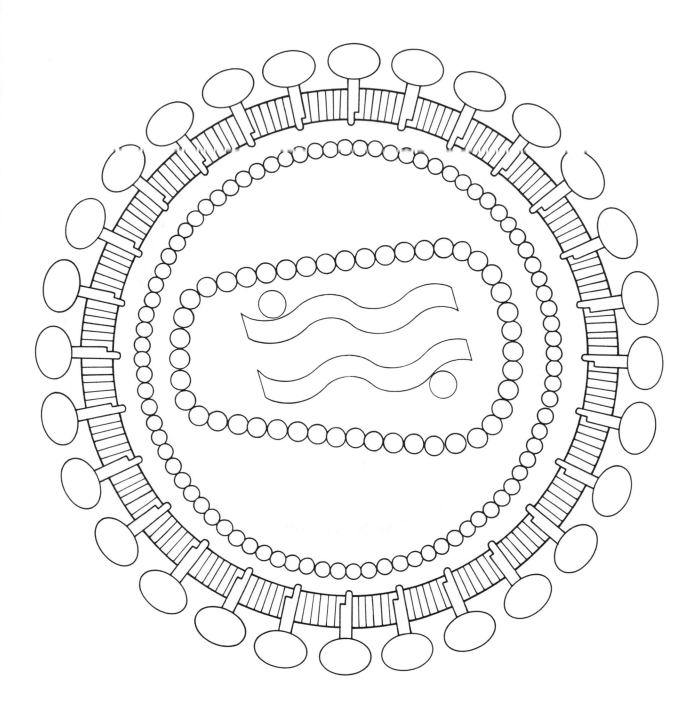

Fig. 16.25 HIV

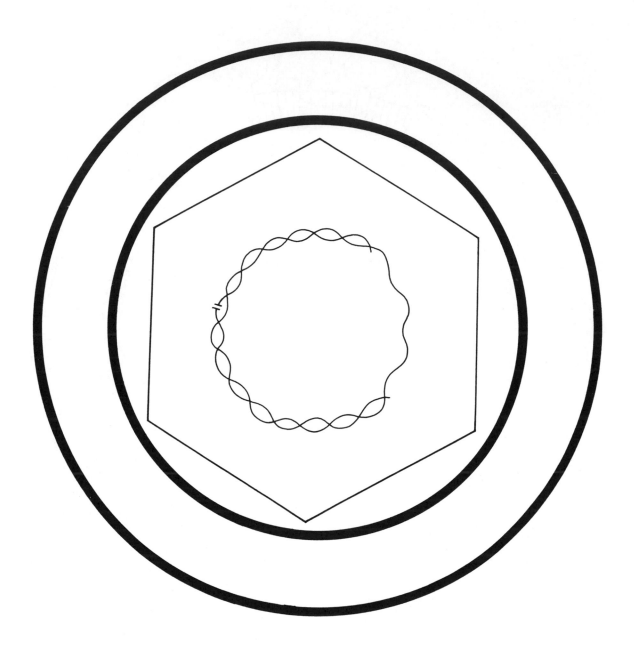

Fig 16.26   HBV

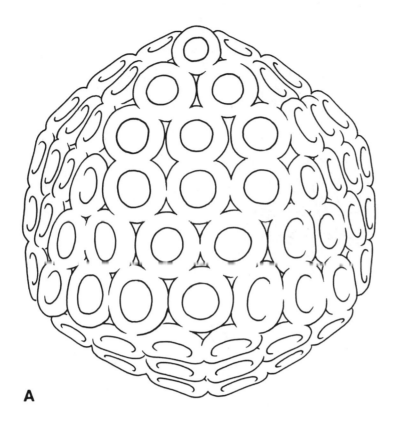

A

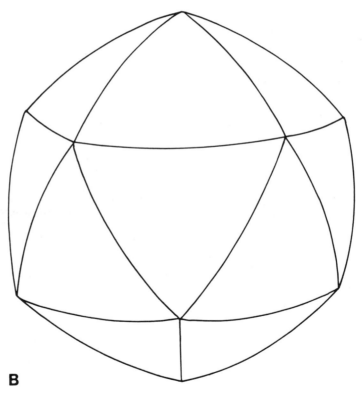

B

Fig 16.27   A - Calicivirus, B - Reovirus

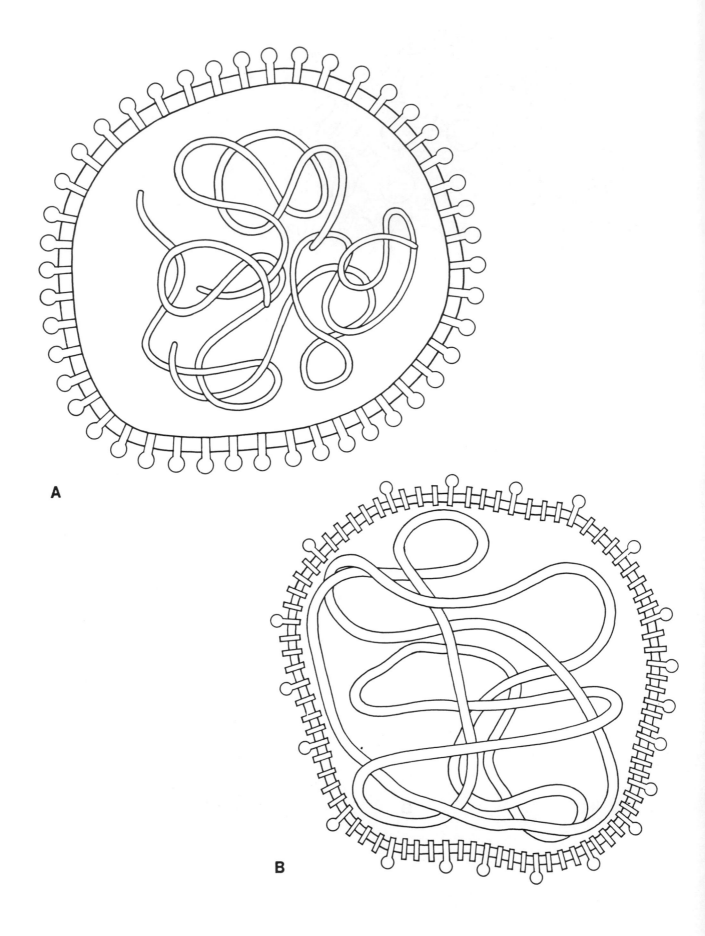

Fig. 16.28   A - Bunyavirus, B - Paramyxovirus

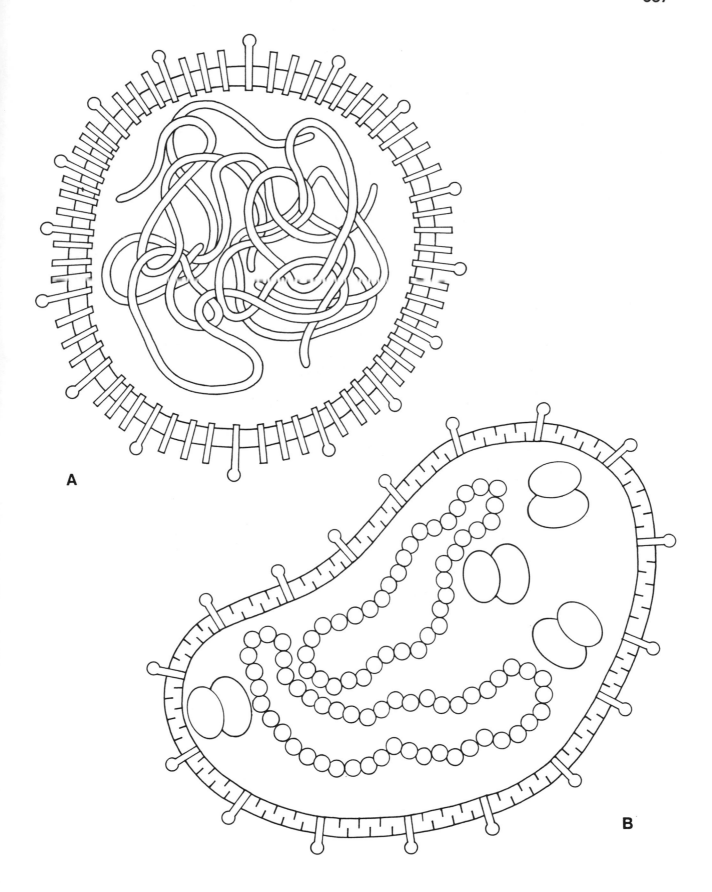

Fig 16.29   A - Orthomyxovirus, B - Arenavirus

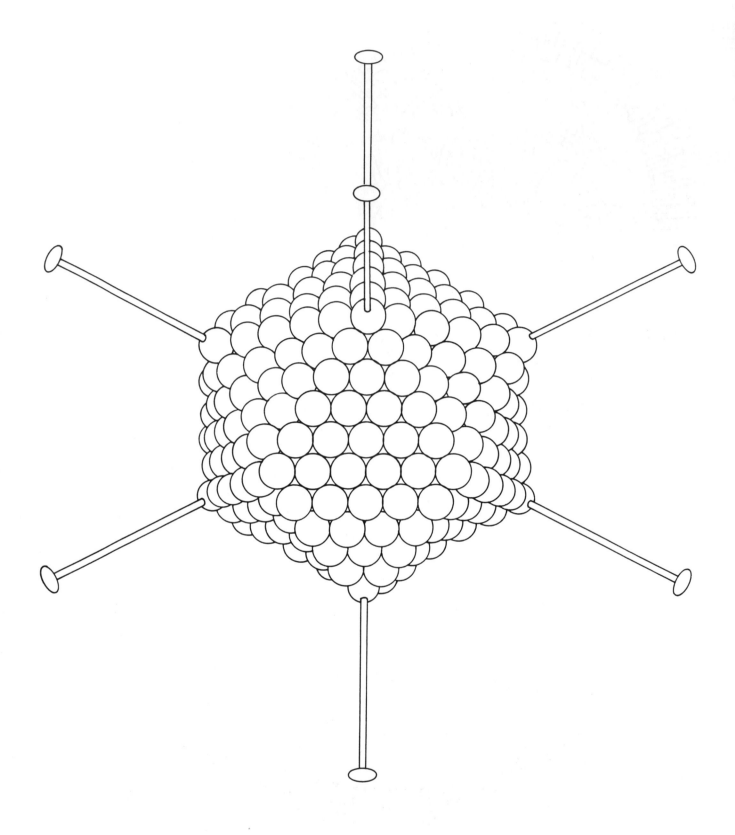

Fig 16.30   Adenovirus

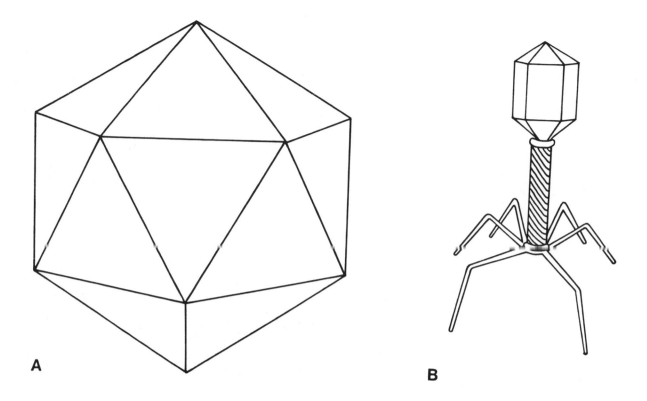

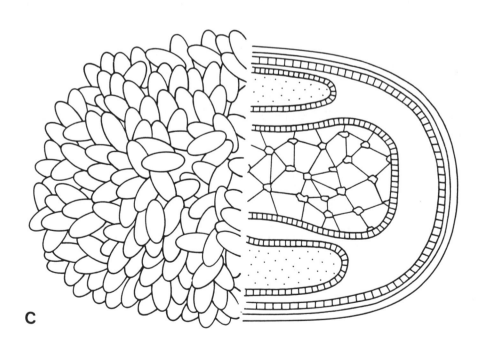

Fig 16.31   A - Toga/Papova/Parvo/Picorna virus, B - Bacteriophage,
C - Pox virus

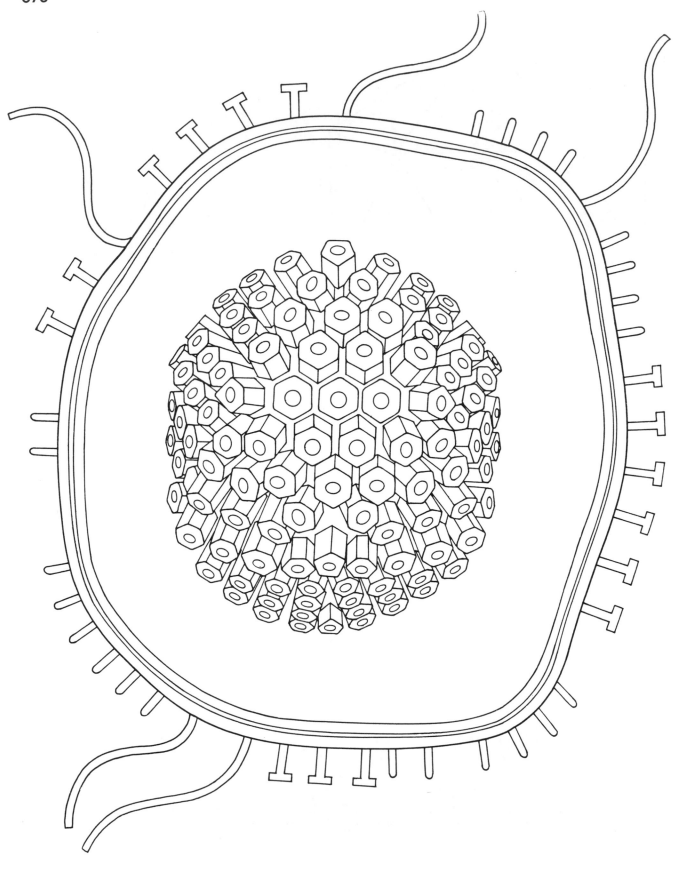

Fig 16.32   Herpes virus

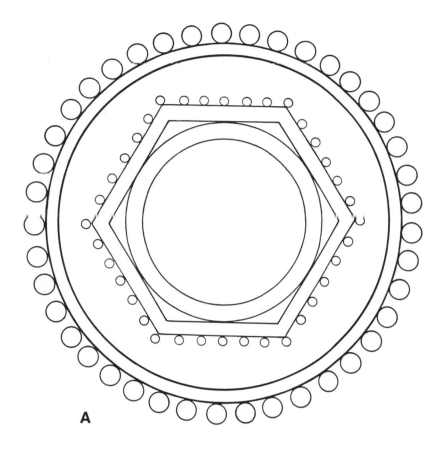

A

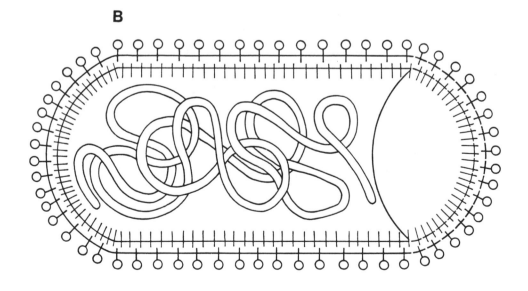

B

Fig 16.33   A - Retrovirus, B - Rhabdovirus

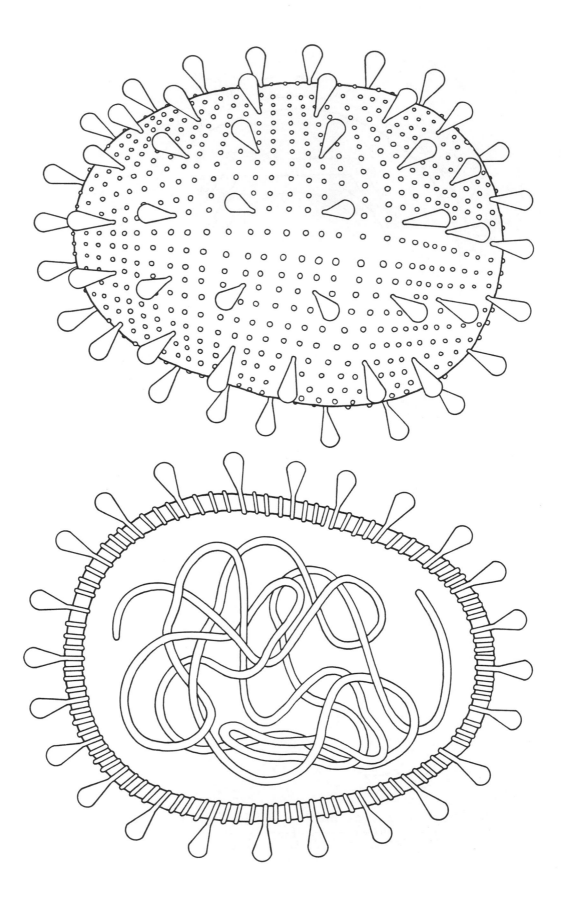

Fig 16.34   Corona virus: capiscid and section

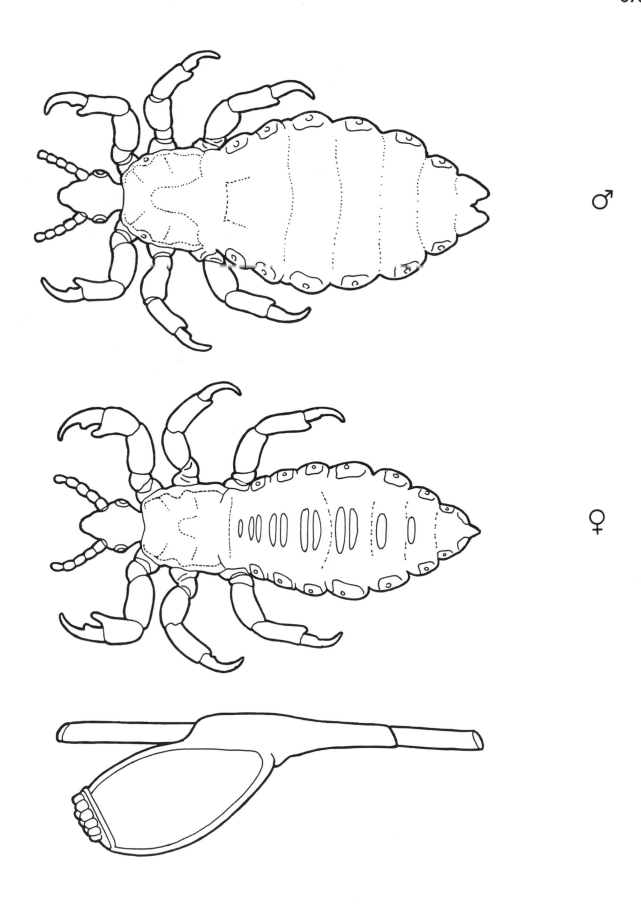

16.35 Human louse, Pediculus humanus humanus, egg and adults

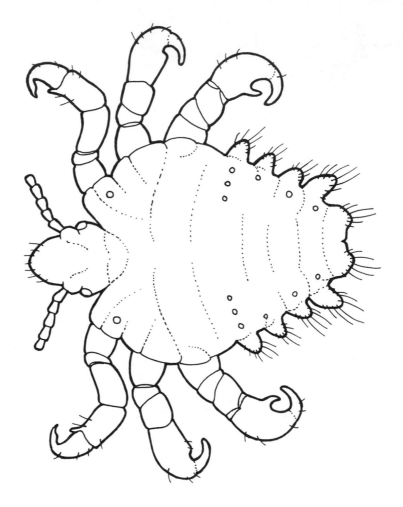

Fig.16.36 Pubic or crab louse, Phthirus pubis

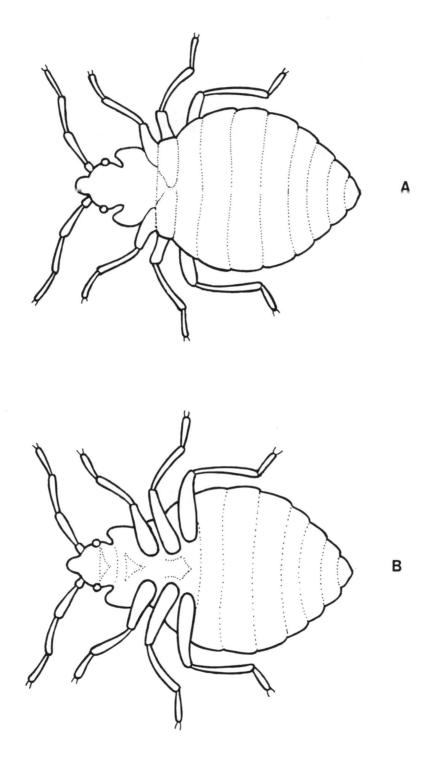

A

B

Fig.16.37 Bedbugs, Cimicidae, dorsal and ventral views

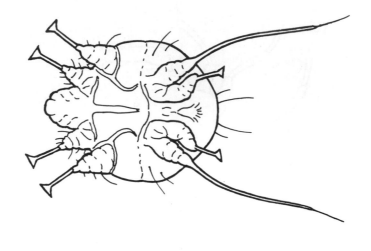

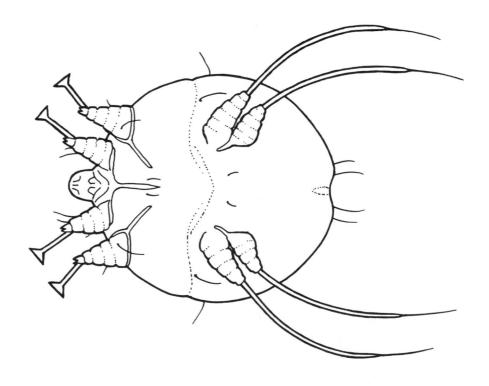

Fig.16.38 Scabies, Sarcoptes scabii

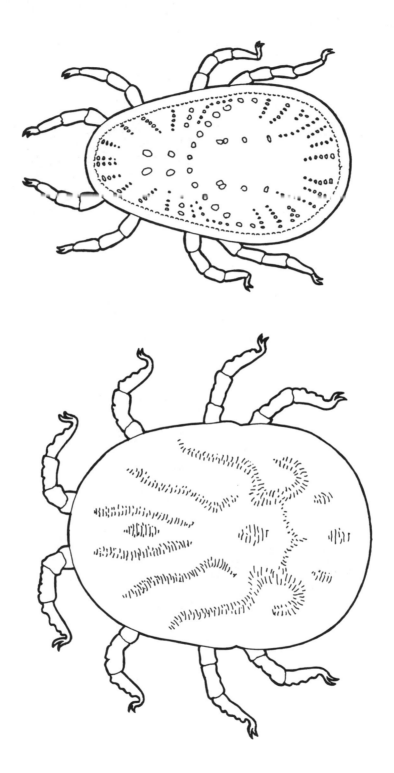

Fig.16.39 Soft ticks, Argas persicus and Ornithodorus moubata

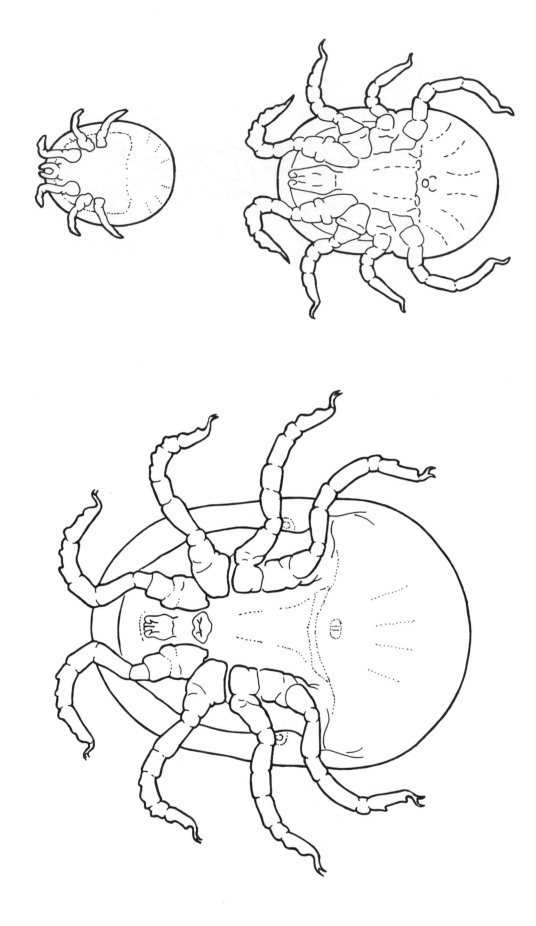

Fig. 16.40 Soft ticks, Ornithodorus moubata, larva, nymph and adult

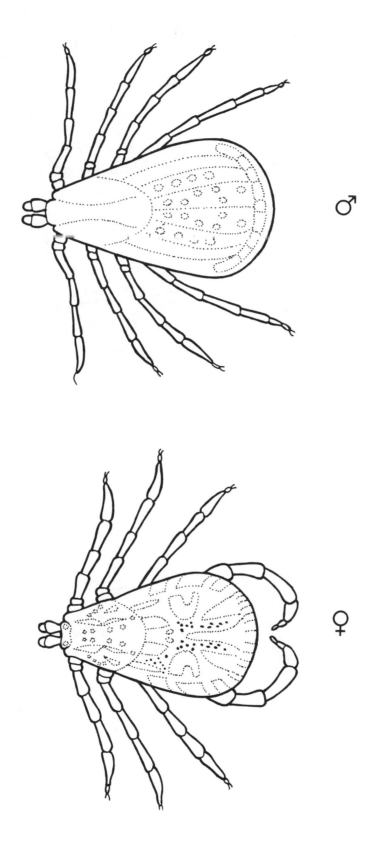

♂

♀

Fig.16.41 Hard ticks, Ixodes

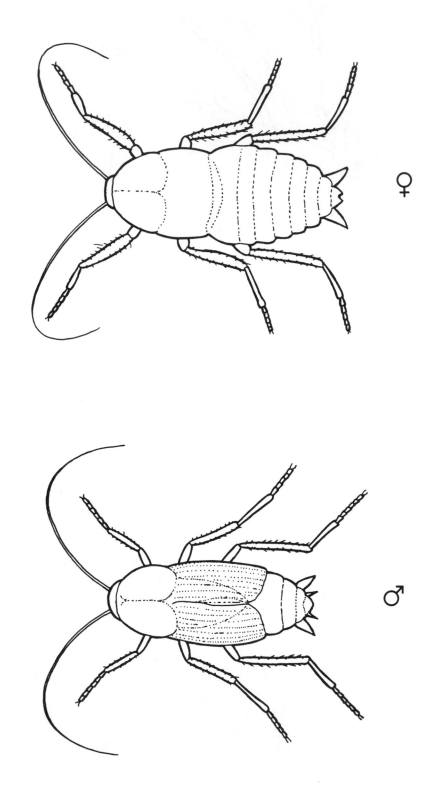

Fig.16.42 Cockroach, Blatella orientalis

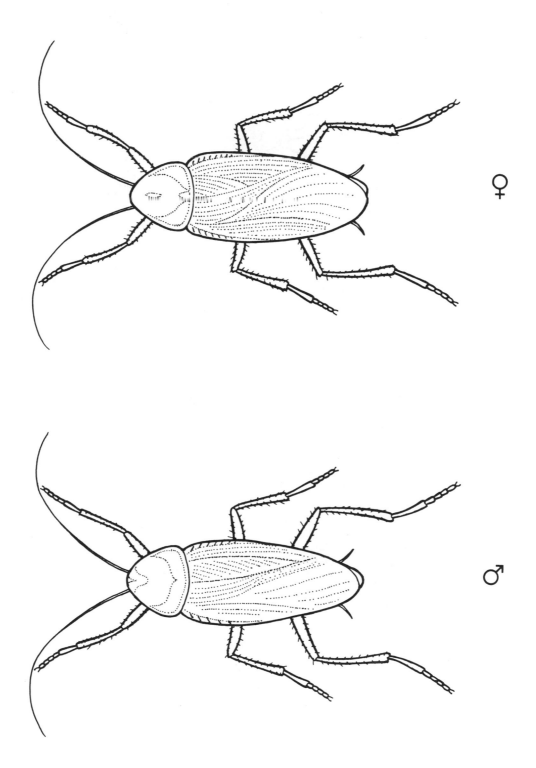

Fig.16.43 Cockroach, Periplaneta americana

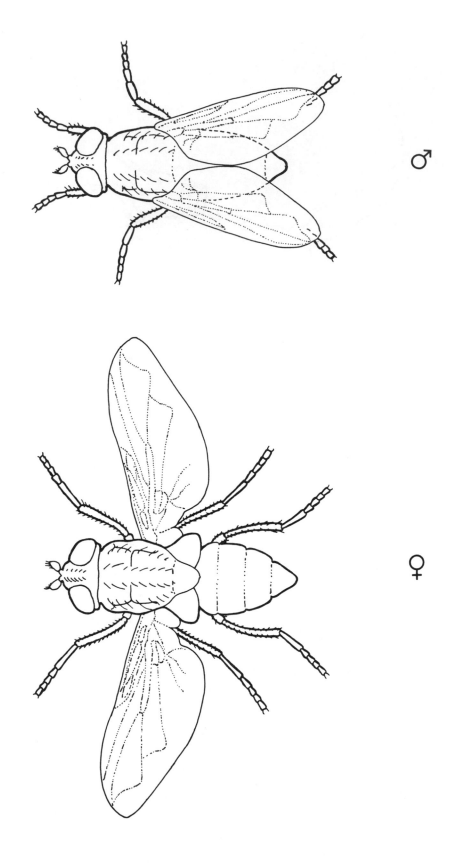

♂

♀

Fig.16.44 Housefly, Musca domestica

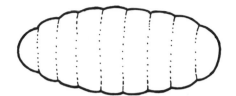

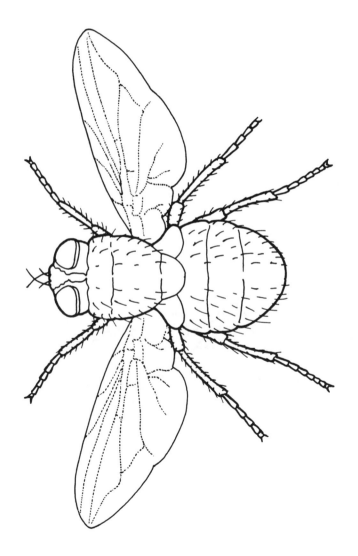

Fig.16.45 Bluebottle, Calliphora, pupa and adult

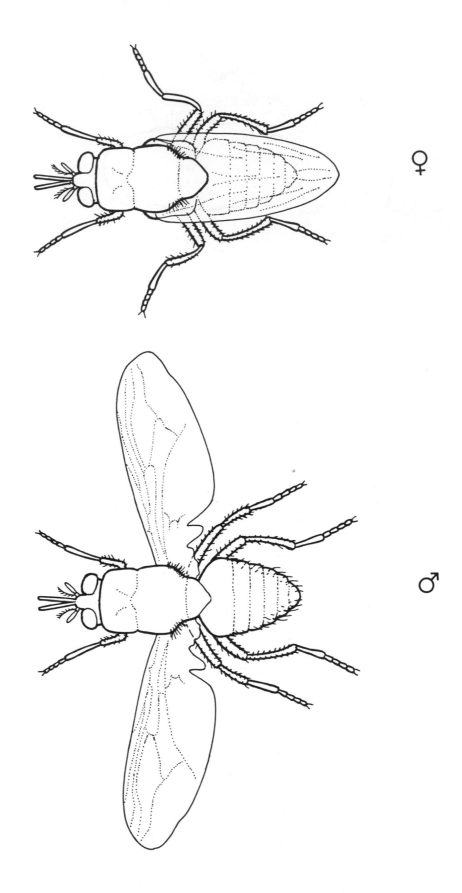

Fig.16.46 Tsetse fly, Glossina

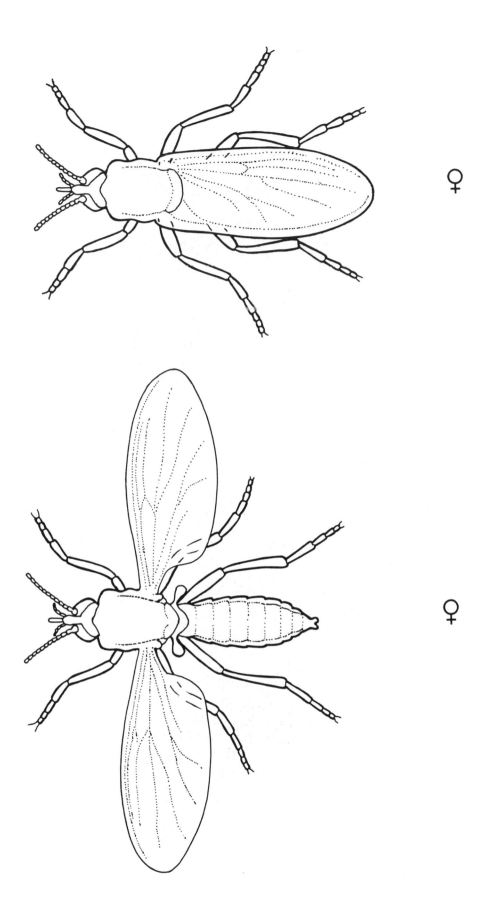

Fig. 16.47 Biting midge, Culicoides

B

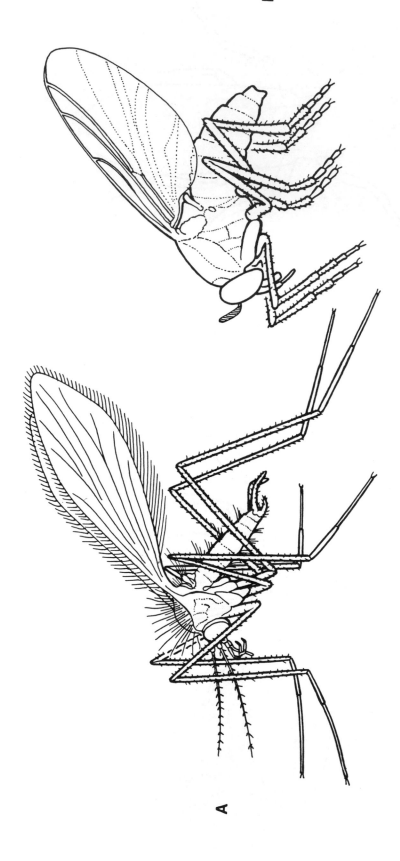

A

Fig.16.48   A - Black fly, Simulium, and B - Sandfly,Phlebotomus

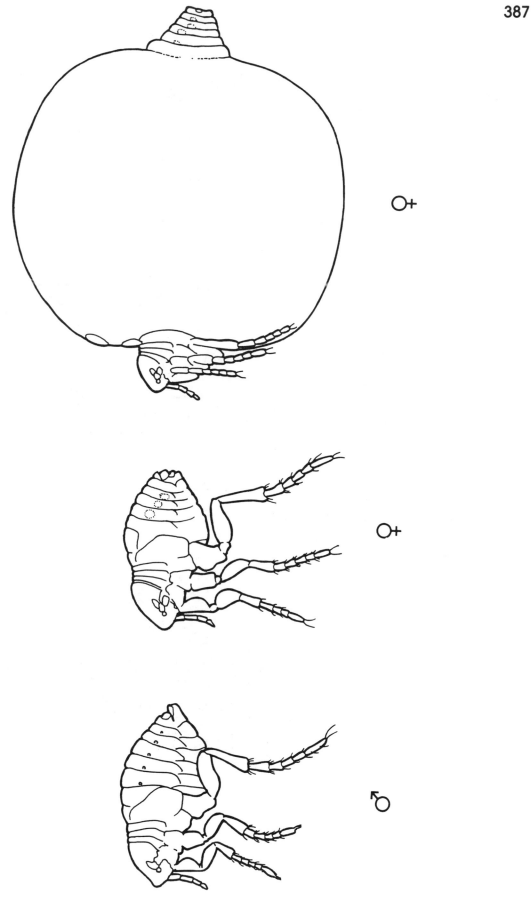

Fig. 16.49 Jigger flea, *Tunga penetrans*, gravid ♀ ♀ and ♂

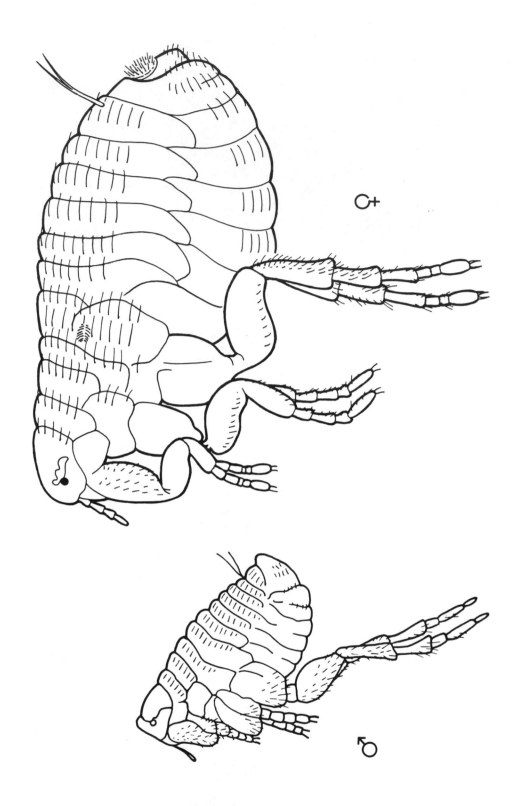

Fig.16.50 Plague flea, Xenopsylla cheopis

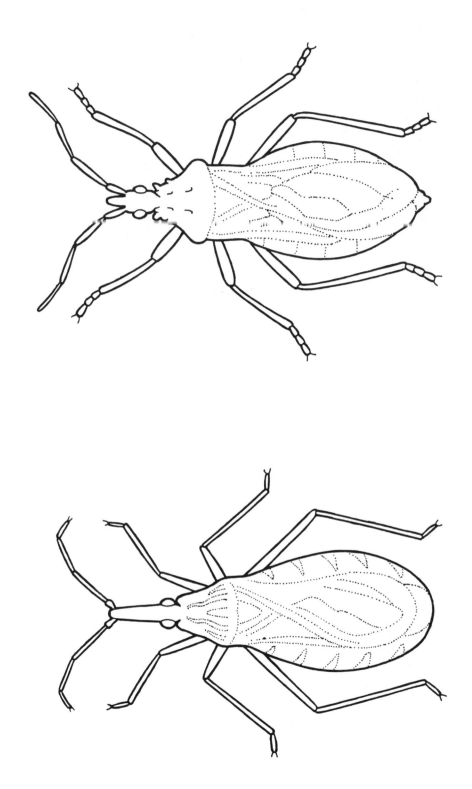

Fig.16.51 Triatomine bugs, Reduviidae

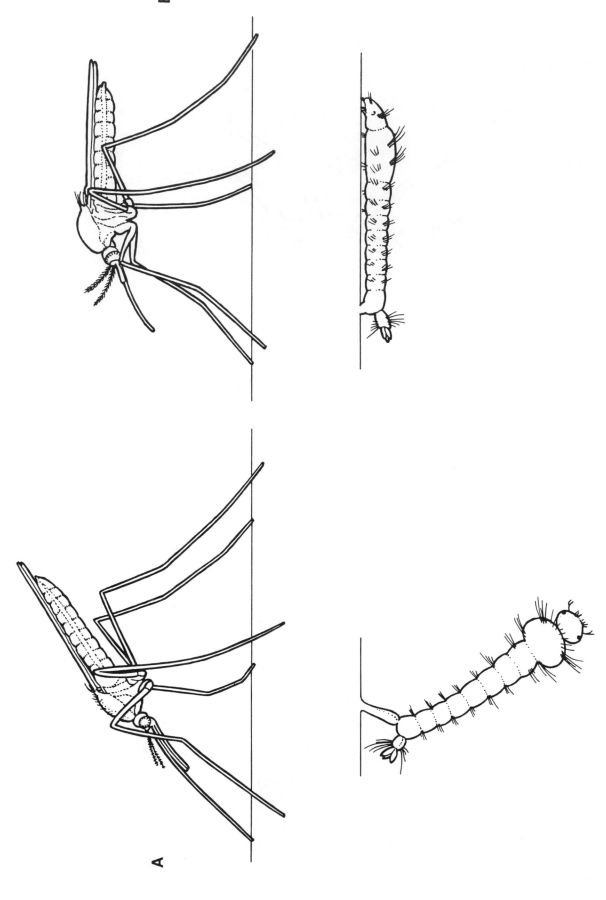

Fig.16.52 Mosquito, A - Anopheles and B - Culicine: larva and adult

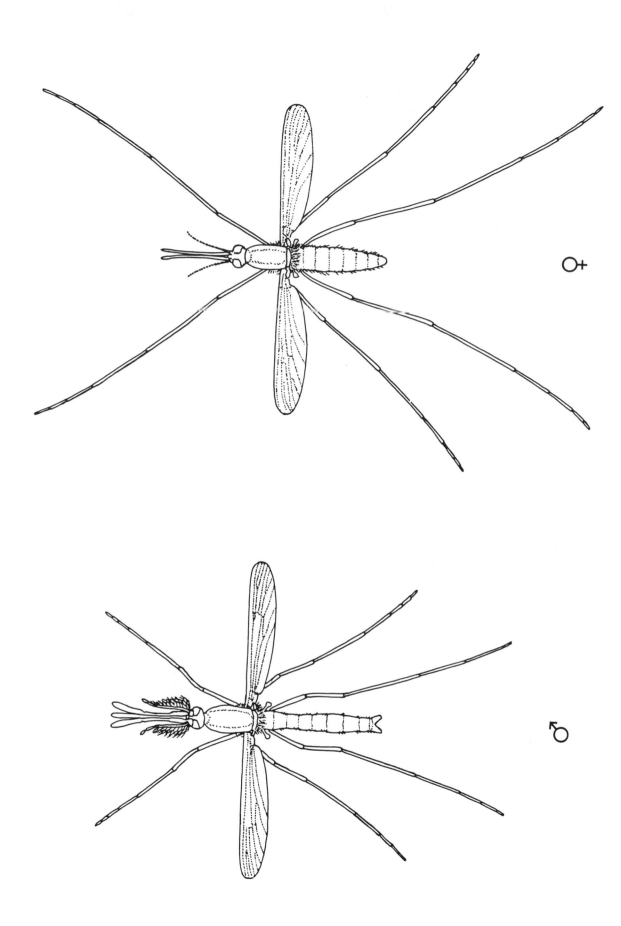

Fig.16.53 Mosquito, Anopheles

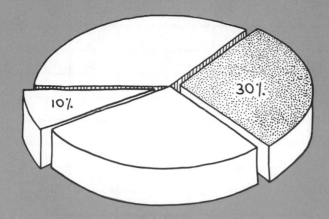

Section 17

Graph, Chart and Layout Guides

In addition to providing the base for constructing graphs, charts, histograms etc. the sheets in this section will also be found useful in a host of other design projects including scheme layouts, floor plans, paste-up guides etc. Use them under tracing paper, or on a light box, or under your OHP trransparencies. Sheet no. 17.11 will help you construct legible tables, charts etc. for slides when using a typewriter as your lettering method.

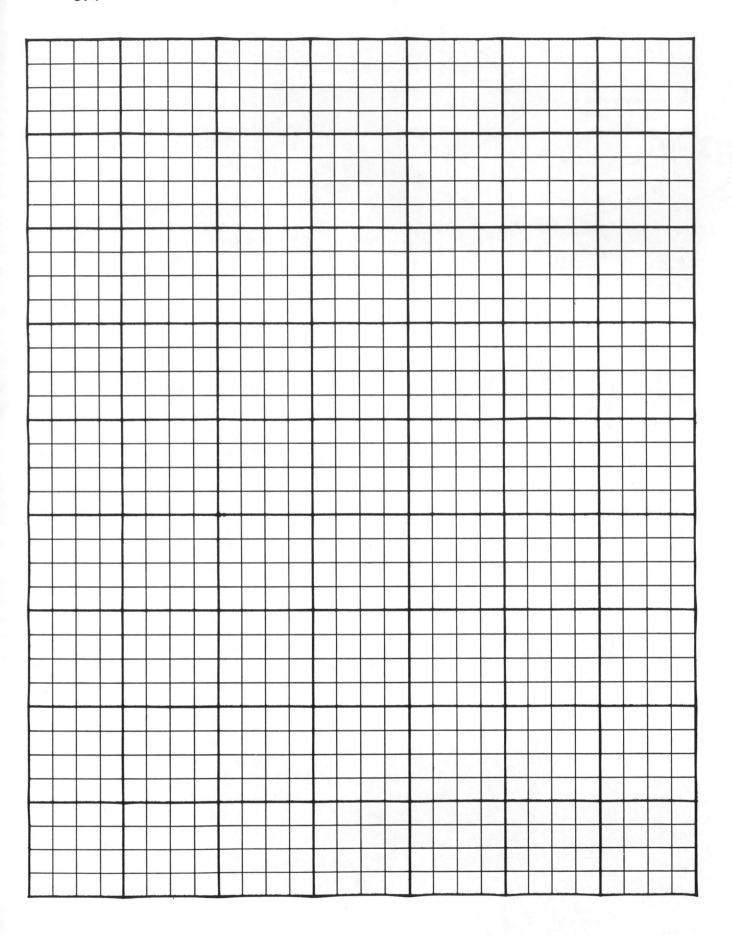

Fig. 17.1   Plan grid 4 to 1 inch

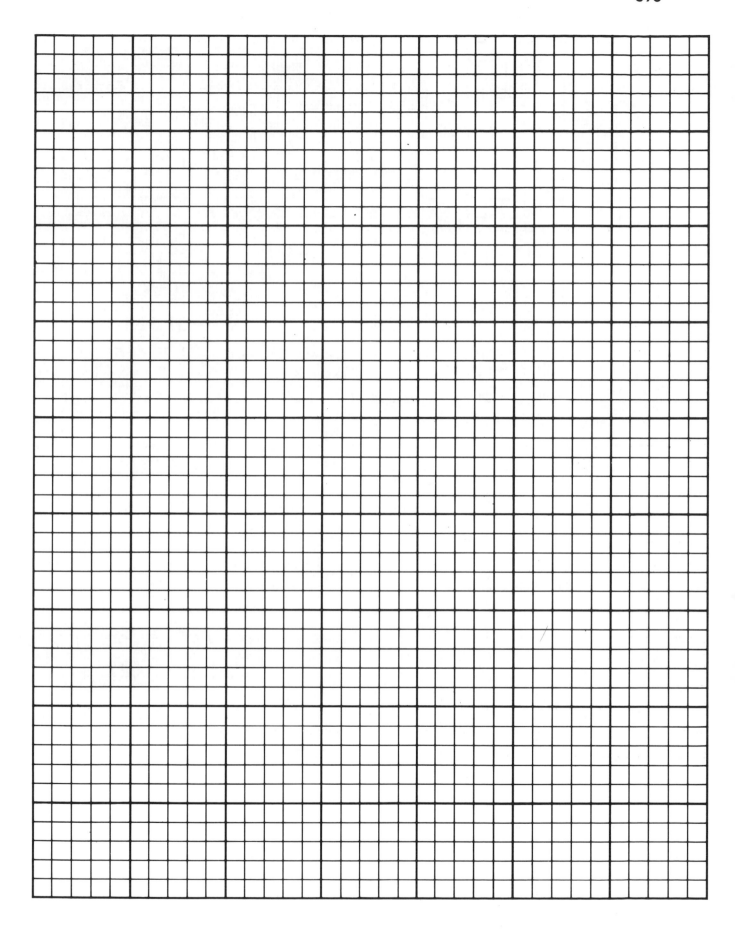

Fig. 17.2   Plan grid 5 to 1 inch

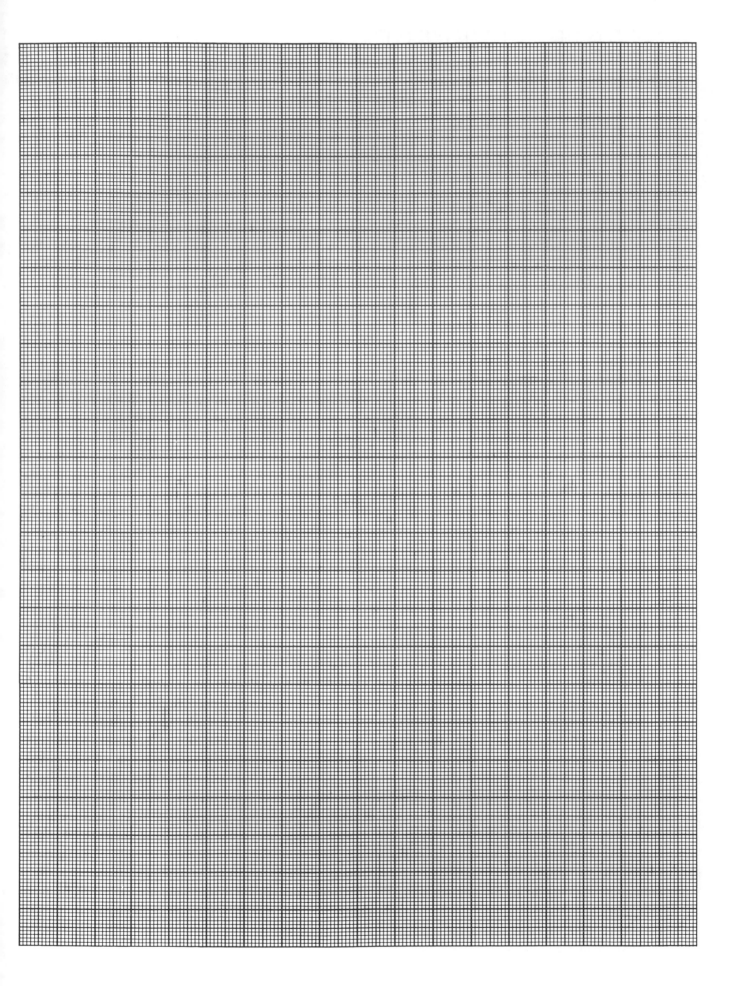

Fig. 17.3   Plan grid 10 to 1 centimetre

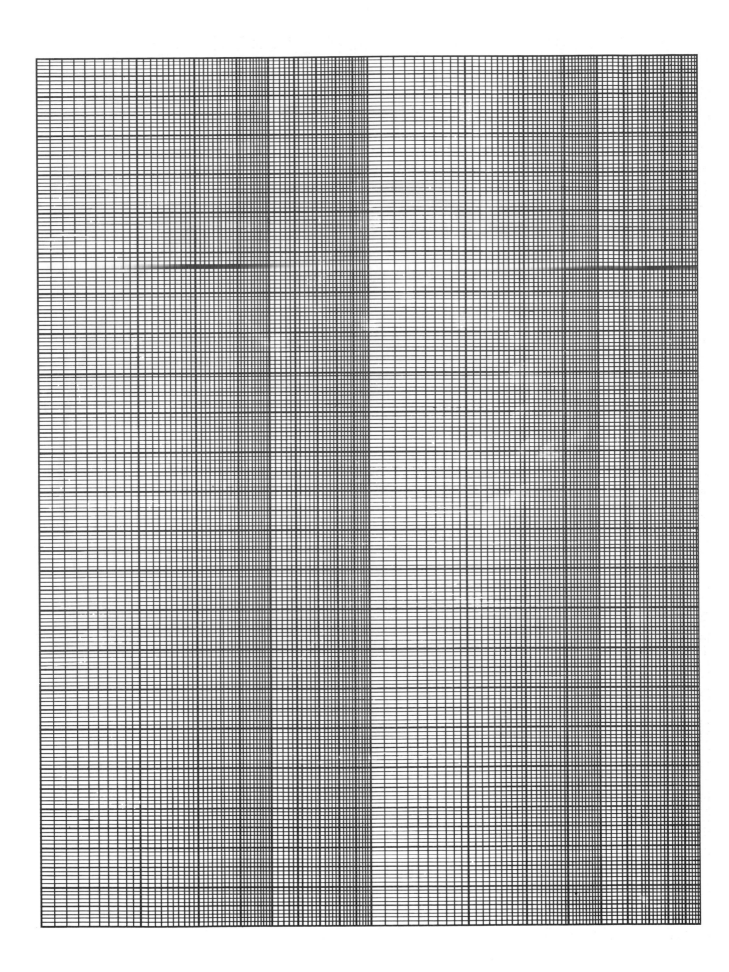

Fig. 17.4   Logarithmic grid

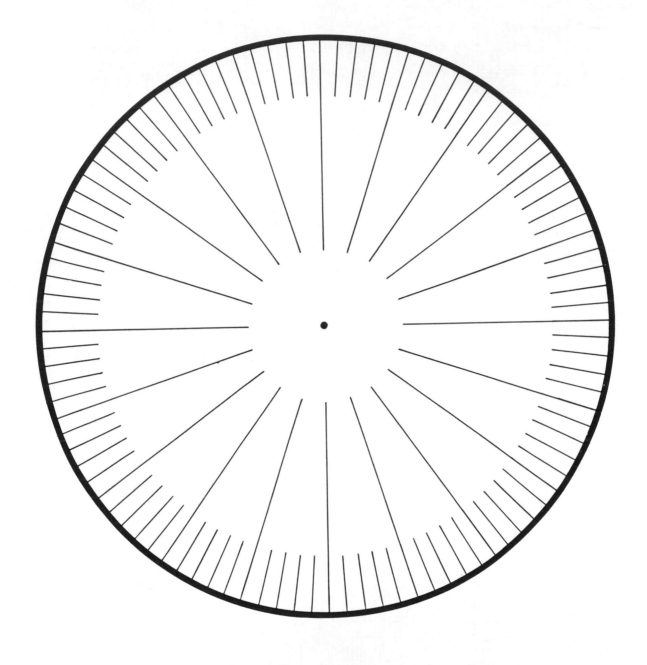

Fig. 17.5   Pie chart guide, 100 divisions

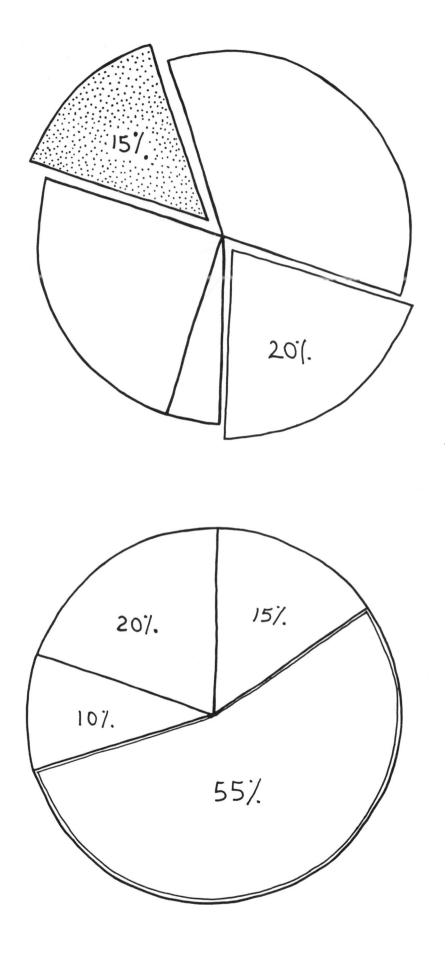

Fig. 17.6   Pie chart examples

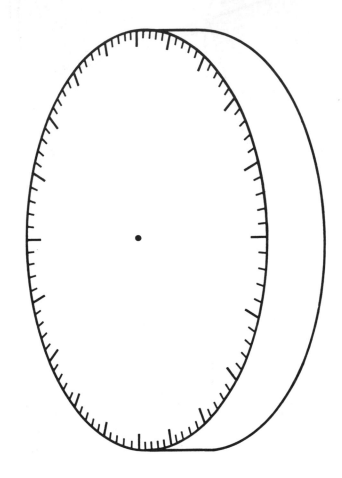

Fig. 17.7   Perspective pie chart, 100 divisions

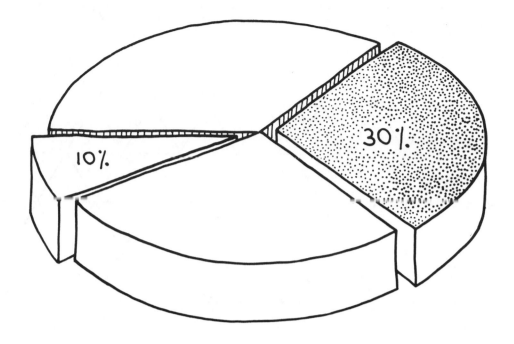

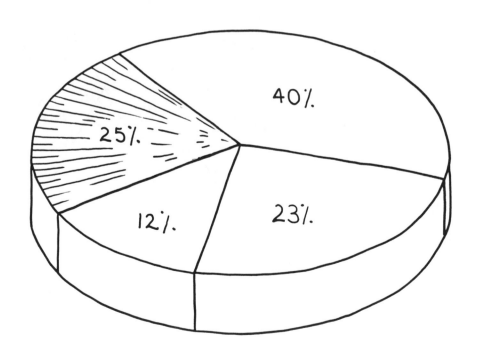

Fig. 17.8   Perspective pie chart examples

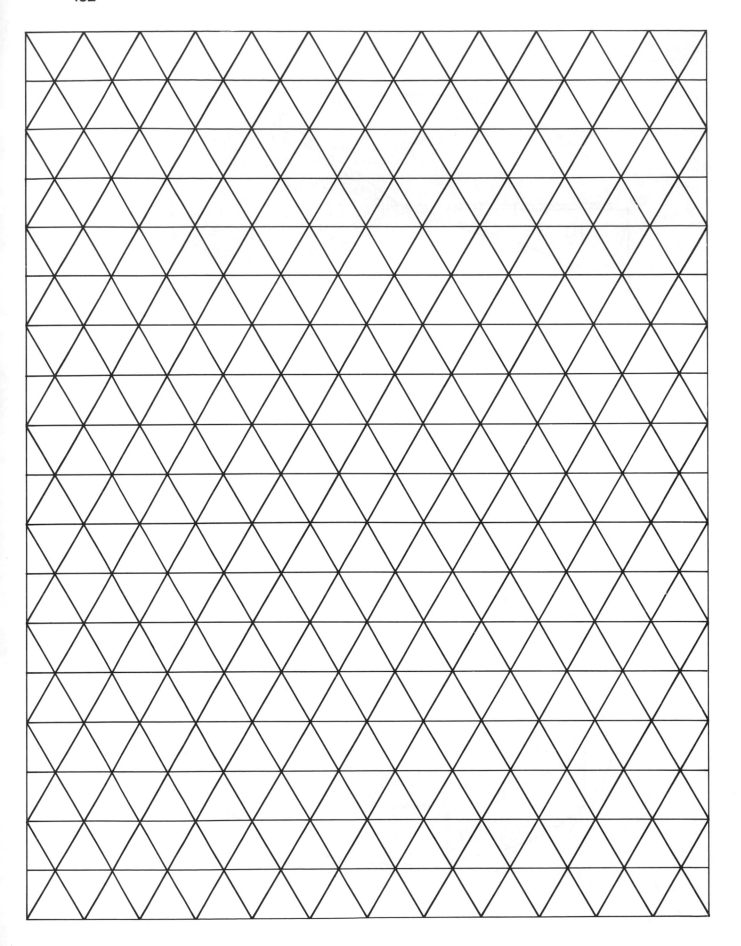

Fig. 17.9   Isometric projection grid

Lay this sheet over grid No 15.9 to see how it was constructed.

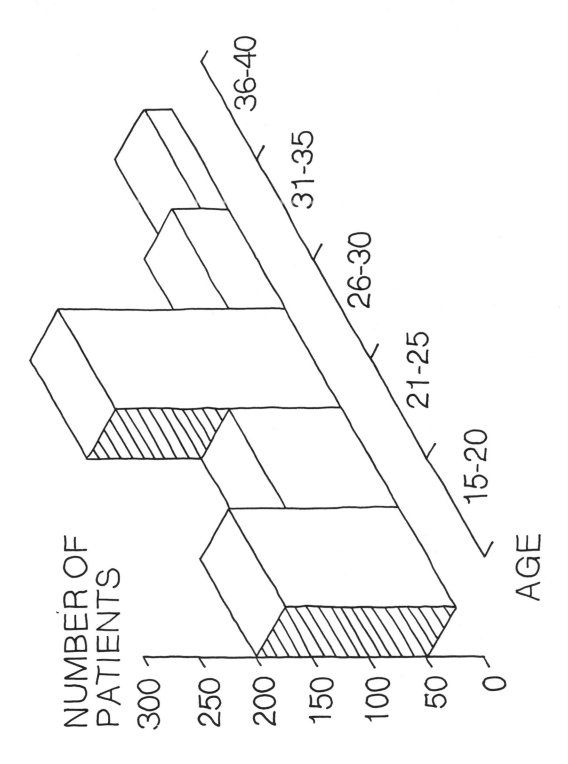

Fig. 17.10   Isometric 3 - dimensional bar chart example

404

When using a typewriter to create lettering in tables, charts, graphs, for 35mm slides the text and graphics should be confined within these outlines. This will ensure that the content is legible when projected on the screen. If you use a lot of material which is typewriter originated you might consider having a stock of good quality paper specially printed with these outlines in very pale blue. The pale blue line disappears in black and white photographic negatives.

Fig. 17.11 Typewriter guide

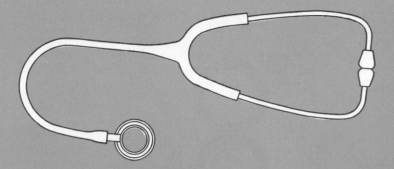

Section 18

Scientific Symbols, Pictograms and Animals

406

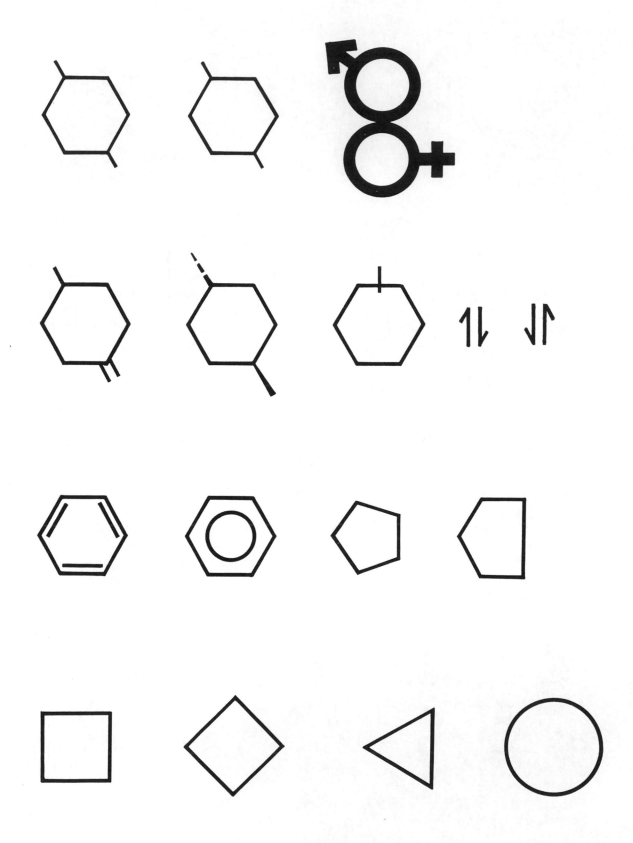

Fig.18.1 Geometric and chemical symbols, and ♂ and ♀

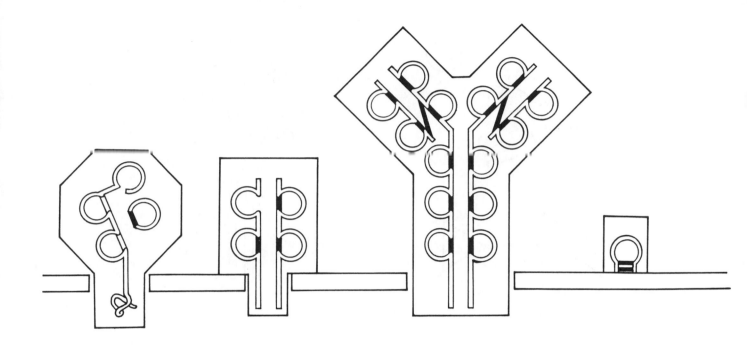

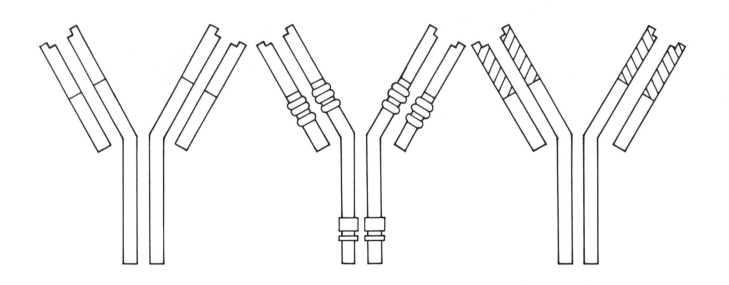

Fig. 18.2   Immunological symbols

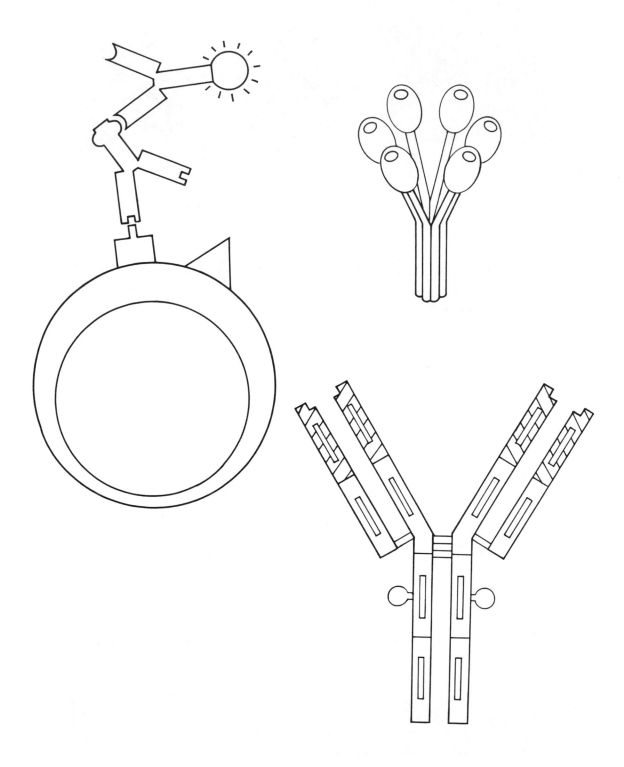

Fig. 18.3   Immunological symbols

409

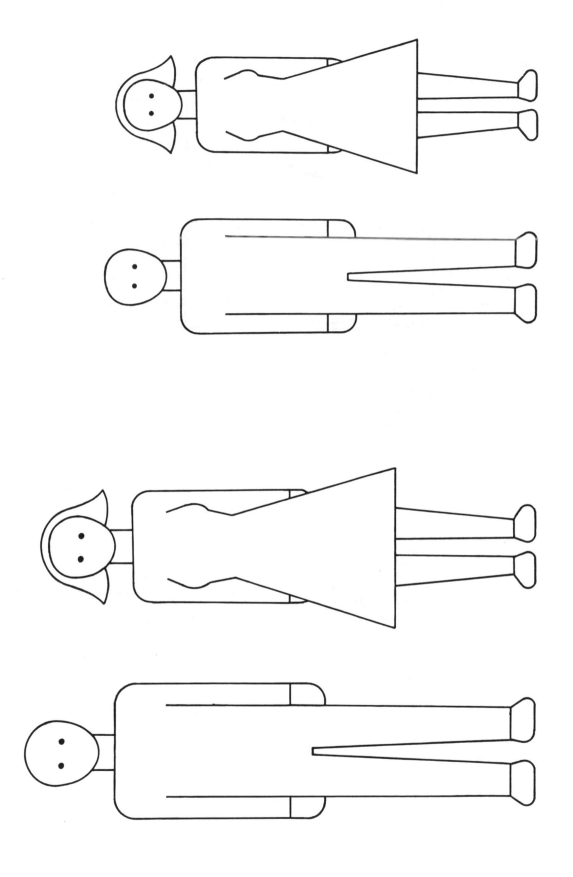

Fig. 18.4   Pictograms: ♂ and ♀ , adult and young

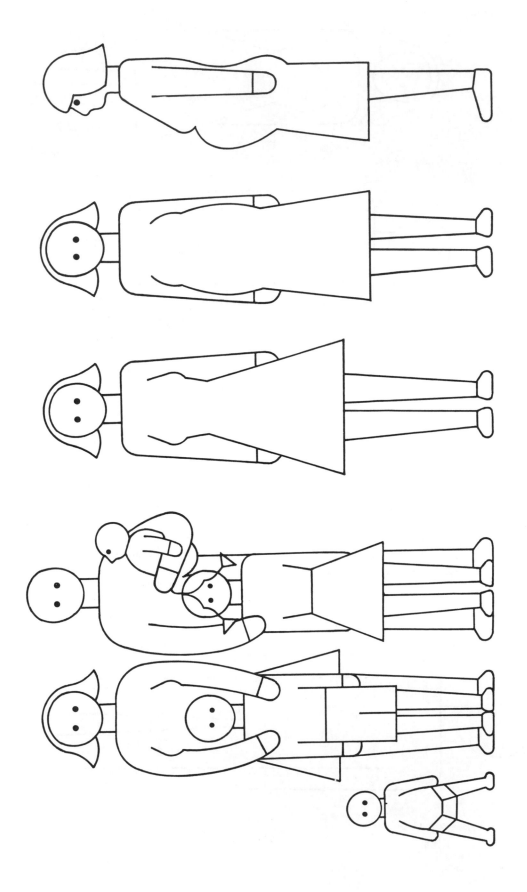

Fig. 18.5   Pictograms: family, ♀ and pregnant ♀

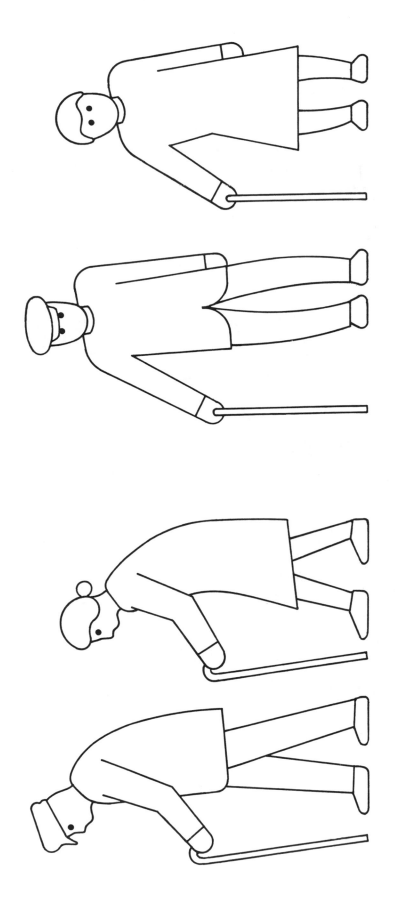

411

Fig. 18.6   Pictograms: ♂ and ♀ , elderly

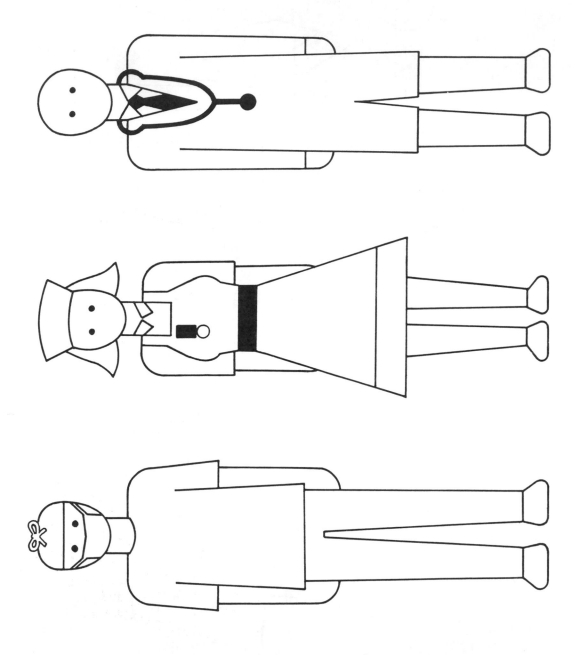

Fig.18.7   Pictograms: Surgeon, nurse, physician

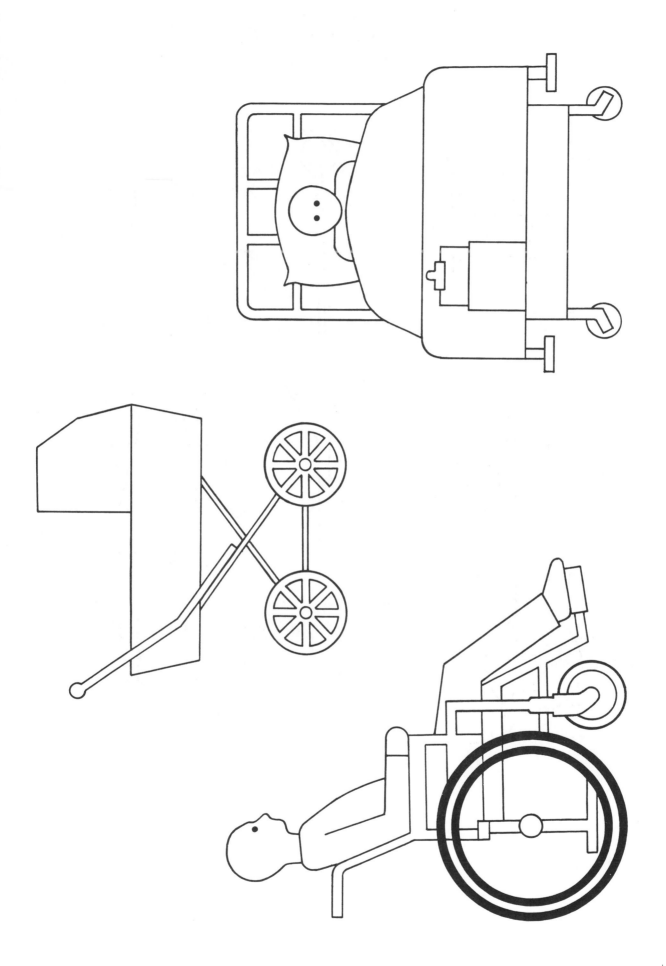

Fig. 18.8   Pictograms: Patient wheelchair, perambulator, patient bed

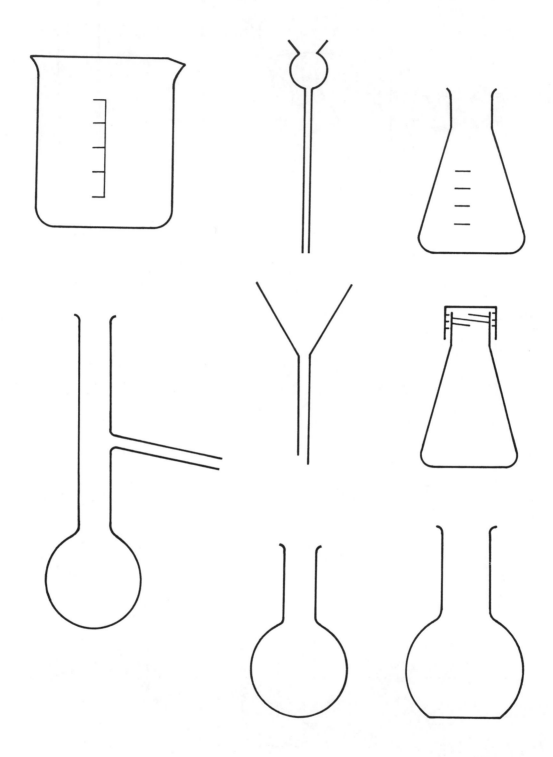

Fig.18.9   Pictograms: Laboratory glassware

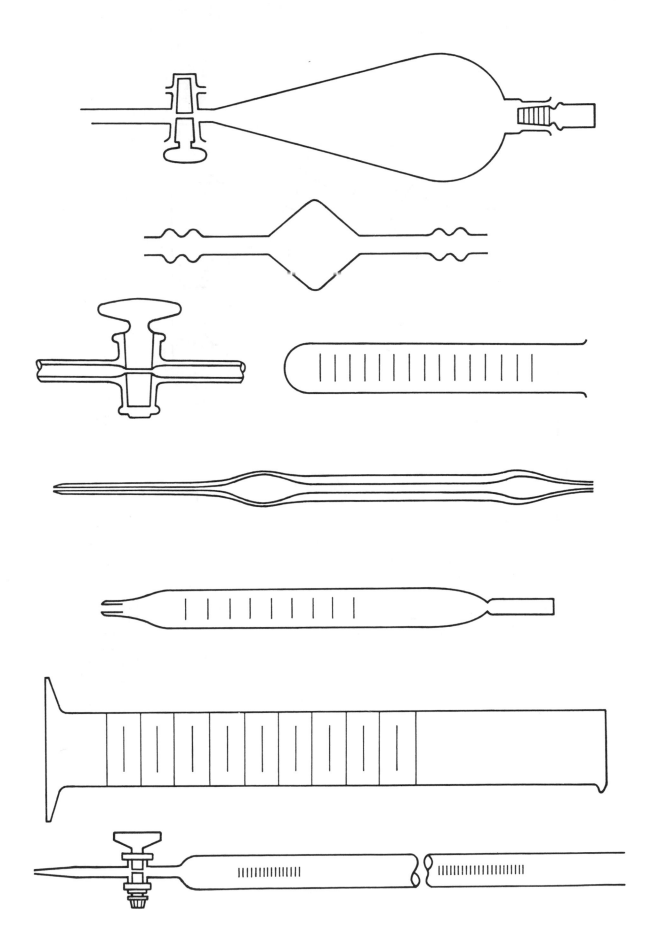

Fig. 18.10 Pictograms: Laboratory glassware

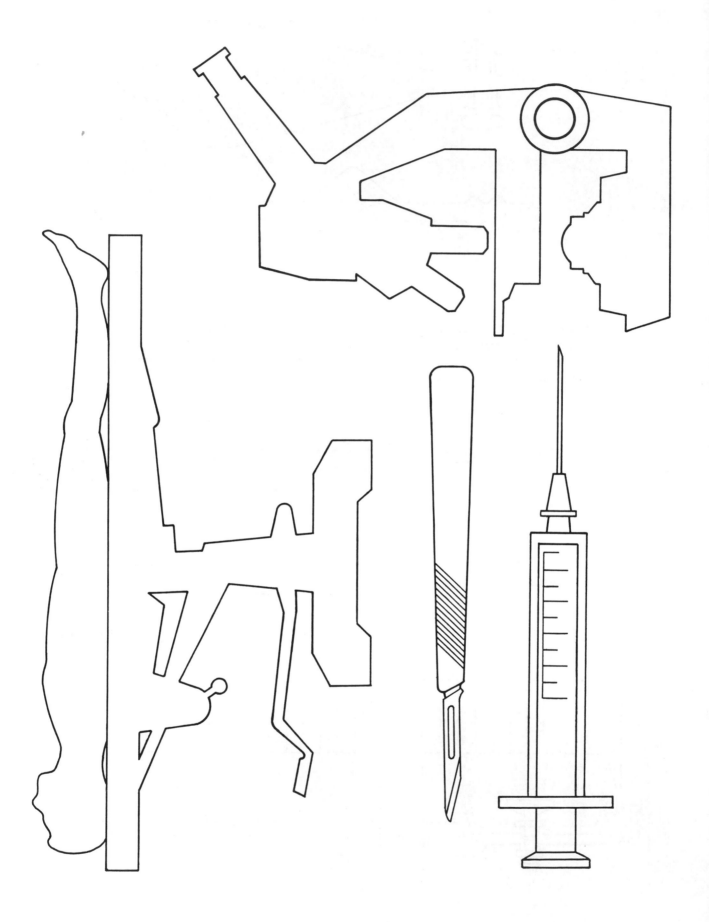

Fig. 18.11 Pictograms: Operating table, scalpel, syringe, microscope

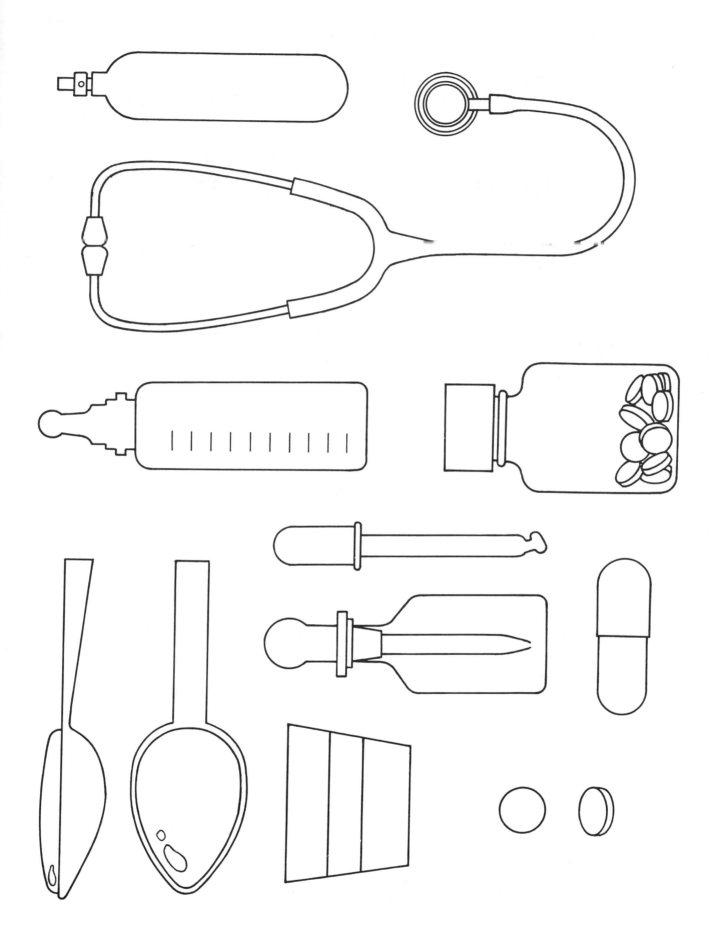

Fig. 18.12 Pictograms: Pharmaceuticals group, feeding bottle, stethoscope, gas cylinder

417

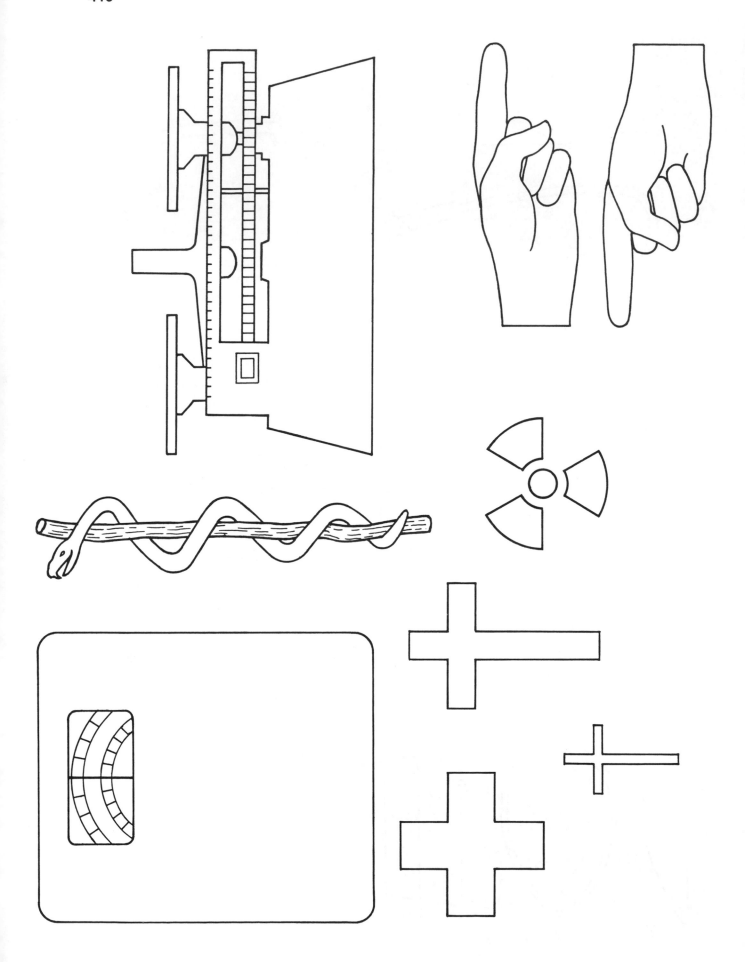

Fig. 18.13 Pictograms: Scales - domestic/laboratory, crosses, radiation, staff/serpent, and pointing hands

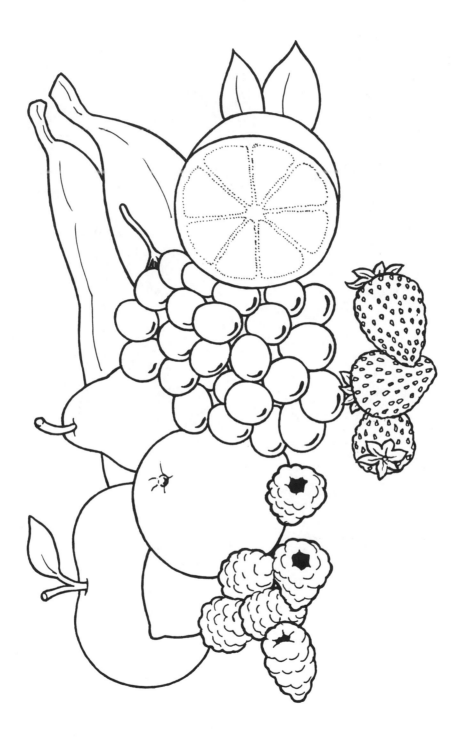

Fig. 18.14 Pictograms: Food group

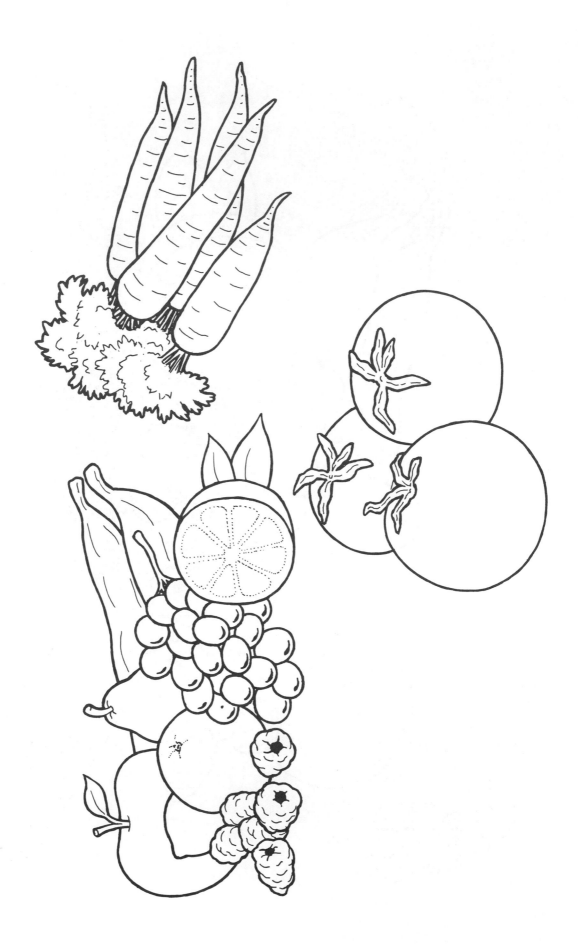

Fig.18.15 Pictograms: Food group

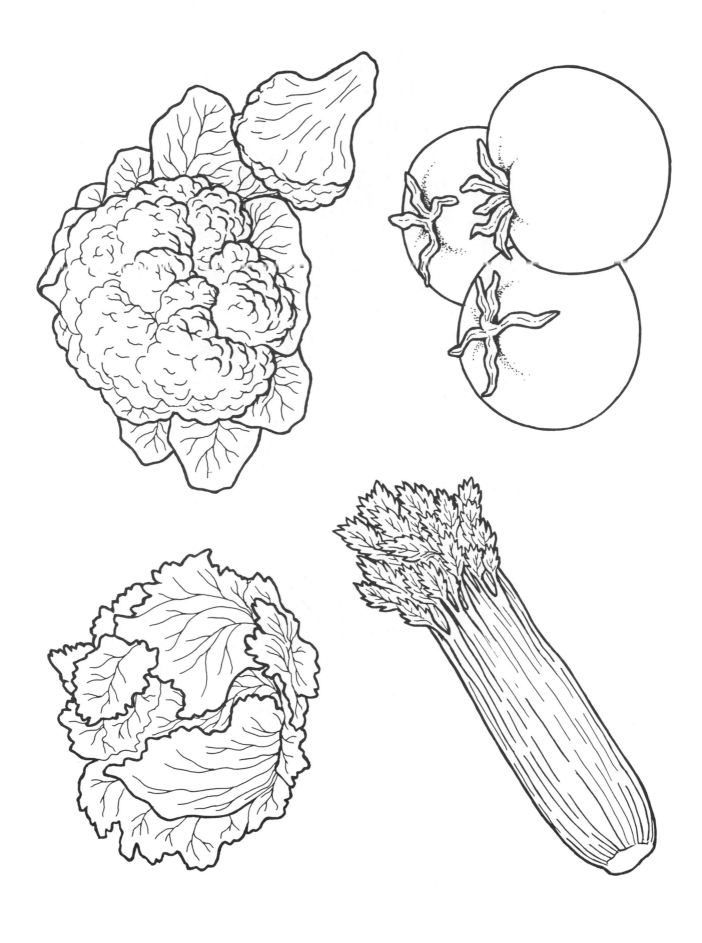

Fig. 18.16 Pictograms: Food group

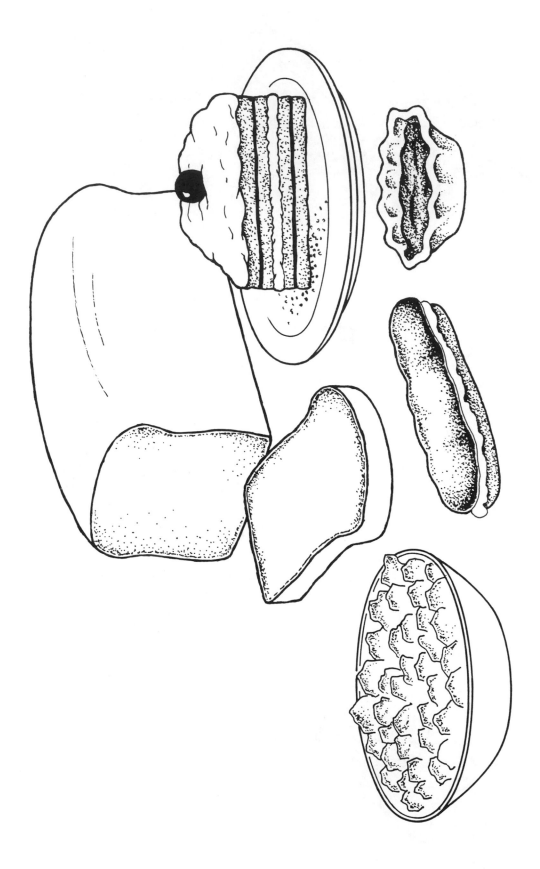

Fig. 18.17 Pictograms: Food group

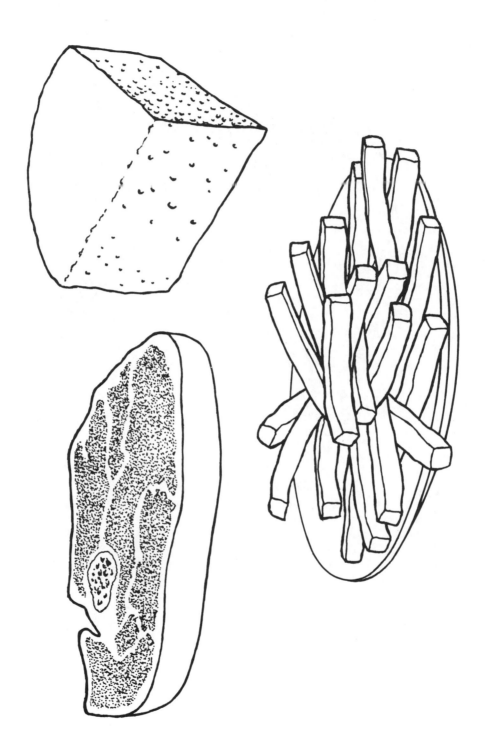

Fig.18.18 Pictograms: Food group

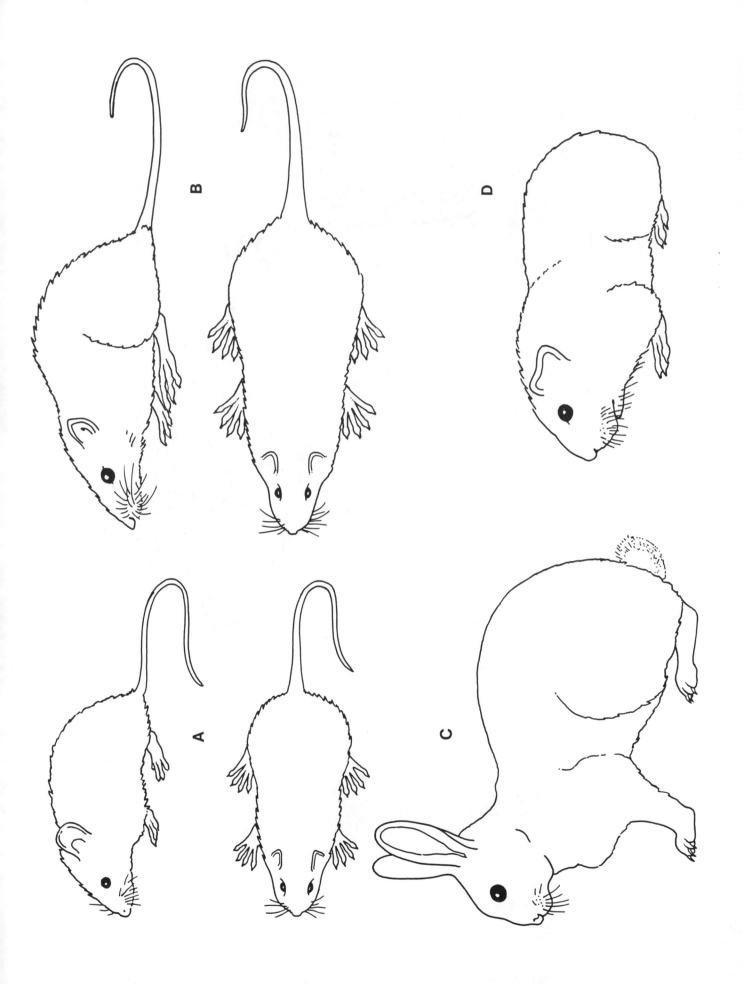

Fig. 18.19 A - mouse, B - rat, C - rabbit, D - guinea pig

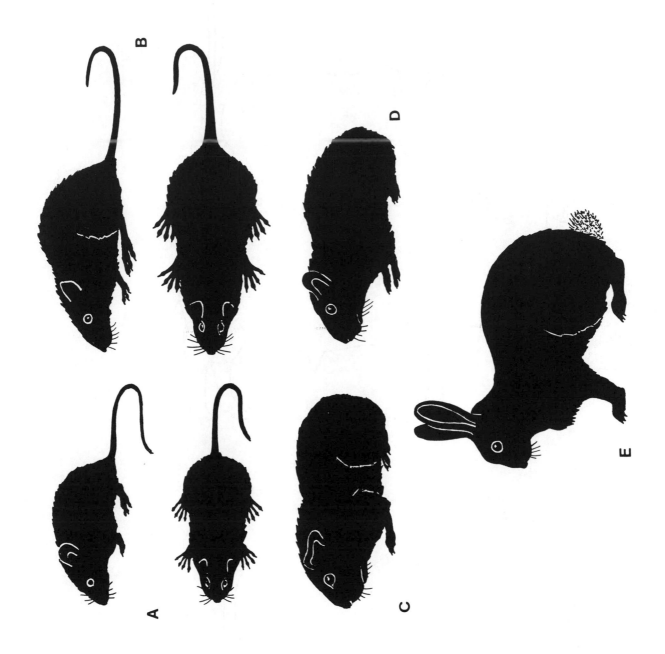

Fig. 18.20 Silhouette: A - mouse, B - rat, C - guinea pig, D - hamster,
E - rabbit

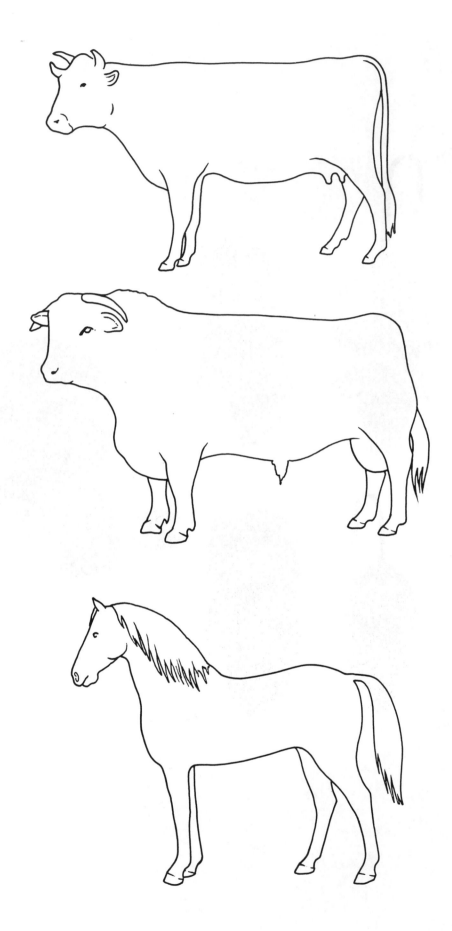

Fig.18.21 Cow, bull, horse

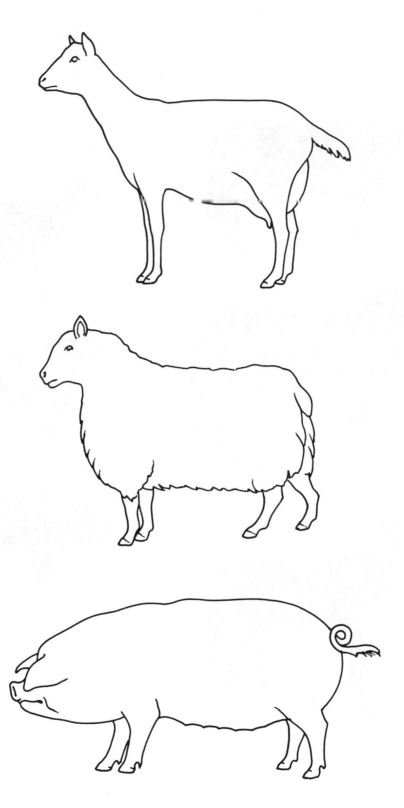

Fig. 18.22 Goat, sheep, pig

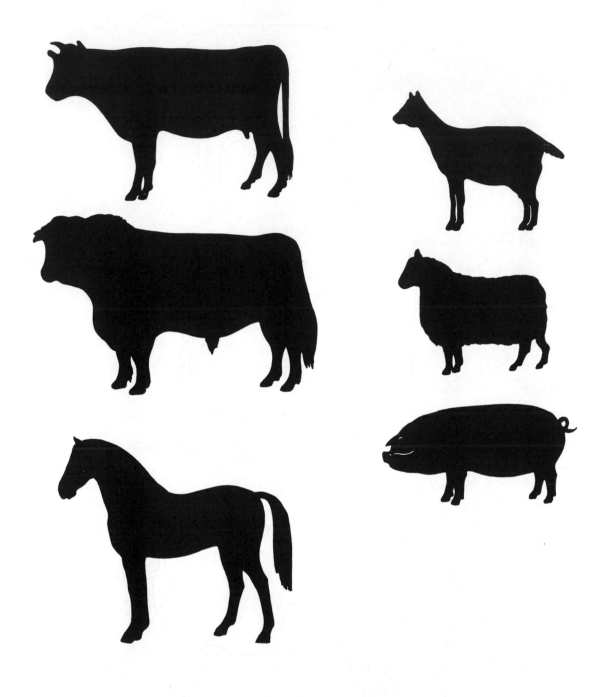

Fig. 18.23 Silhouette: cow, bull, horse, goat, sheep, pig

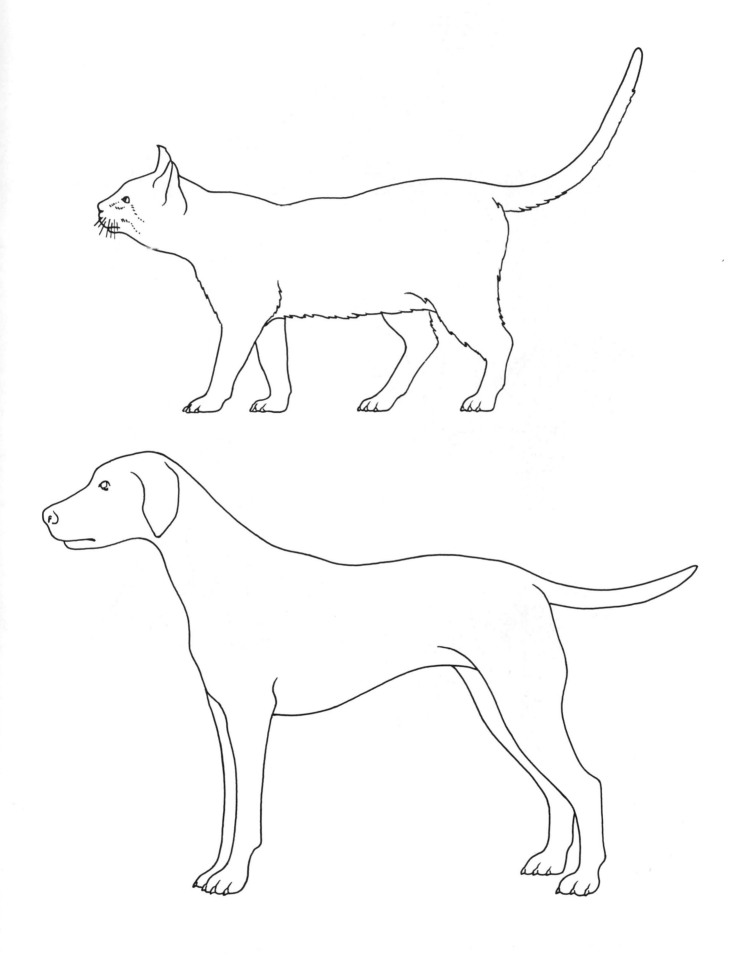

Fig. 18.24 Cat, dog

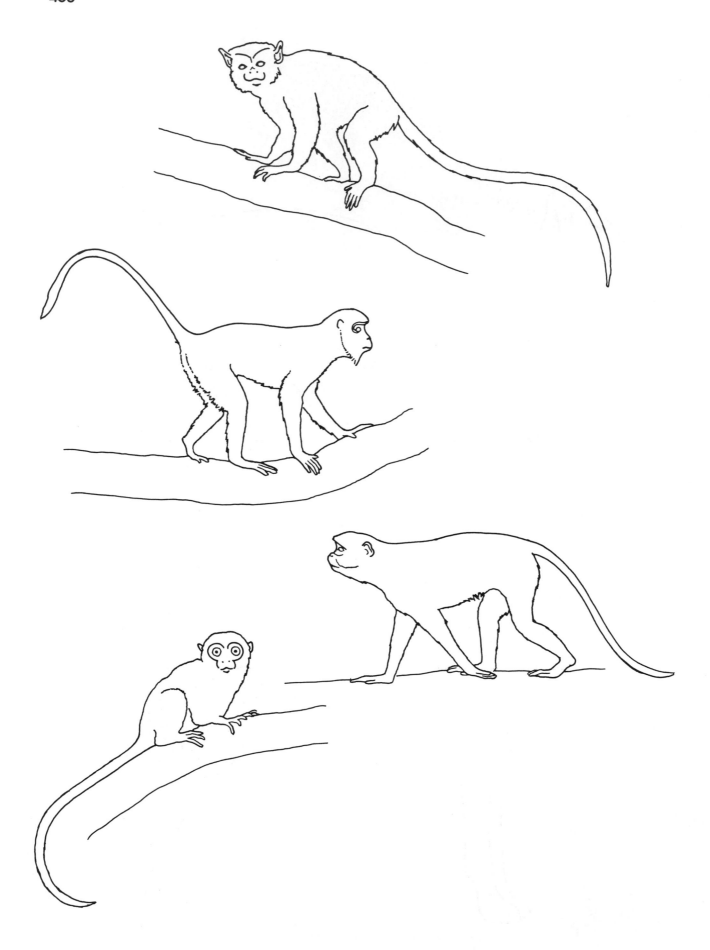

Fig.18.25 Monkeys: Black and Red Tamarin, Red Colobus,
Allen's Swamp, Pygmy Marmoset

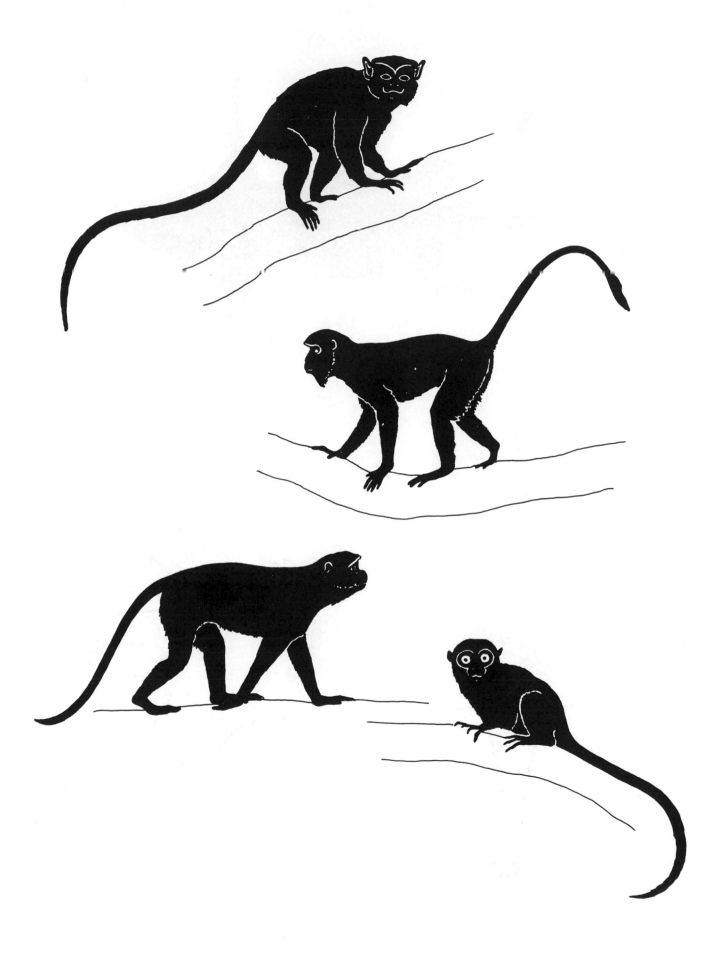

Fig.18.26 Silhouette: Monkeys: Black and Red Tamarin, Red Colobus, Allen's Swamp, Pygmy Marmoset

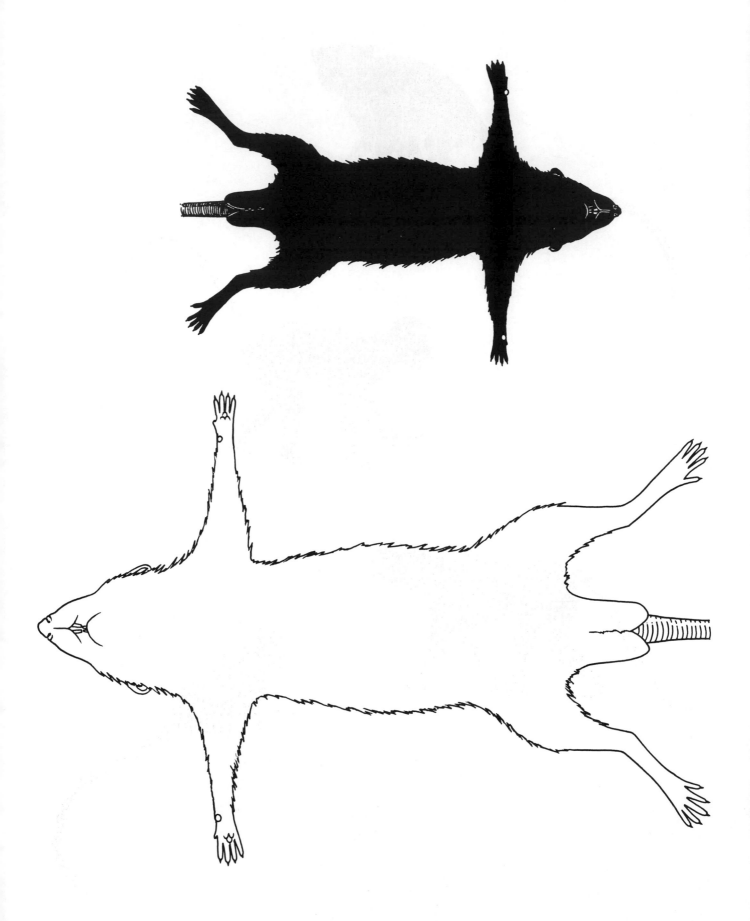

Fig. 18.27 Rat: ventral, silhouette and outline

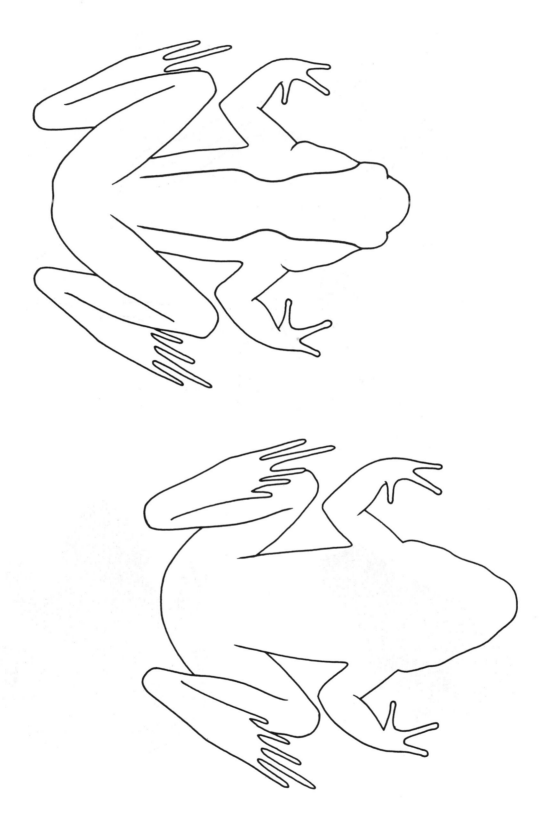

Fig. 18.28 Frog: dorsal and ventral

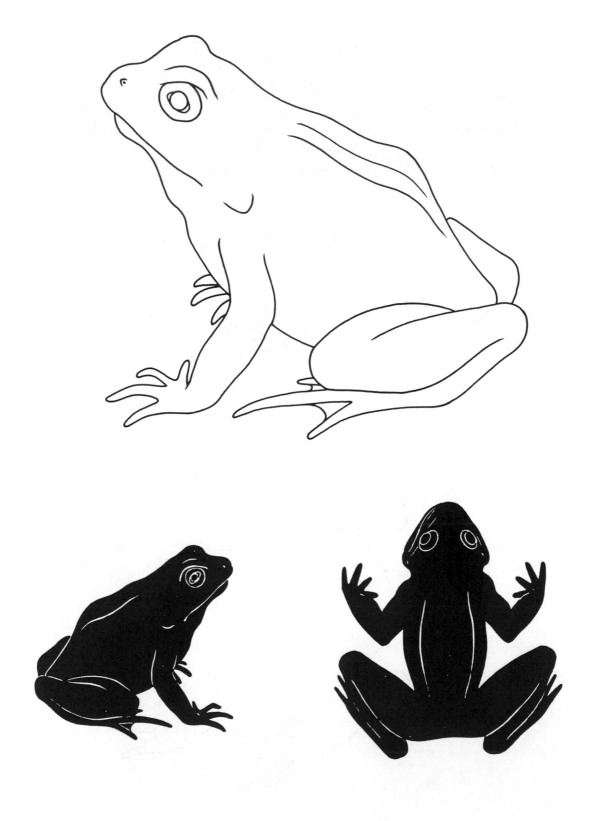

Fig. 18.29 Toad, lateral, silhouettes lateral and dorsal

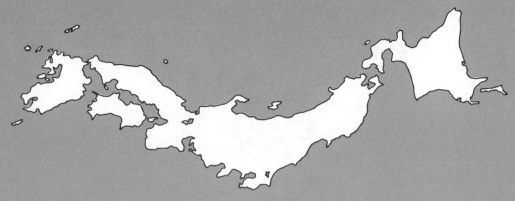

Section 19

Maps

436

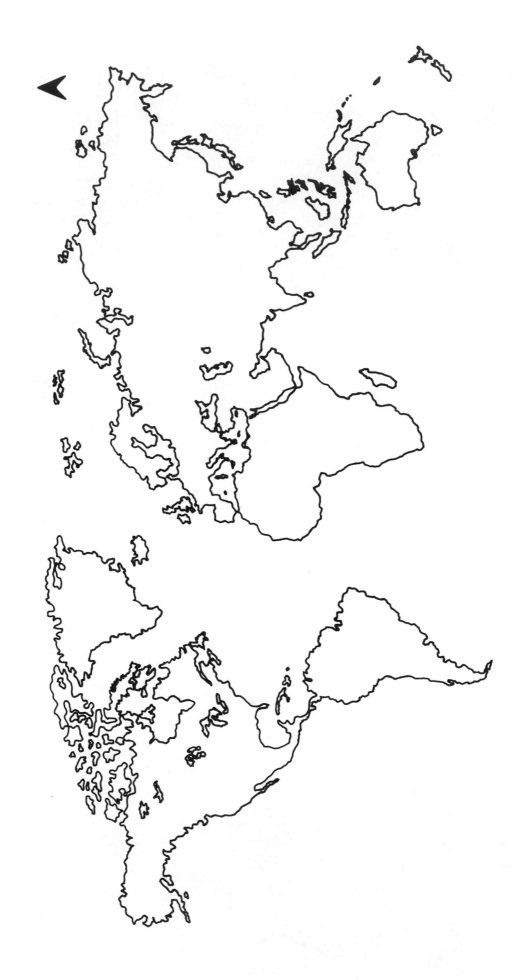

Fig. 19.1   Map, World

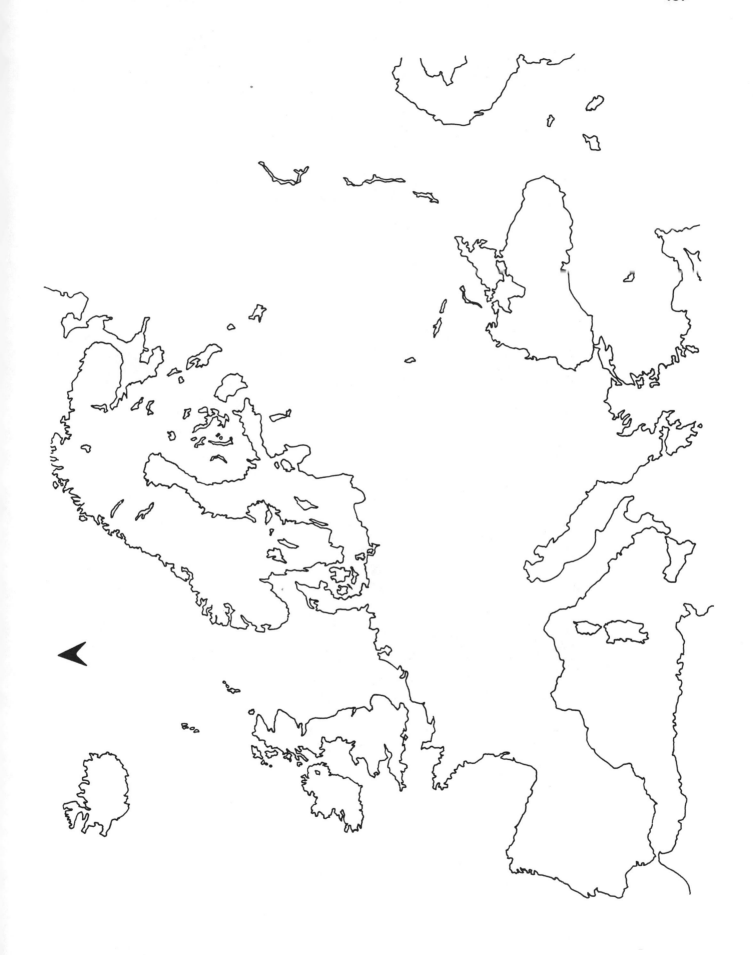

Fig. 19.2   Europe

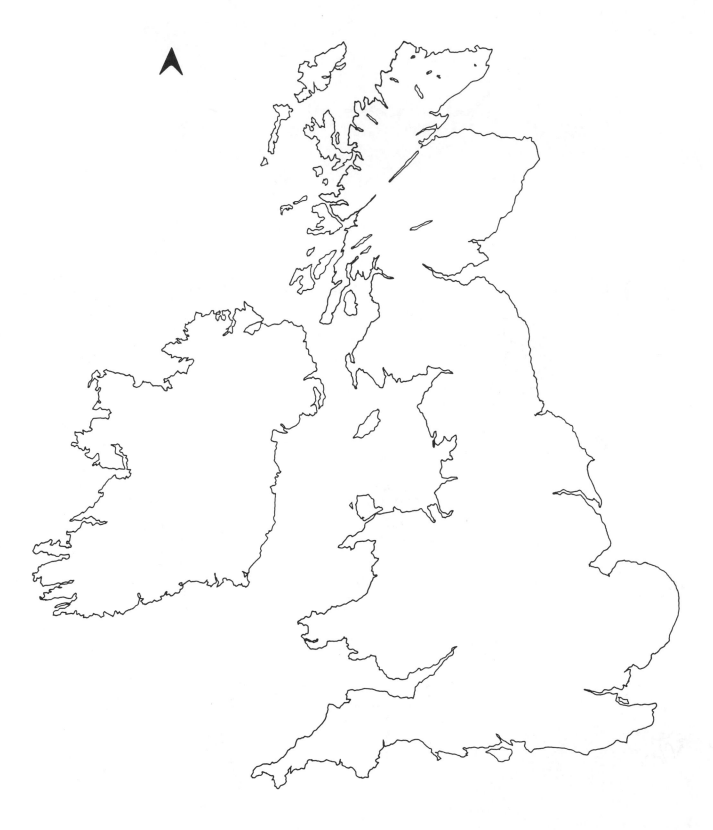

Fig. 19.3   UK/Ireland

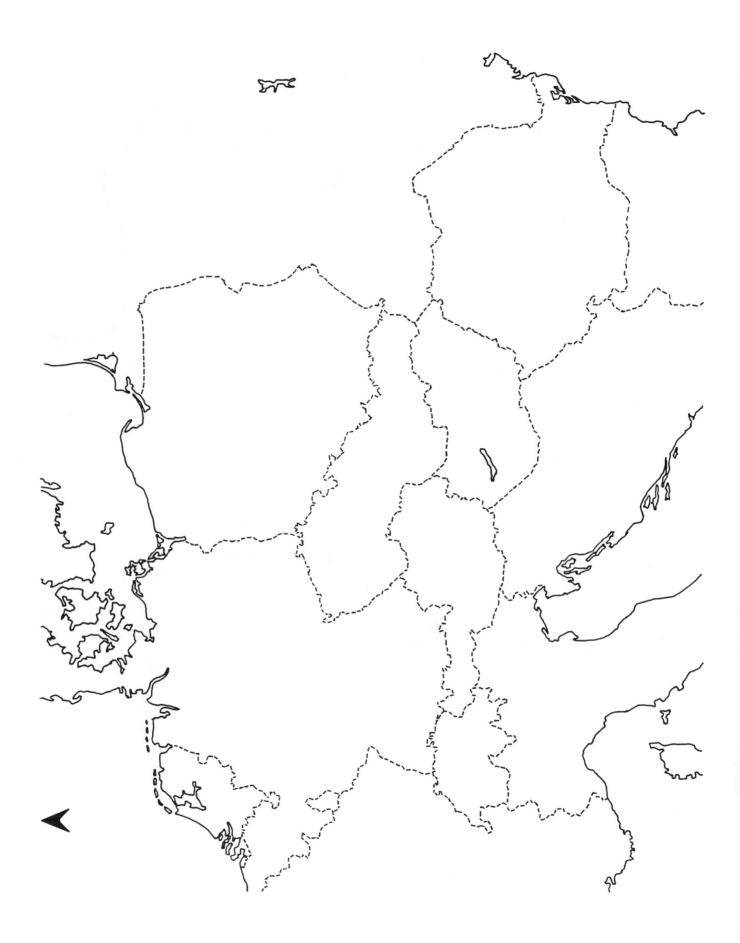

Fig. 19.4   Central Europe

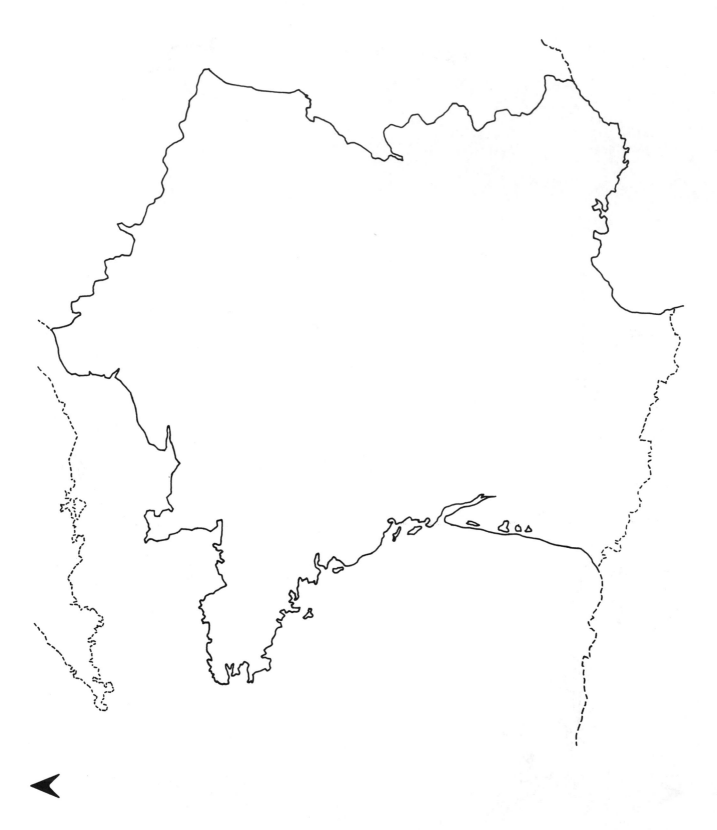

Fig. 19.5   France

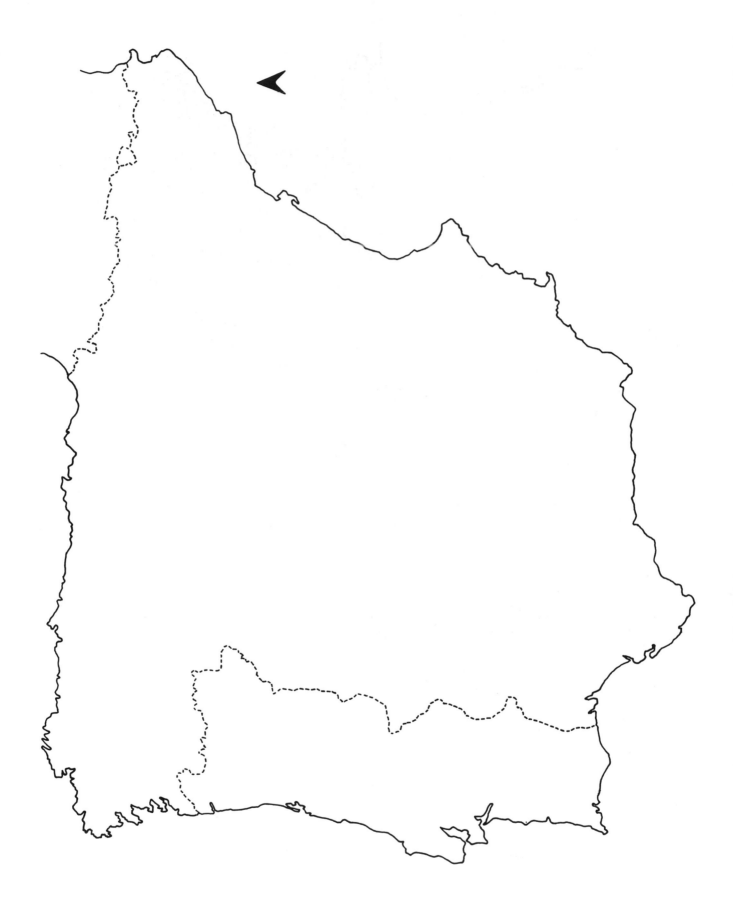

Fig. 19.6   Spain/Portugal

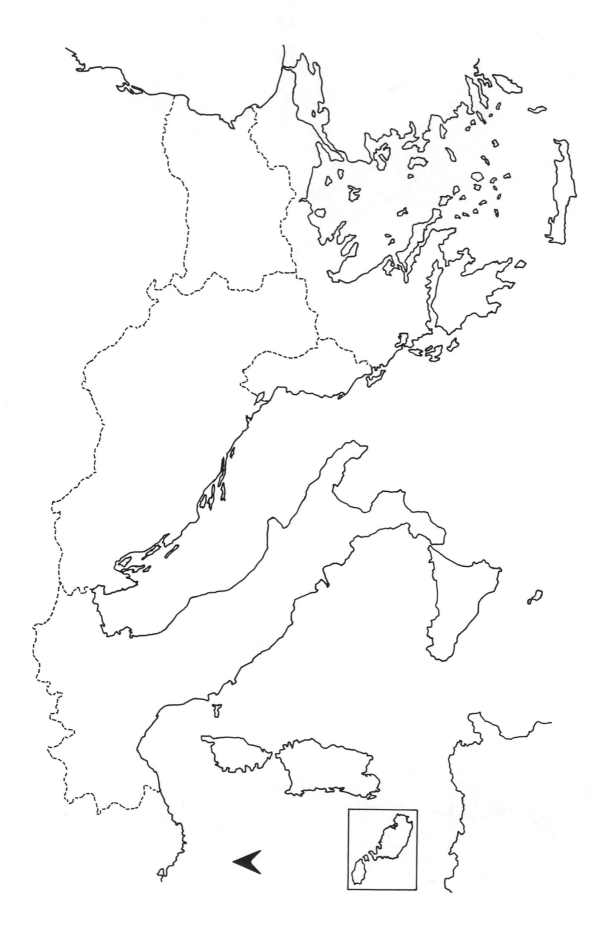

Fig. 19.7   Italy/Balkan States

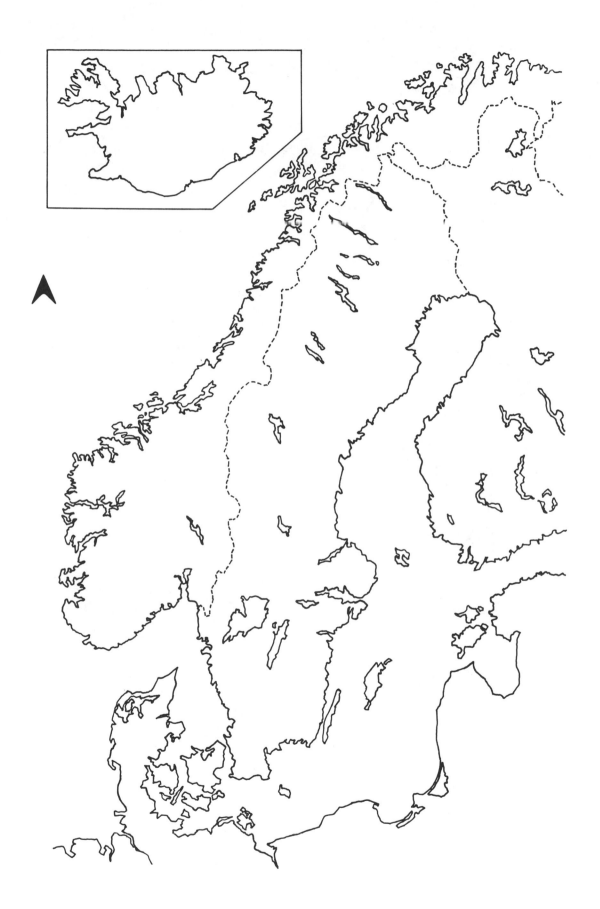

Fig. 19.8   Scandinavia/Iceland

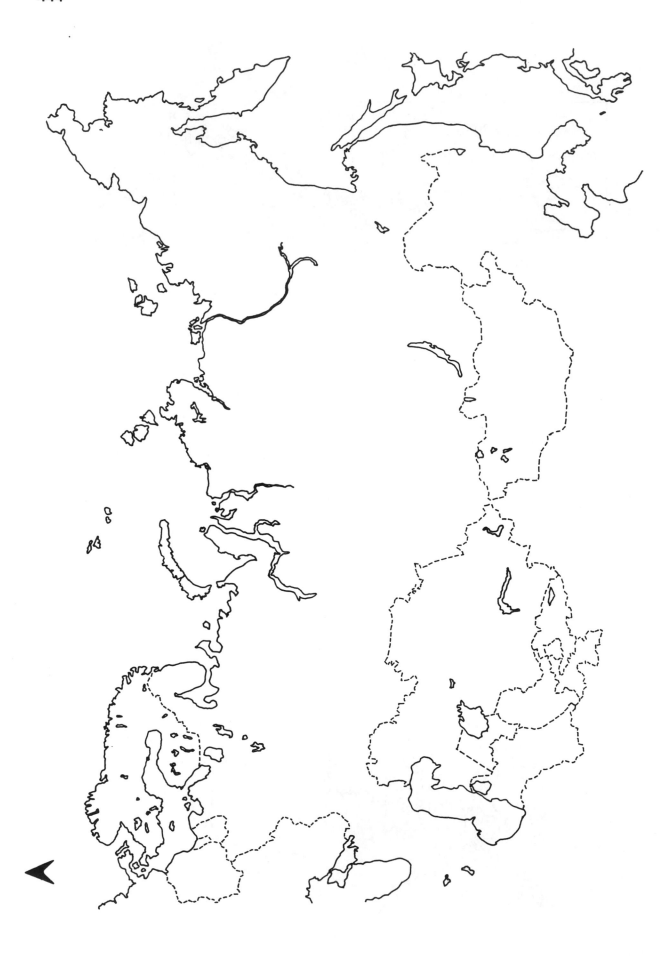

Fig. 19.9   USSR

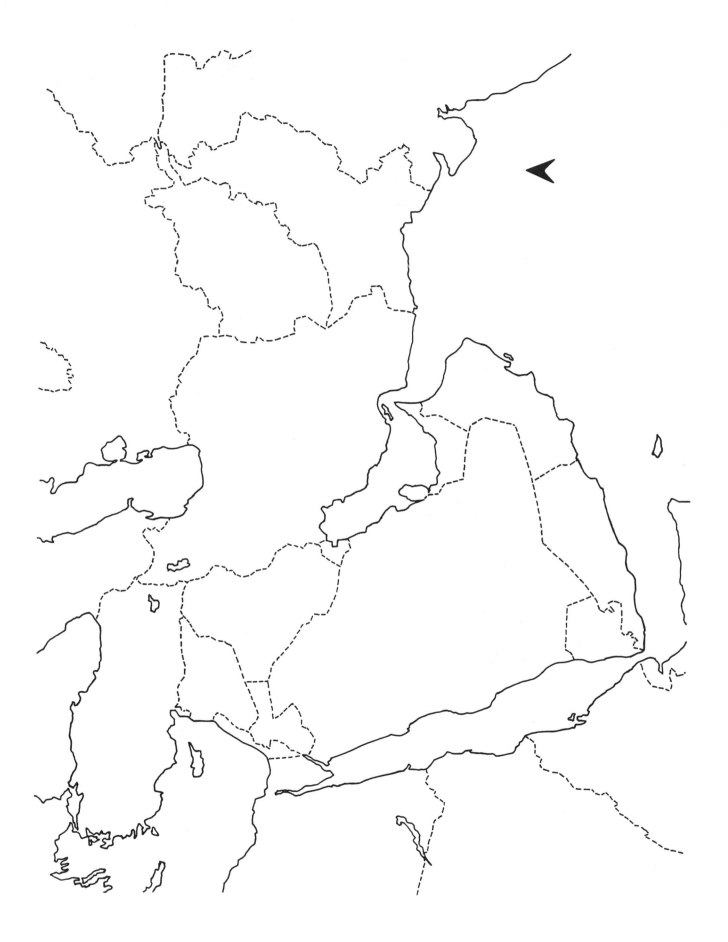

Fig. 19.10 S.W. Asia

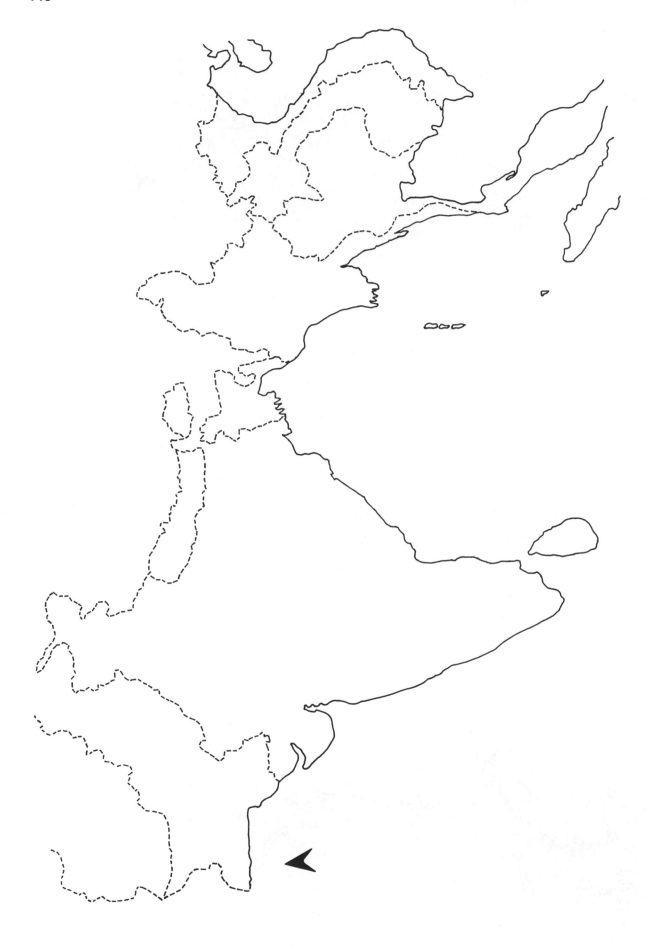

Fig. 19.11 S. Asia

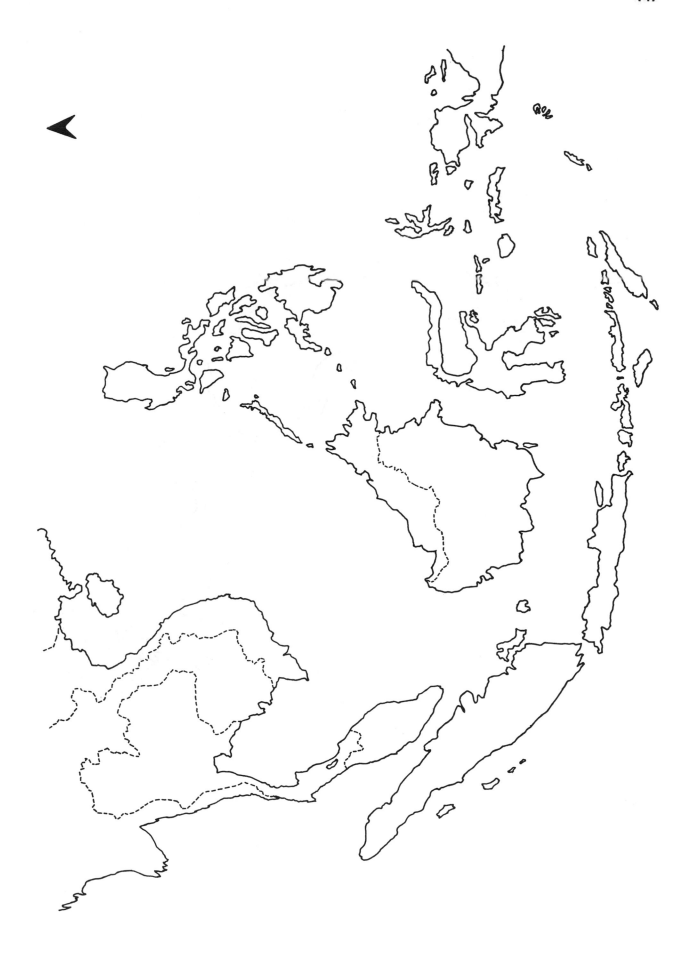

Fig. 19.12 S.E. Asia

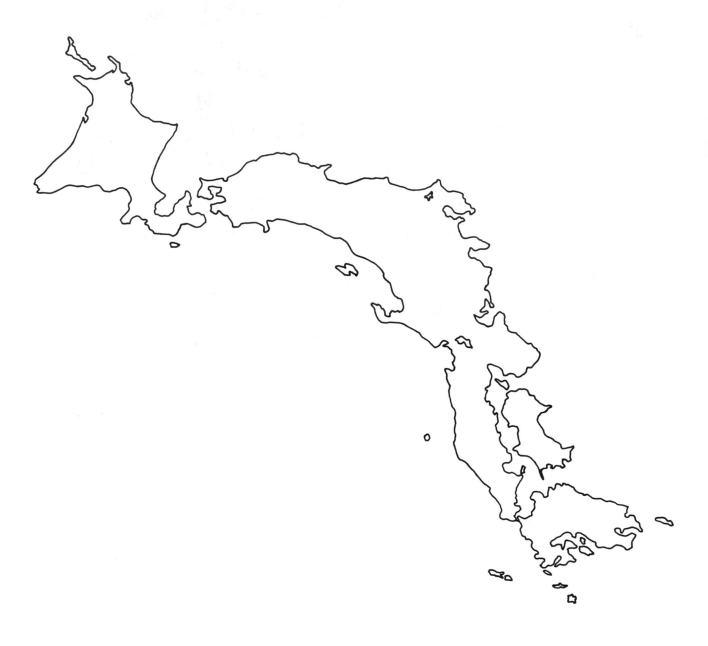

Fig. 19.13 Japan

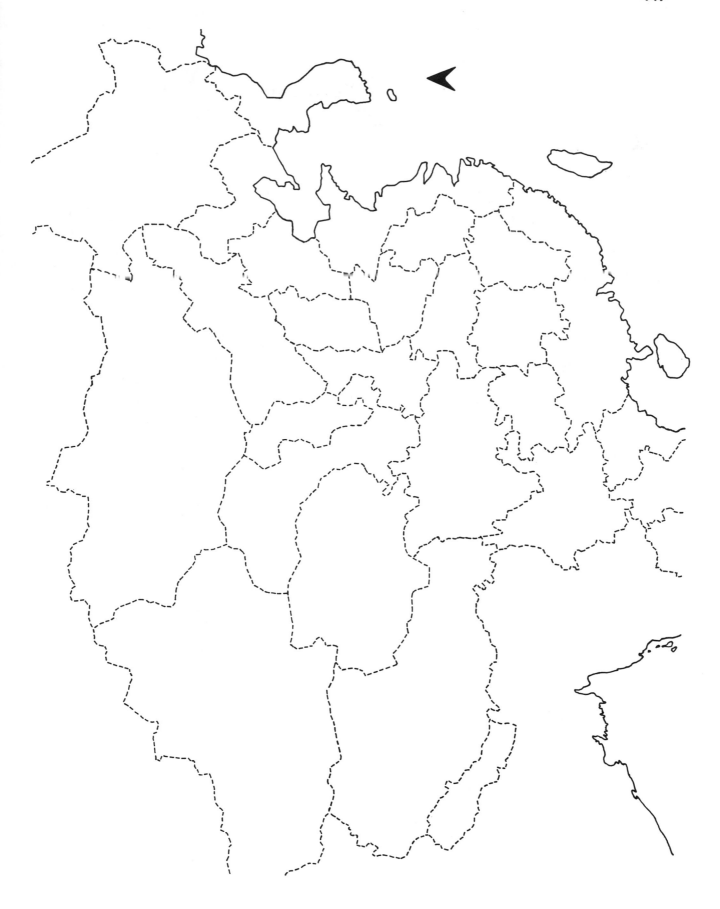

Fig. 19.14 China

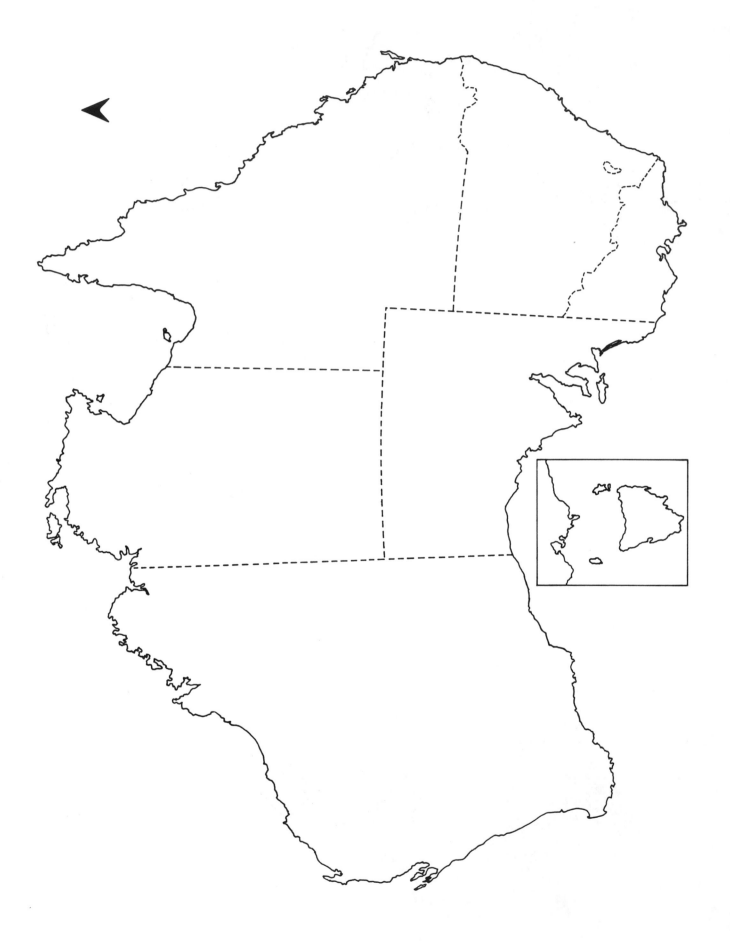

Fig. 19.15 Australia

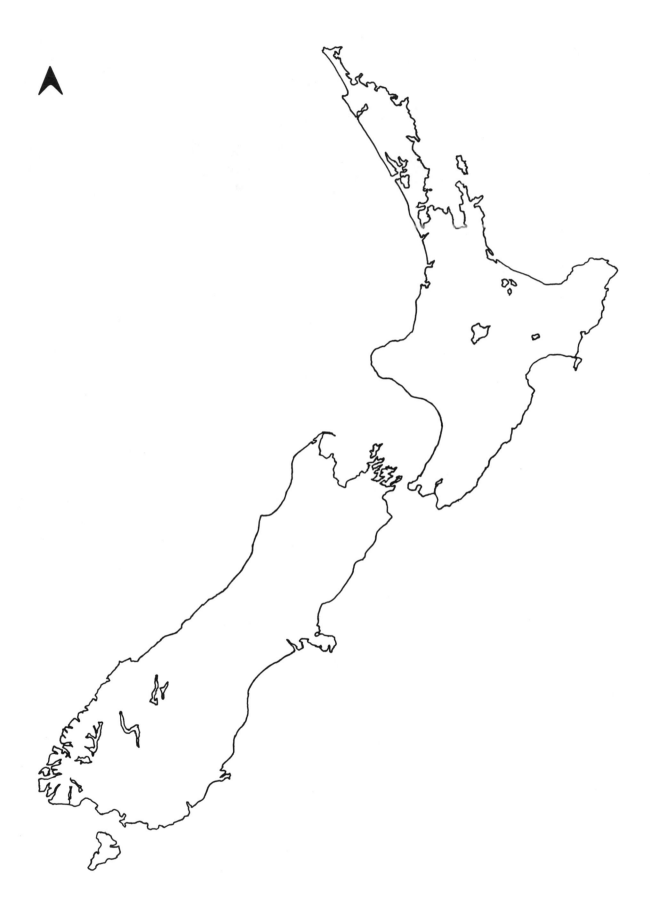

Fig. 19.16 New Zealand

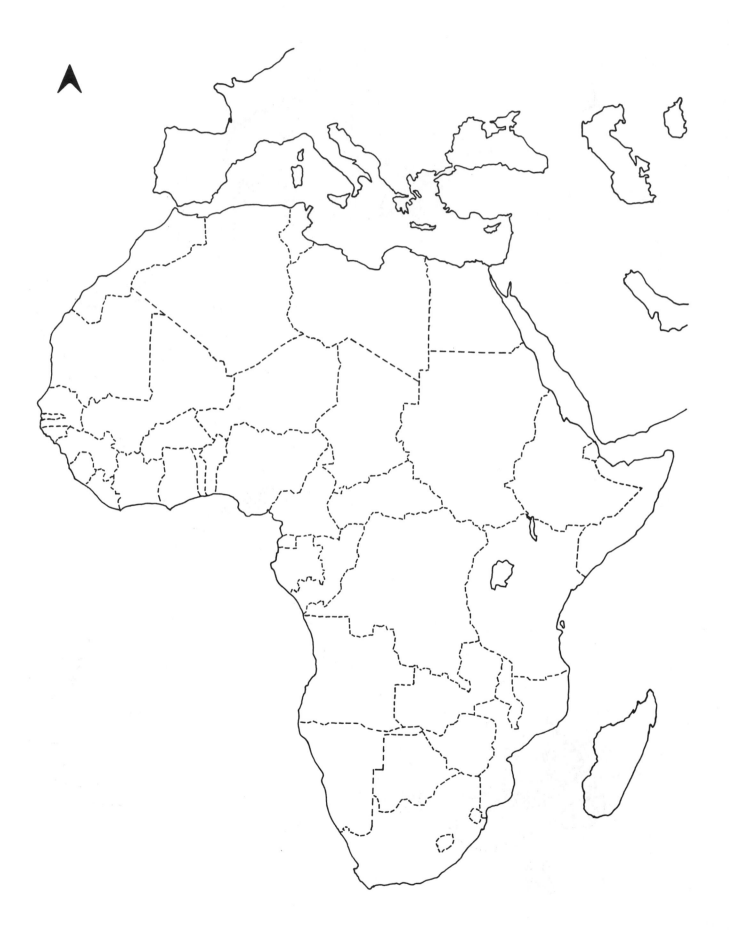

Fig. 19.17 Africa

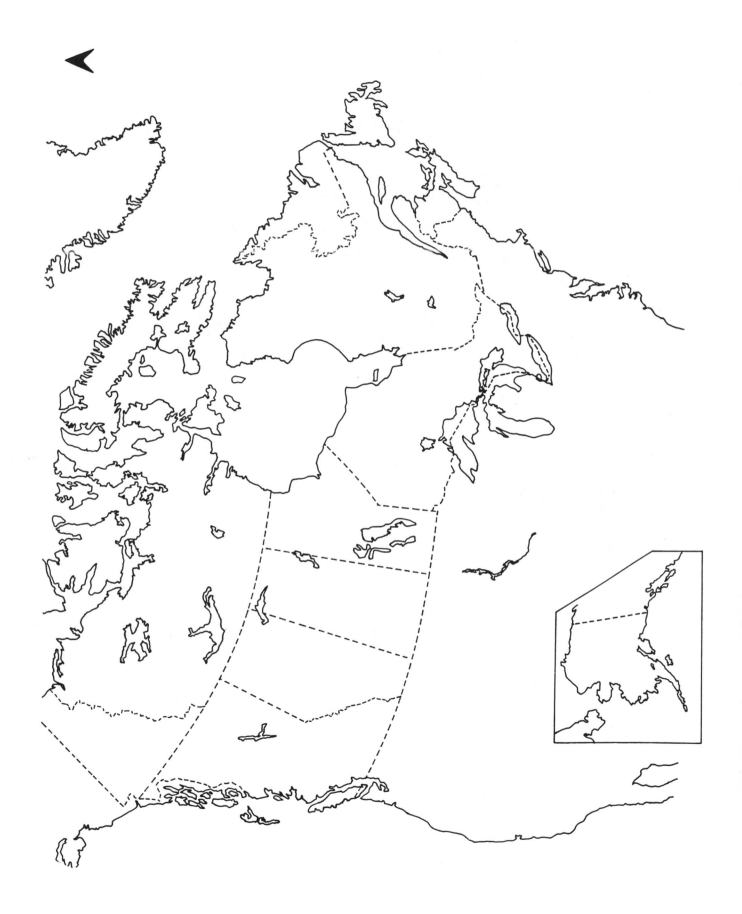

Fig. 19.18 Canada

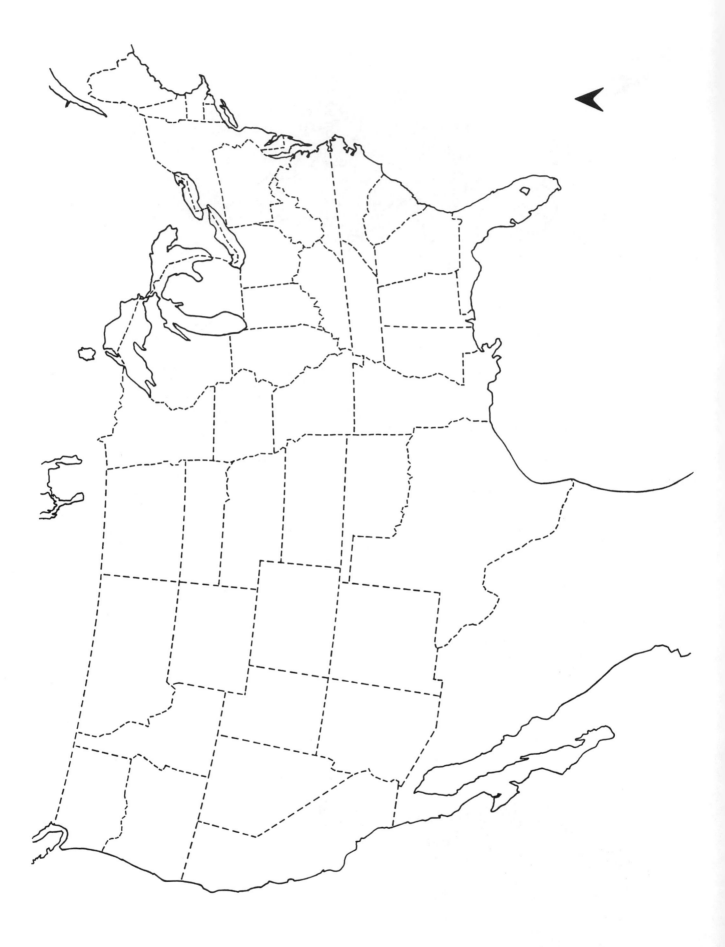

Fig. 19.19 United States

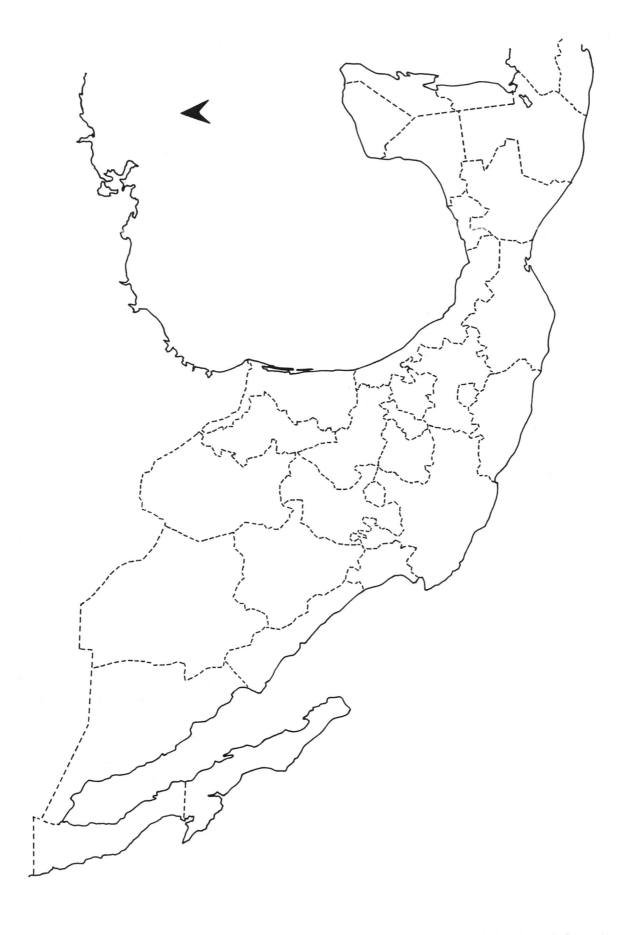

Fig. 19.20 Mexico

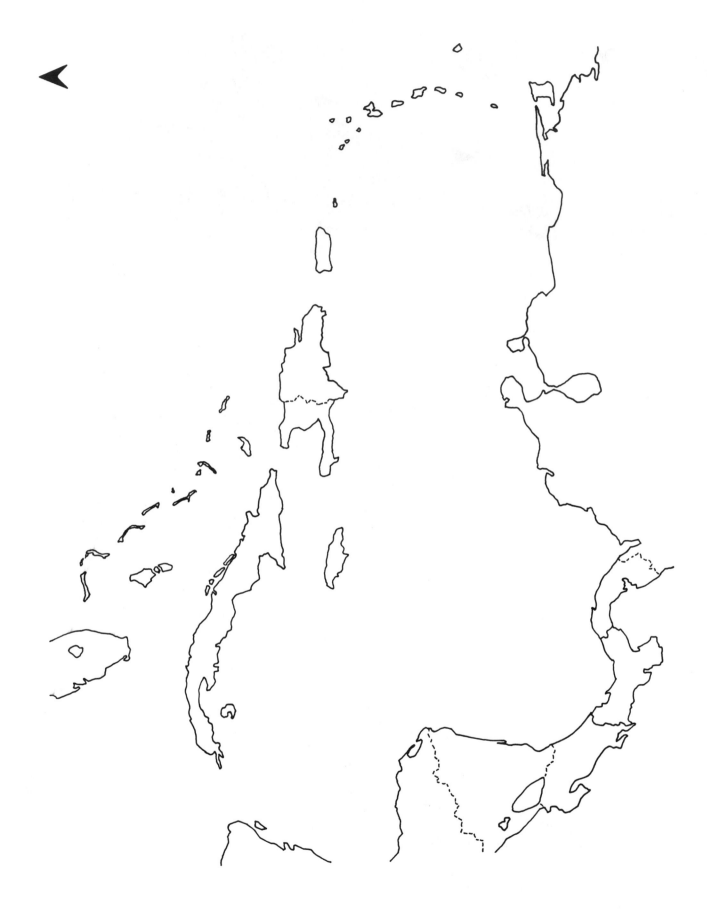

Fig. 19.21 West Indies

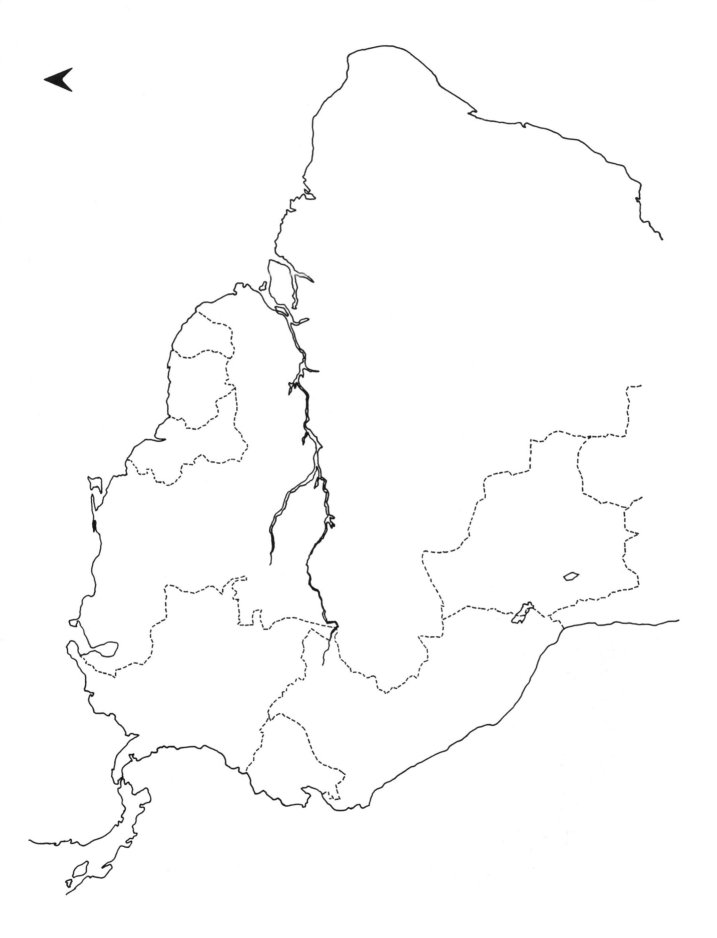

Fig. 19.22 N. South America

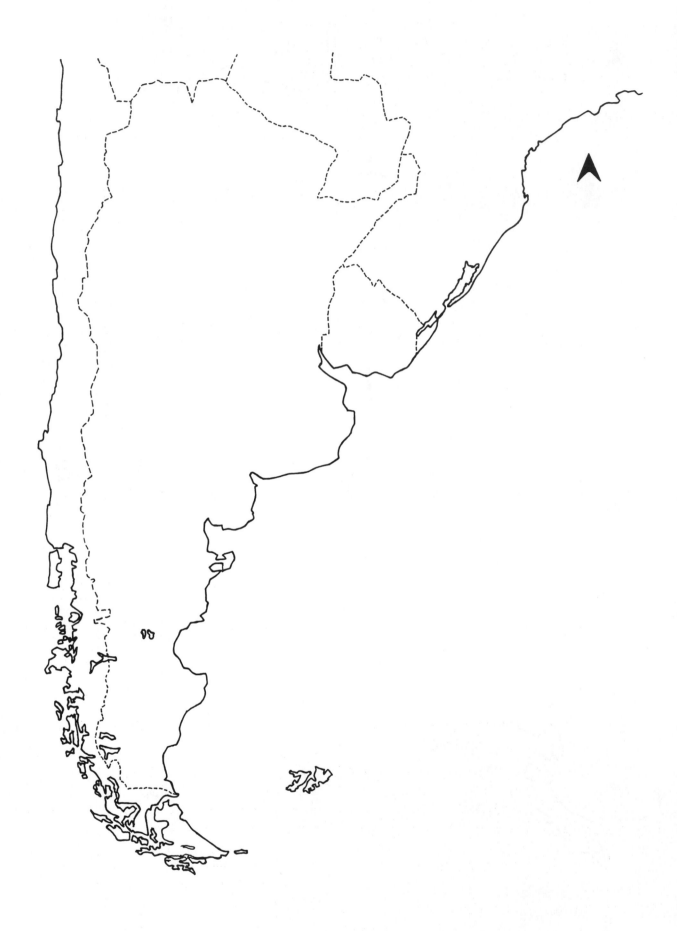

Fig. 19.23 S. South America

abc defg

Section 20

Freehand Lettering Guides

The examples of lettering included here are intended to act as guides to the formation and shape of letters drawn freehand. They are not designed to be traced, though of course you may if you wish. The style of most is similar to the Univers/Helvetica family of typefaces which give clean legible text. Remember that a combination of upper and lower case letters is more legible than upper case capitals alone.

20.1   6mm lettering grid no. 1
20.2   6mm lettering examples. Standard, Bold, Condensed, Italic
20.3   7mm lettering grid no. 2
20.4   7mm lettering examples. Standard, Bold, Condensed, Italic
20.5   8mm lettering grid no. 3
20.6   8mm lettering examples. Standard, Bold
20.7   8mm lettering examples. Condensed, Italic
20.8   10mm lettering grid no. 4
20.9   10mm lettering examples. Standard, Bold
20.10 10mm lettering examples. Condensed, Italic
20.11 13mm lettering grid no. 5
20.12 13mm lettering examples. Standard, Bold
20.13 13mm lettering examples. Condensed, Italic
20.14 15mm lettering grid no. 6
20.15 15mm lettering example. Standard
20.16 15mm lettering example. Bold
20.17 15mm lettering example. Condensed
20.18 15mm lettering example. Italic
20.19 15mm lettering example. Standard plus serifs
20.20 15mm lettering example. Outline Bold
20.21 15mm lettering example. Script
20.22 15mm lettering example. Standard plus outline

The grids may be placed under your OHP transparency or tracing material to keep your text straight and the lines correctly distanced. The guidelines also ensure that the capitals and lower case letters are correctly proportioned.

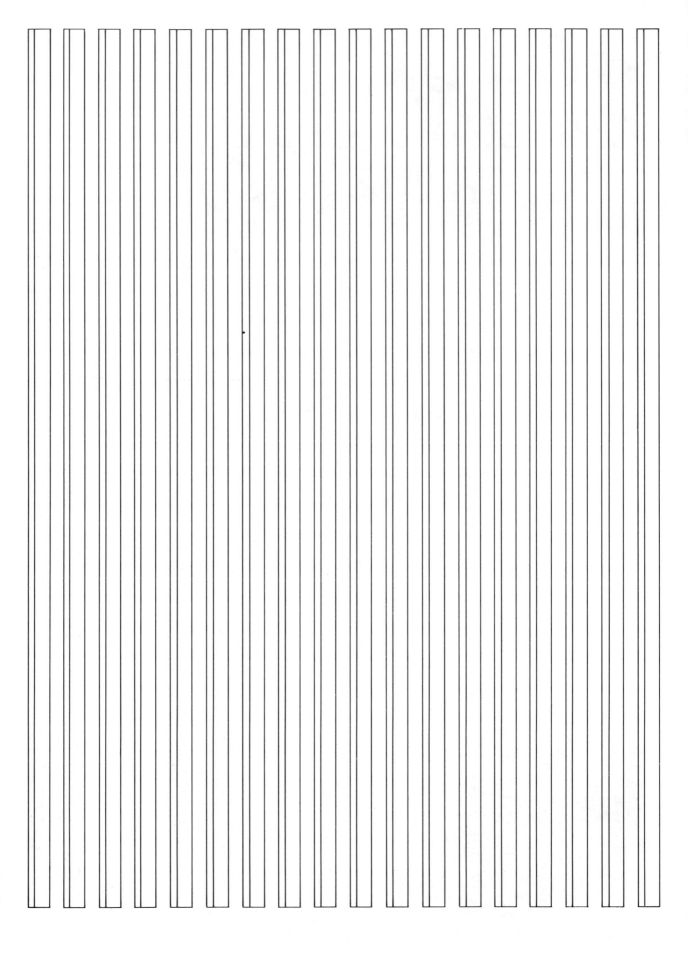

Grid number 1

Fig. 20.1   6mm lettering grid no. 1

Lettering for use with grid number 1

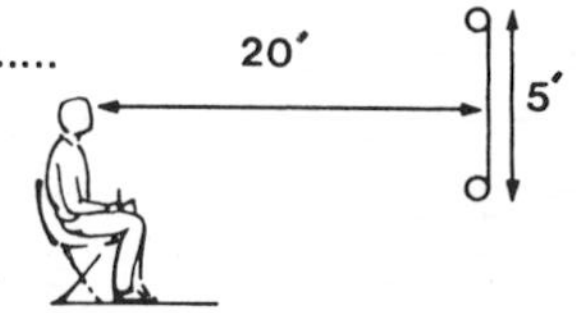

Legible at..... 20' 5'

Standard

abcdefghijklmnopqrstuvwxyz
ABCDEFGHIJKLMNOPQRSTUVWXYZ
1234567890

Bold

abcdefghijklmnopqrstuvwxyz
ABCDEFGHIJKLMNOPQRSTUVWXYZ
1234567890

Condensed

abcdefghijklmnopqrstuvwxyz
ABCDEFGHIJKLMNOPQRSTUVWXYZ
1234567890

Italic

abcdefghijklmnopqrstuvwxyz
ABCDEFGHIJKLMNOPQRSTUVWXYZ
1234567890

Fig. 20.2 6mm lettering examples. Standard, Bold, Condensed, Italic

Grid number 2

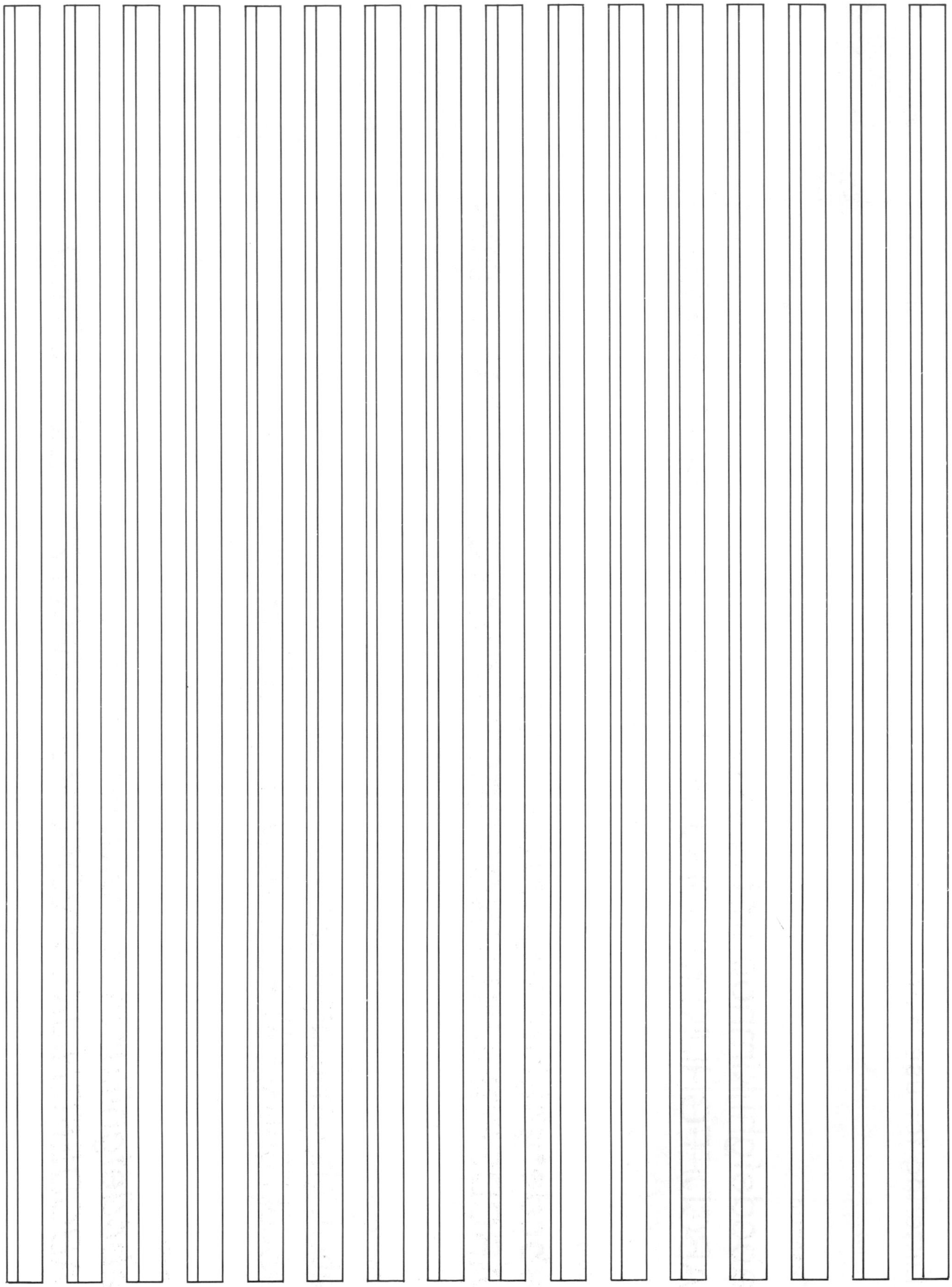

Fig. 20.3   7mm lettering grid no. 2

Legible at.... 30' 5'

Lettering for use with grid number 2

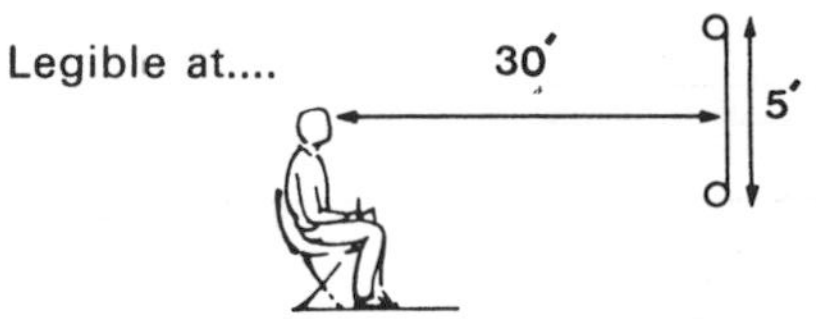

Standard

abcdefghijklmnopqrstuvwxyz
ABCDEFGHIJKLMNOPQRSTUVWXYZ
1234567890

Bold

abcdefghijklmnopqrstuvwxyz
ABCDEFGHIJKLMNOPQRSTUVWXYZ
1234567890

Condensed

abcdefghijklmnopqrstuvwxyz
ABCDEFGHIJKLMNOPQRSTUVWXYZ
1234567890

Italic

abcdefghijklmnopqrstuvwxyz
ABCDEFGHIJKLMNOPQRSTUVWXYZ
1234567890

Fig. 20.4   7mm lettering examples. Standard, Bold, Condensed, Italic

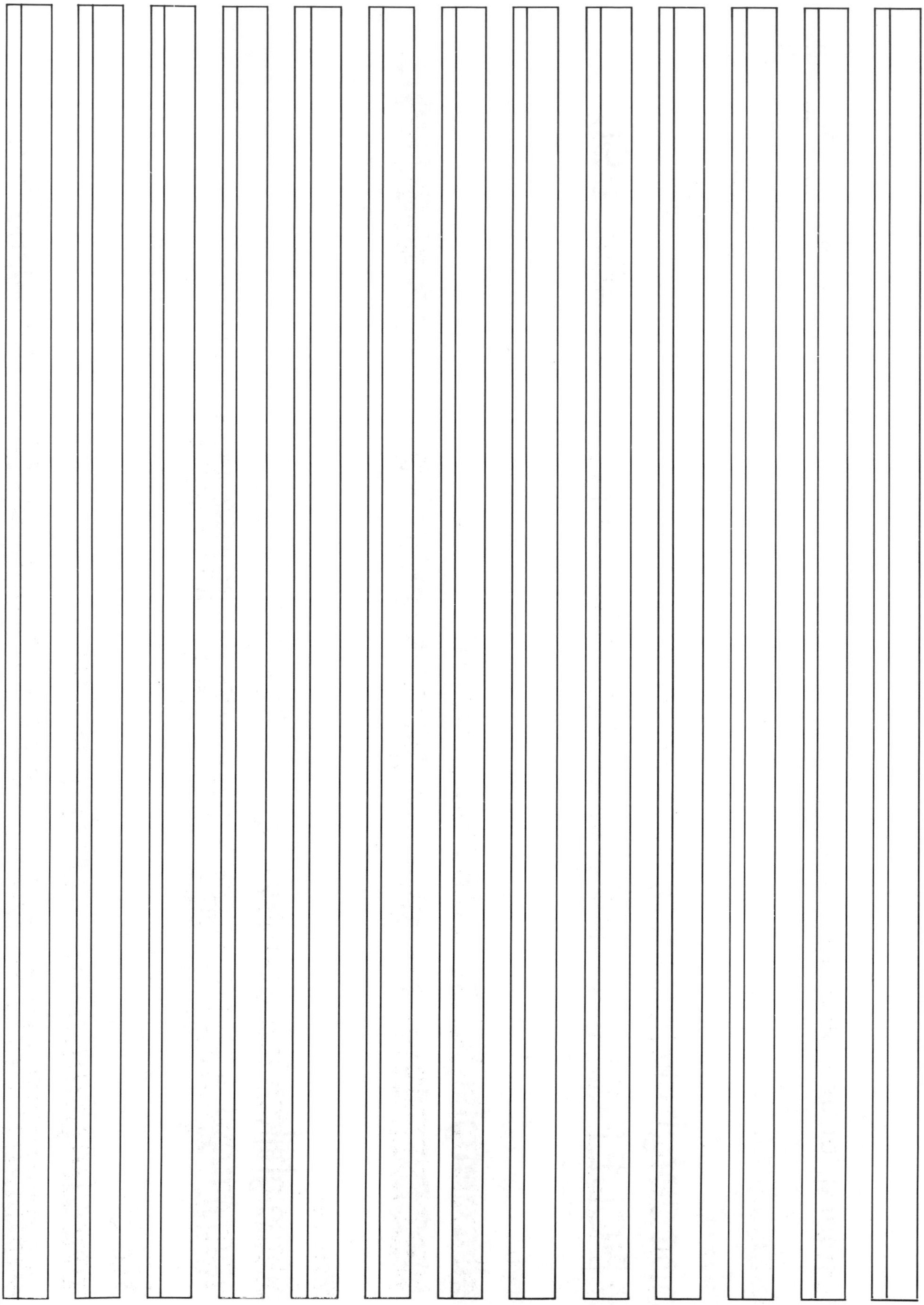

Grid number 3

Fig. 20.5 8mm lettering grid no. 3

Lettering for use with grid number 3

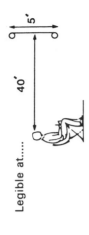

Legible at.....

40'

5'

Standard

abcdefghijklmnopqrstuvwxyz
ABCDEFGHIJKLMNOPQRSTUVWXYZ
1234567890

Bold

abcdefghijklmnopqrstuvwxyz
ABCDEFGHIJKLMNOPQRSTUVWXYZ
1234567890

Fig. 20.6 8mm lettering examples. Standard, Bold

Legible at...... 40' 5'

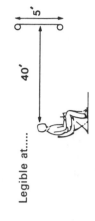

Lettering for use with grid number 3

Condensed

abcdefghijklmnopqrstuvwxyz
ABCDEFGHIJKLMNOPQRSTUVWXYZ
1234567890

Italic

abcdefghijklmnopqrstuvwxyz
ABCDEFGHIJKLMNOPQRSTUVWXYZ
1234567890

Fig. 20.7 8mm lettering examples. Condensed, Italic

Grid number 4

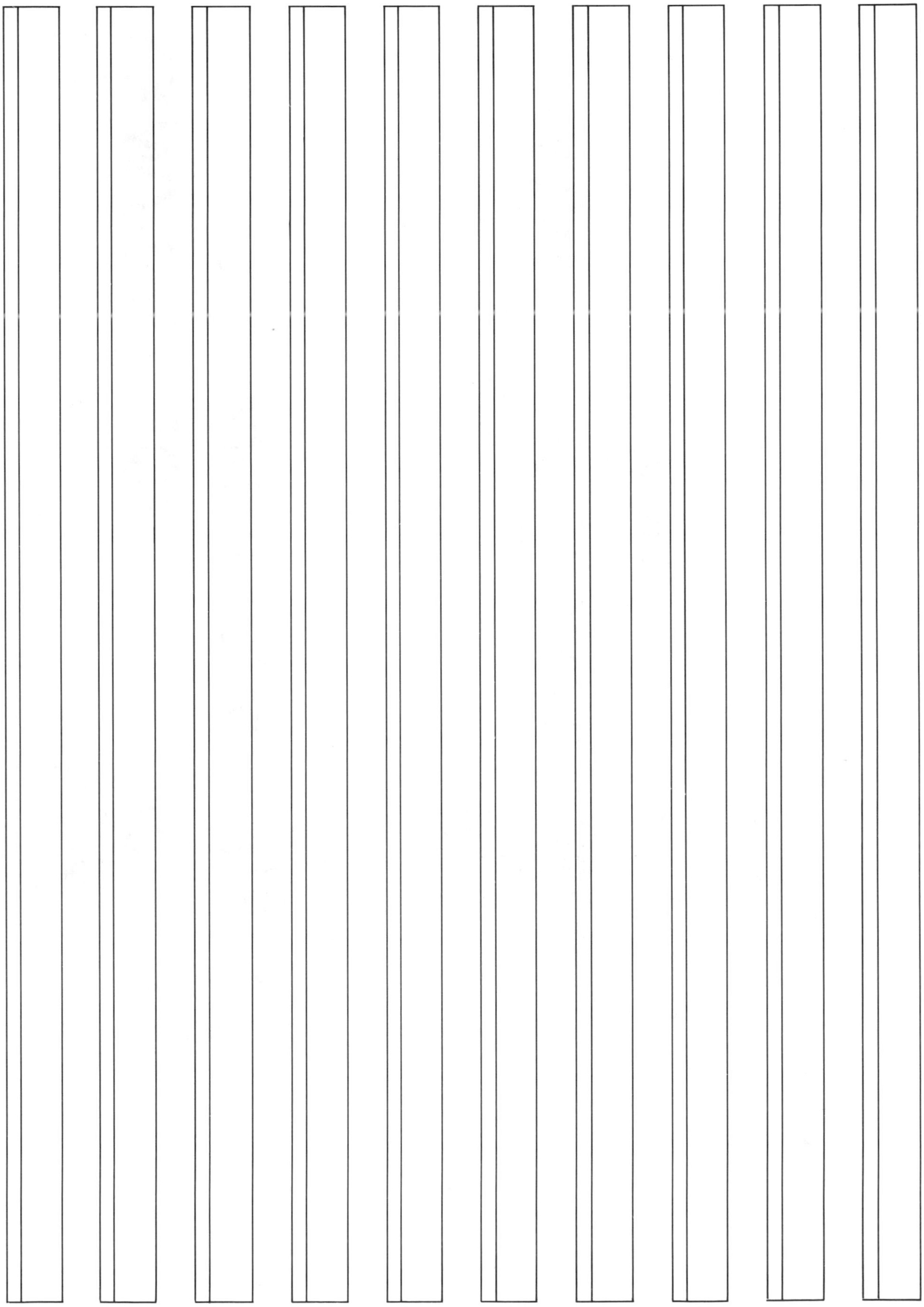

Fig. 20.8   10mm lettering grid no. 4

468

Lettering for use with grid number 4

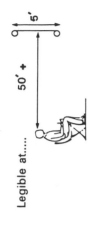

Legible at..... 50' +   5'

Standard

abcdefghijklmnopqrstuvwxyz
ABCDEFGHIJKLMNOPQRSTUVWXY
Z   1234567890

Bold

abcdefghijklmnopqrstuvwxyz
ABCDEFGHIJKLMNOPQRSTUVWXY
Z   1234567890

Fig. 20.9   10mm lettering examples. Standard, Bold

Lettering for use with grid number 4

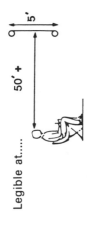

Legible at..... 50'+ 5'

Condensed

abcdefghijklmnopqrstuvwxyz
ABCDEFGHIJKLMNOPQRSTUVWXYZ
1234567890

Italic

abcdefghijklmnopqrstuvwxyz
ABCDEFGHIJKLMNOPQRSTUVWXYZ
1234567890

Fig.20.10 10mm lettering examples. Condensed, Italic

Grid number 5

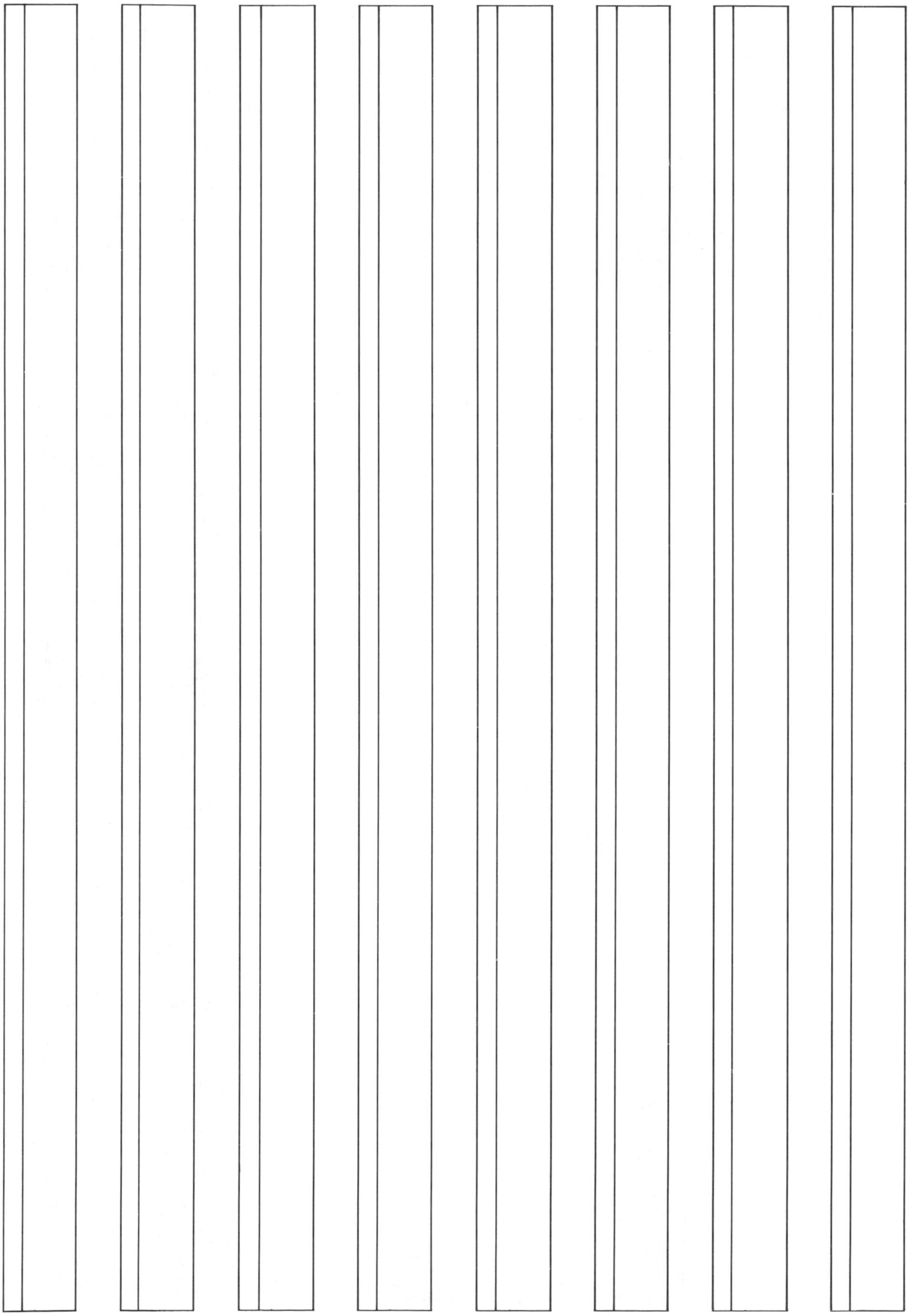

Fig. 20.11 13mm lettering grid no. 5

Lettering for use with grid number 5

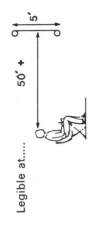

Legible at......   50' +   5'

Standard

abcdefghijklmnopqrstuvvwxyz
ABCDEFGHIJKLMNOPQRST
UVWXYZ 1234567890

Bold

abcdefghijklmnopqrstuvvwxy
z ABCDEFGHIJKLMNOPQRS
TUVWXYZ 1234567890

Fig. 20.12 13mm lettering examples. Standard, Bold

472

Lettering for use with grid number 5

Legible at..... 50' +   5'

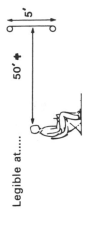

Condensed

abcdefghijklmnopqrstuvwxyz
ABCDEFGHIJKLMNOPQRSTUVWXYZ
1234567890

Italic

abcdefghijklmnopqrstuvwxyz
ABCDEFGHIJKLMNOPQRST
UVWXYZ
1234567890

Fig. 20.13 13mm lettering examples. Condensed, Italic

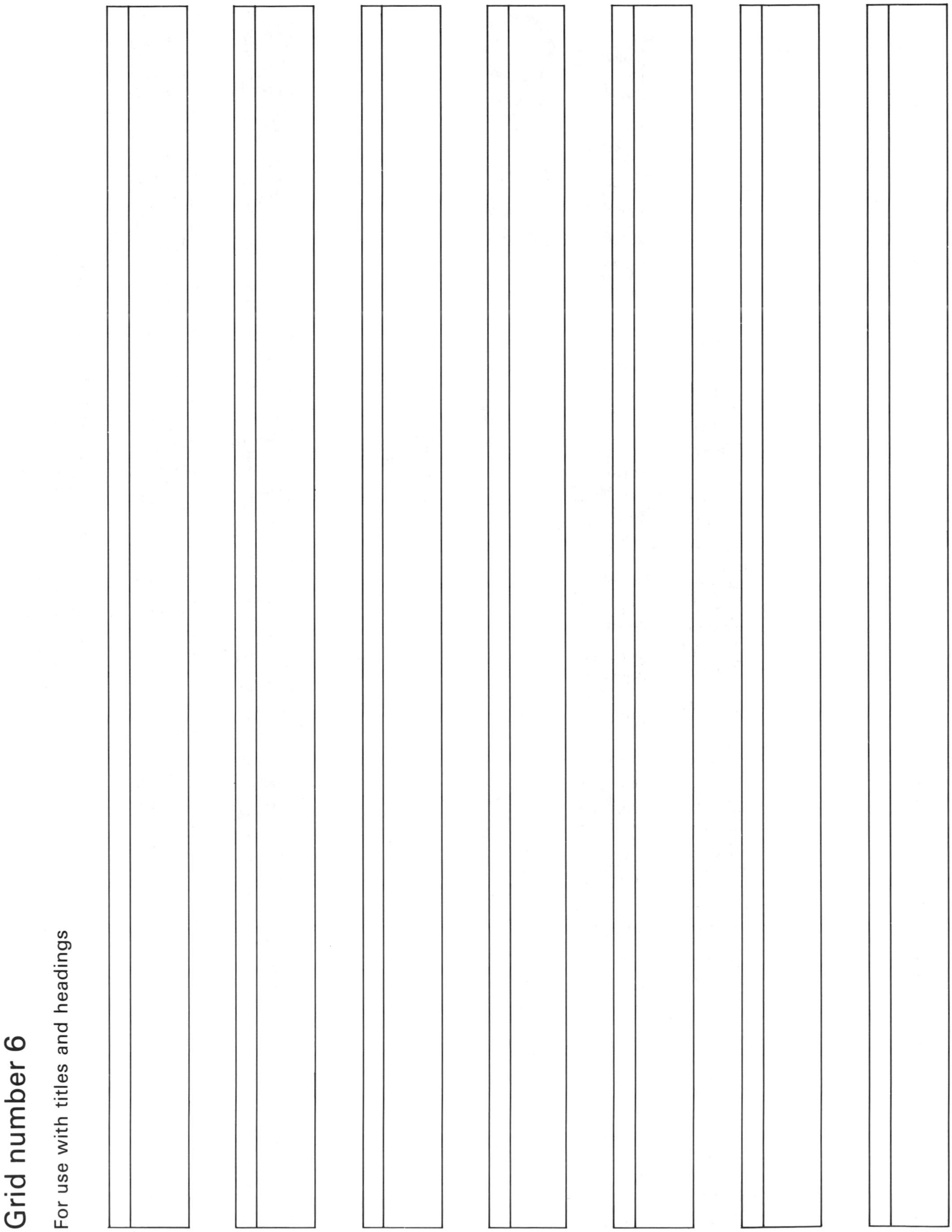

Grid number 6

For use with titles and headings

Fig. 20.14   15mm lettering grid no. 6

Lettering for use with grid number 6

Standard

Legible at..... 50' +

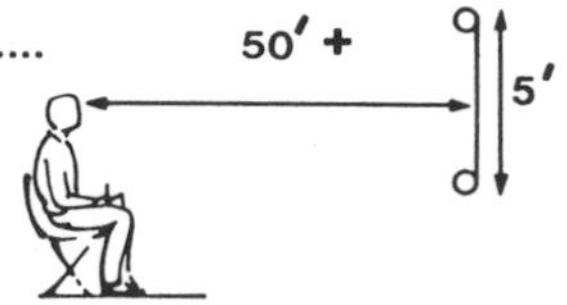

abcdefghijklmnopqrstuvw
xyz ABCDEFGHIJKLMNO
PQRSTUVWXYZ
1234567890

Fig. 20.15 15mm lettering example. Standard

Lettering for use with grid number 6

Bold

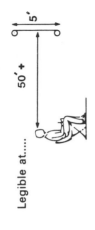

Legible at..... 50´+ 5´

abcdefghijklmnopqrstuv
wxyz ABCDEFGHIJKLM
NOPQRSTUVWXYZ
1234567890

Fig. 20.16 15mm lettering example. Bold

476

Lettering for use with grid number 6

Condensed

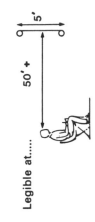

Legible at......

50' +

5'

abcdefghijklmnopqrstuvwxyz

ABCDEFGHIJKLMNOPQRSTUVW

XYZ 1234567890

Fig. 20.17 15mm lettering example. Condensed

Lettering for use with grid number 6

Italic

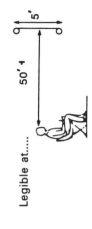

Legible at..... 50' 5'

abcdefghijklmnopqrstuv
wxyz ABCDEFGHIJKLM
NOPQRSTUVWXYZ
1234567890

Fig. 20.18 15mm lettering example. Italic

Lettering for use with grid number 6

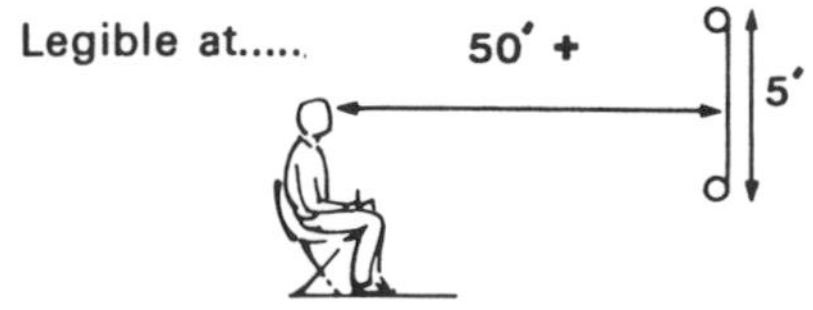

Embelishing standard lettering by adding serifs

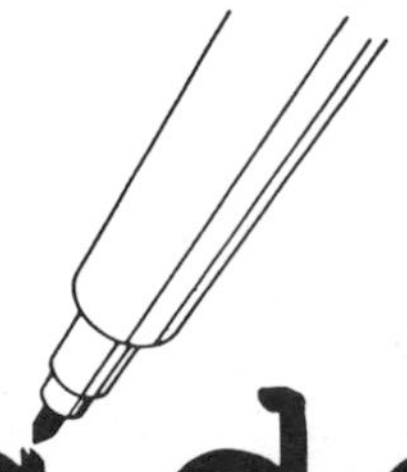

Legible at..... 50' + 5'

abc abc defghijklmno
pqrstuvwxyz
ABCDEFGHIJKLMN OPQRST
UVWXYZ
1234567890

Fig. 20.19 15mm lettering example. Standard plus serifs

Lettering for use with grid number 6

Outlining bold lettering

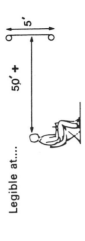

Legible at.... 50' + 5'

ab ab ab

abcdefghijklmnopqrst
uvwxyz

ABCDEFGHIJKL
MNOPQRSTUVWXYZ

1234567890

Fig. 20.20 15mm lettering example. Outline Bold

480

Lettering for use with grid number 6

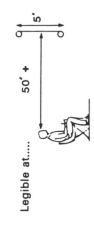

Script

abcdefghijklmnopqrstuvwx
yz ABCDEFGHIJKLMNOPQRST
UVWXYZ 1234567890

Fig. 20.21   15mm lettering example. Script

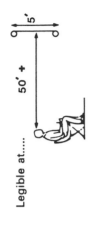

Lettering for use with grid number 6

Adding outline to standard lettering

a a a a a a

abcdefghijklmn
opqrstuvwxyz
ABCD
EFGHIJKLMNOPQRS
TUVWXYZ
1234567890

Fig. 20.22 15mm lettering example. Standard plus outline

Legible at..... 50' + 5'

481